Manual of
Histological Techniques

Manual of
Histological Techniques

Santosh Kumar Mondal MD (Pathology)
Associate Professor
Department of Pathology
Bankura Sammilani Medical College
Bankura, West Bengal, India
Ex-Associate Professor
Department of Pathology
Medical College
Kolkata, West Bengal, India

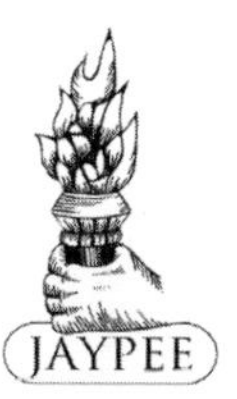

The Health Sciences Publisher
New Delhi | London | Philadelphia | Panama

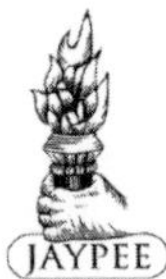

Jaypee Brothers Medical Publishers (P) Ltd

Headquarters
Jaypee Brothers Medical Publishers (P) Ltd
4838/24, Ansari Road, Daryaganj
New Delhi 110 002, India
Phone: +91-11-43574357
Fax: +91-11-43574314
Email: jaypee@jaypeebrothers.com

Overseas Offices

J.P. Medical Ltd
83 Victoria Street, London
SW1H 0HW (UK)
Phone: +44 20 3170 8910
Fax: +44 (0)20 3008 6180
Email: info@jpmedpub.com

Jaypee-Highlights Medical Publishers Inc
City of Knowledge, Bld. 235, 2nd Floor, Clayton
Panama City, Panama
Phone: +1 507-301-0496
Fax: +1 507-301-0499
Email: cservice@jphmedical.com

Jaypee Medical Inc
325 Chestnut Street
Suite 412, Philadelphia, PA 19106, USA
Phone: +1 267-519-9789
Email: support@jpmedus.com

Jaypee Brothers Medical Publishers (P) Ltd
17/1-B Babar Road, Block-B, Shaymali
Mohammadpur, Dhaka-1207
Bangladesh
Mobile: +08801912003485
Email: jaypeedhaka@gmail.com

Jaypee Brothers Medical Publishers (P) Ltd
Bhotahity, Kathmandu
Nepal
Phone: +977-9741283608
Email: kathmandu@jaypeebrothers.com

Website: www.jaypeebrothers.com
Website: www.jaypeedigital.com

Inquiries for bulk sales may be solicited at: jaypee@jaypeebrothers.com

Manual of Histological Techniques

First Edition: **2017**

ISBN: 978-93-86261-19-9

Printed at Rajkamal Electric Press, Plot No. 2, Phase-IV, Kundli, Haryana.

Dedicated to

My parents,
Mr Nitai Chandra Mondal
and
Ms Jyotsna Mondal

Preface

The relentless progresses of medical technology have brought into its wake novel methods of investigations and treatments, rendering many older methods obsolete. Pathological investigations remain cornerstone of medical diagnosis. Histotechnology plays a pivotal role to make a diagnosis of surgical specimens.

With the advent of newer diagnostic techniques like molecular diagnostic methods, a quick but very reliable diagnosis is possible, even from small amount of tissue. In this manual, I have included the molecular techniques, immunohistochemistry, cell blocks, and immunofluorescence along with the conventional techniques. For students' easy understanding; many figures, charts, diagrams and tables have been included. At the same time, the volume of the book has been restricted; so that students do not become overburdened during preparation of examination. Specialists and consultants who are working in a surgical pathology laboratory will also find it useful.

I am indebted to my parents Mr Nitai Chandra Mondal and Smt Jyotsna Mondal for their value-based guidance, blessings and constant support that I have received throughout my life. I thank my son Soumyadeep, brother Monotosh and wife Shampa, for their continuous encouragement during preparation of this manual. I also thank postgraduates of pathology (MD, PGT), especially Dr Saikat Mandal and Dr Debasish Bhattacharya, for their help during preparation of this book. I am thankful to my friend Dr Sanjib Pattari, for supplying a few special stained slides.

Despite my best efforts, some mistakes might have crept in. So, I request all readers to kindly bring it to my notice. Your constructive criticism, appreciation and suggestions are most welcome.

Santosh Kumar Mondal
E-mail: dr_santoshkumar@hotmail.com

Contents

PLATE 1

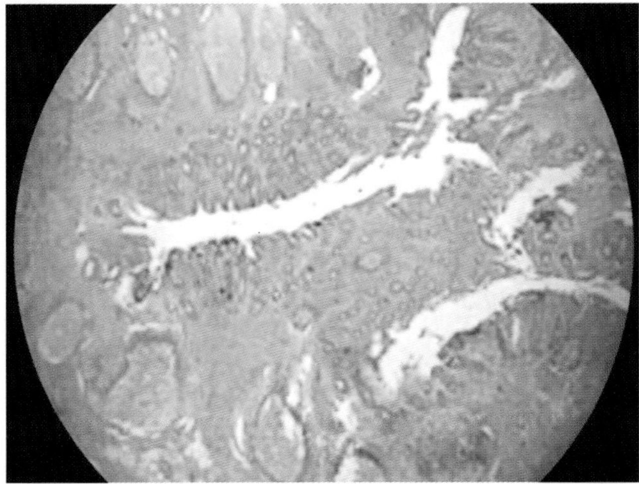

Fig. 1: Photomicrograph showing mucosal glands of appendix and lymphoid aggregates forming lymphoid follicles (H and E, low power view,100×) *(Chapter 5)*

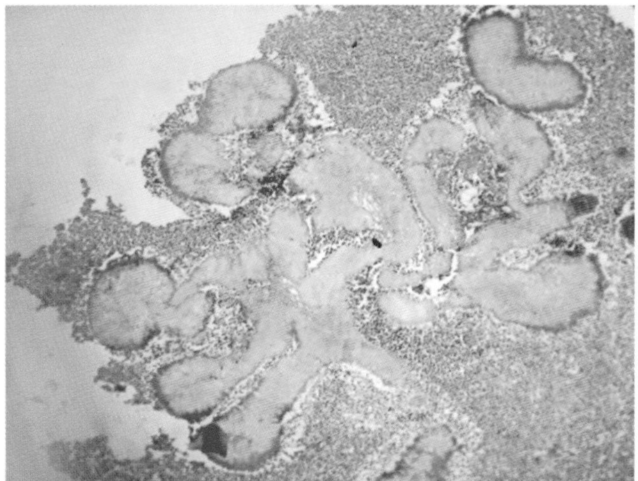

Fig. 2: Microphotograph showing fungal mycetoma (eumycetoma) or 'madura foot'. Multiple aggregates of fungal hyphae and sulfur granules, surrounded by neutrophils/microabscess (H and E, low power view,100×) *(Chapter 5)*

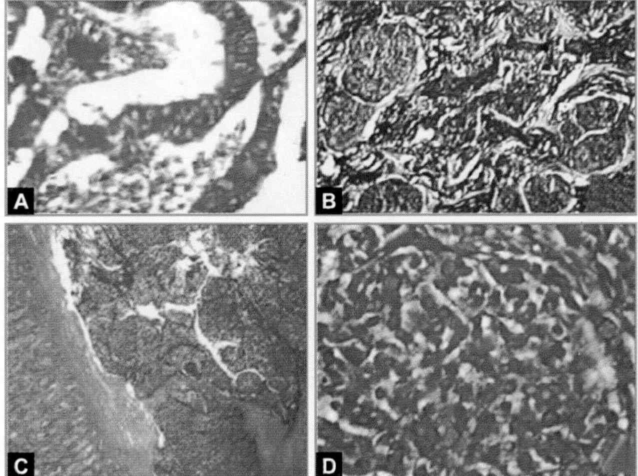

Figs 1A to D: (A) Adenocarcinoma of colon showing malignant cells with neutral mucins (PAS,400×); (B) Mucinous carcinoma showing pools of acidic mucin (Alcian blue,400×); (C) Mucinous carcinoma showing acidic and neutral mucins (Combined Alcian blue and PAS,100×); (D) Signet ring cell carcinoma showing neutral mucin (Combined Alcian blue and PAS, 400×) *(Chapter 6)*

PLATE 2

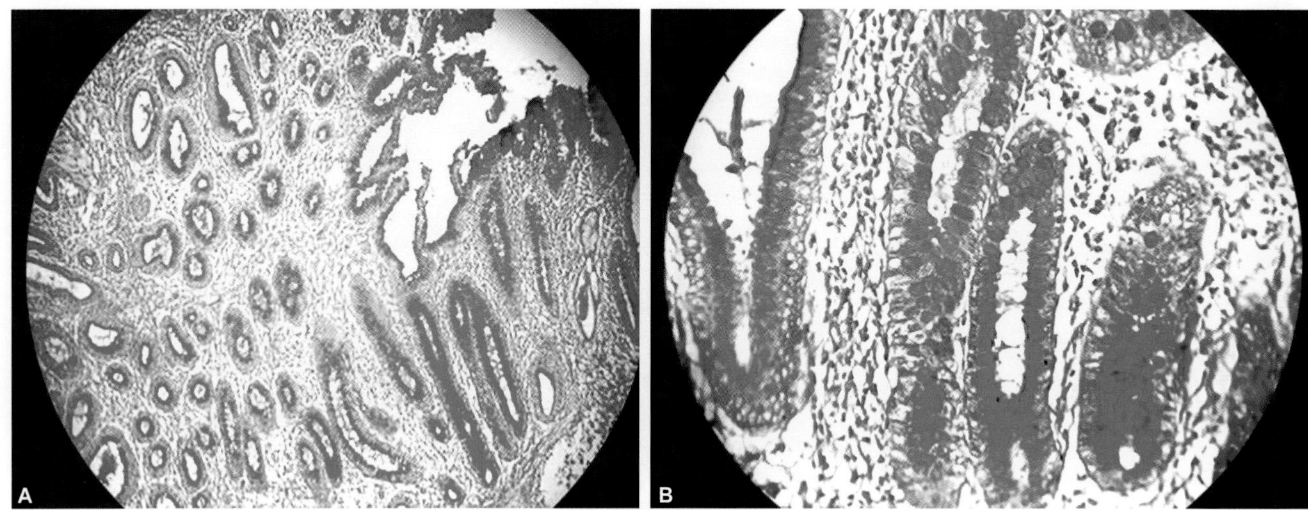

Figs 2A and B: PAS positive materials (mucin) are stained as magenta/bright red: (A) PAS: Appendix, low power; (B) PAS: Appendix, high power *(Chapter 6)*

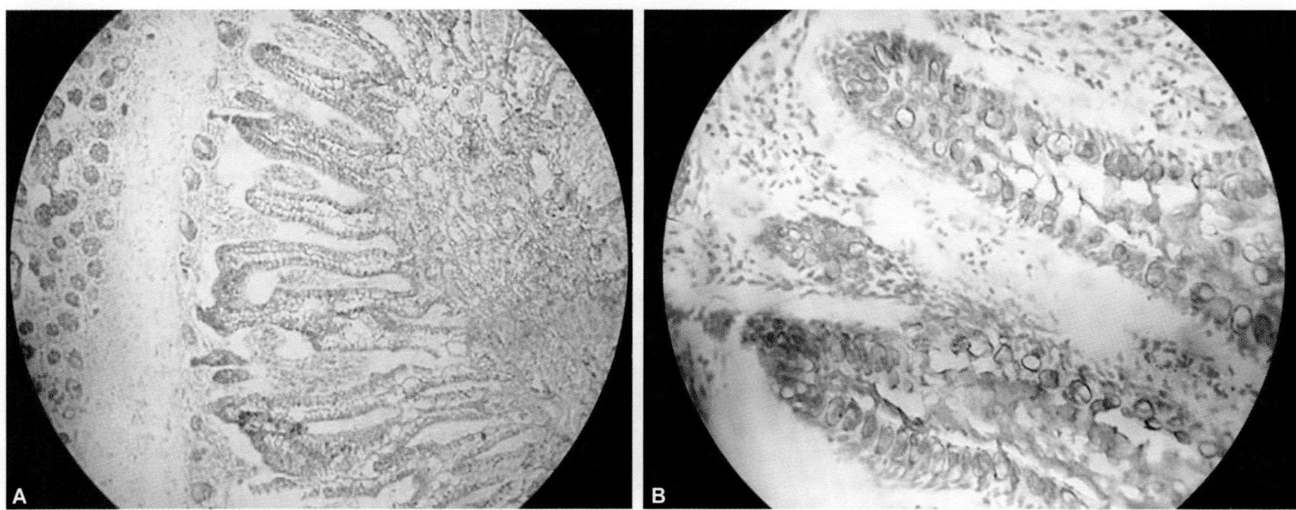

Figs 3A and B: Alcian blue, intestine, low and high power. Alcian blue stains acid mucins as blue *(Chapter 6)*

PLATE 3

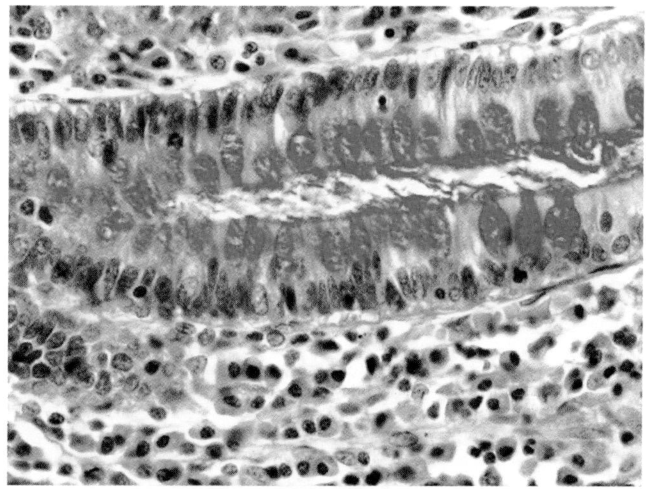

Fig. 4: Mucicarmine stains strongly sulfated or acid mucin as red *(Chapter 6)*

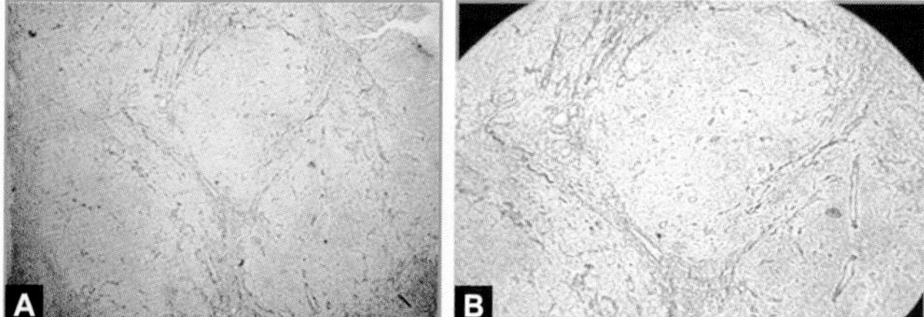

Figs 1A and B: (A) Microphotograph showing reticulin fibers in cirrhotic nodules of liver (Reticulin stain, low power view, 100×); (B) Microphotograph showing retculin fibers in a cirrhotic nodule (Reticulin stain, high power view, 400×) *(Chapter 9)*

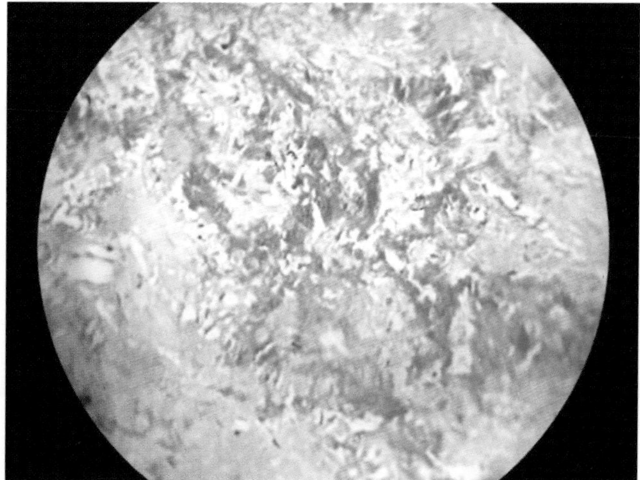

Fig. 1: Congo red stain, high power. Amyloids are stained by Congo red stain as deep pink to red *(Chapter 13)*

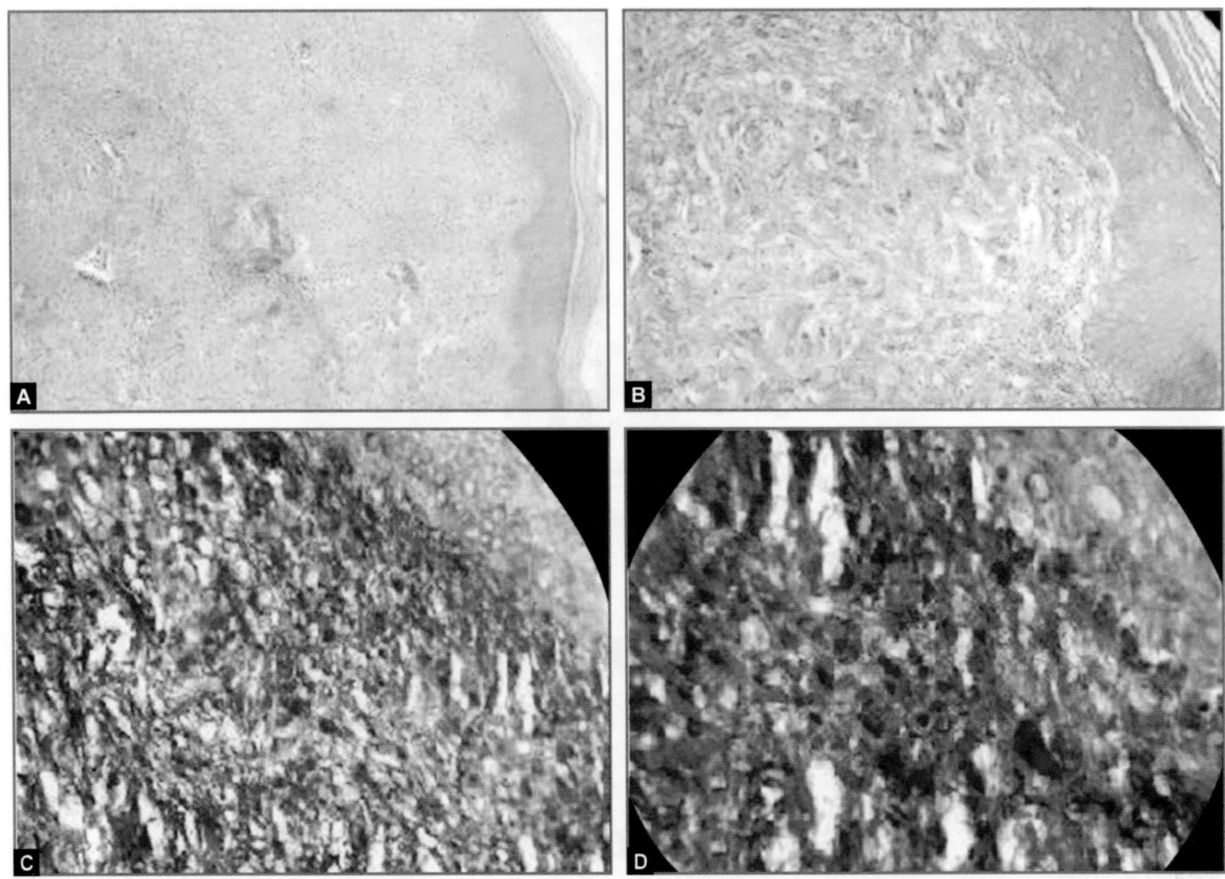

Figs 2A to D: (A) Low power view of skin lesion in lepromatous leprosy (H & E, ×100); (B) High power view showing sheets of foamy macrophages in dermis (H & E, ×400); (C) Modified Wade-Fite stain showing numerous red-colored lepra bacilli in dermis (×400); (D) Modified Wade-Fite stain showing red-colored lepra bacilli arranged in clusters and singly within foamy macrophages in dermis (×1000) *(Chapter 13)*

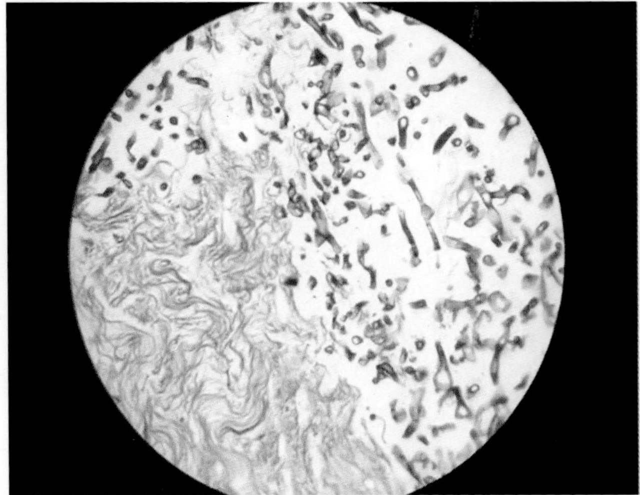

Fig. 1: Photomicrograph showing broad aseptate, ribbon-like hyphae of mucormycosis (Grocott silver methenamine stain, ×400) *(Chapter 14)*

PLATE 5

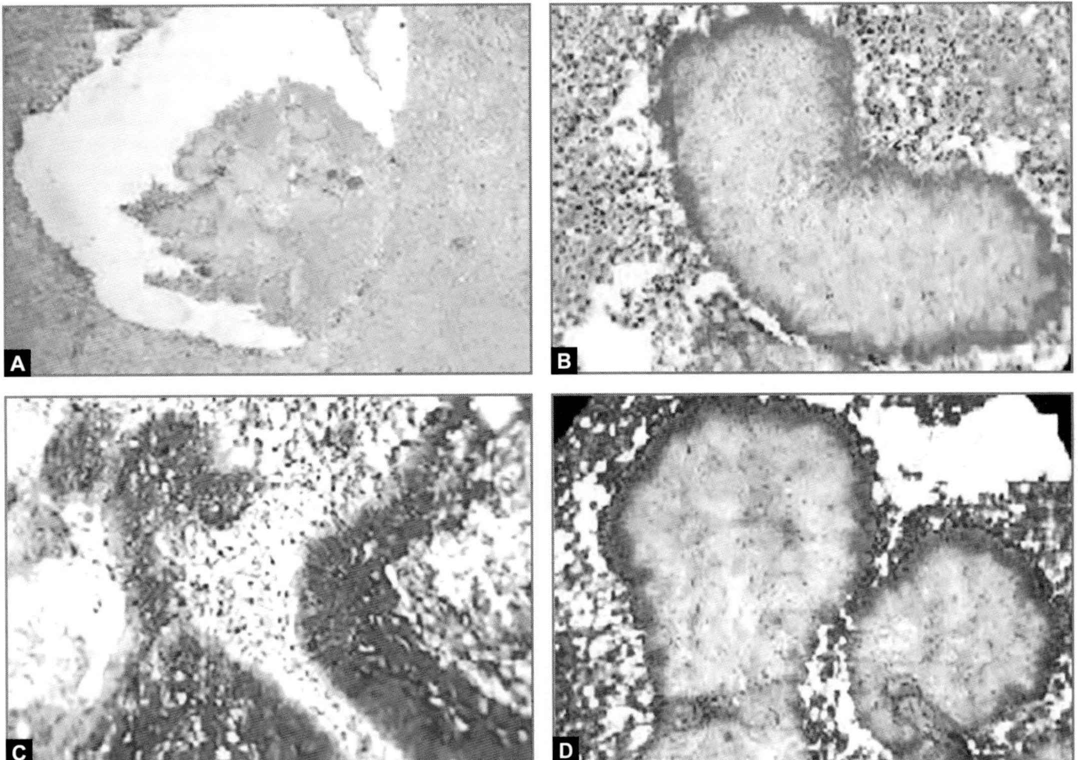

Figs 2A to D: (A) Microphotograph showing fungal mycetoma (eumycetoma) or "madura foot" (H & E, scanner view, 40×); (B) Microphotograph showing aggregates of fungal hyphae surrounded by neutrophils or microabscess and sulfur granules (PAS, low power view, ×100); (C) Microphotograph showing broader aseptate hyphae surrounded by neutrophils (PAS, high power view, 400×); (D) Microphotograph showing gram-negative organism/fungal element (Gram stain, high power view, 400×) *(Chapter 14)*

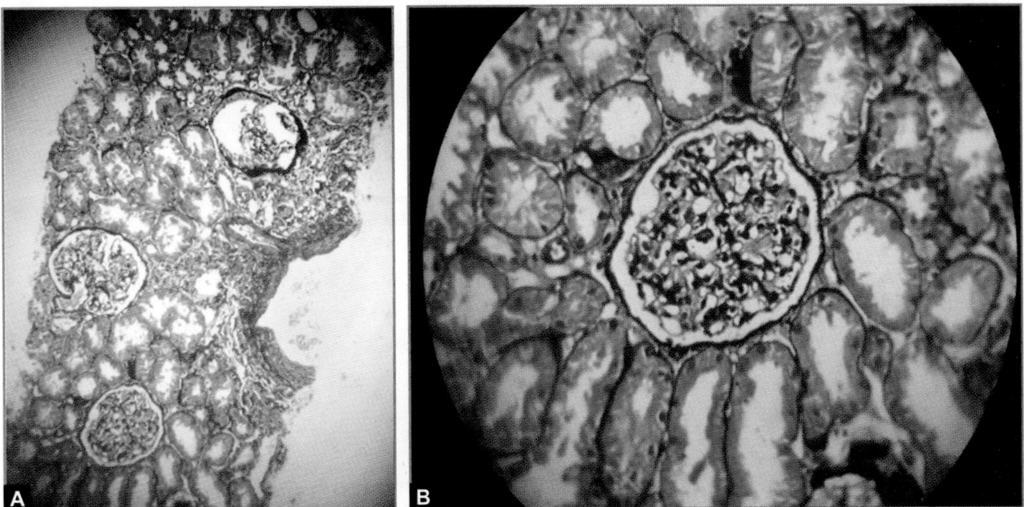

Figs 3A and B: Combined PAS and Jone's methenamine silver (JMS stain); kidney biopsy, low power and high power. PAS stains tubules as pink whereas JMS stains basement membrane surrounding Bowman's space and glomerular capillaries as black *(Chapter 14)*

PLATE 6

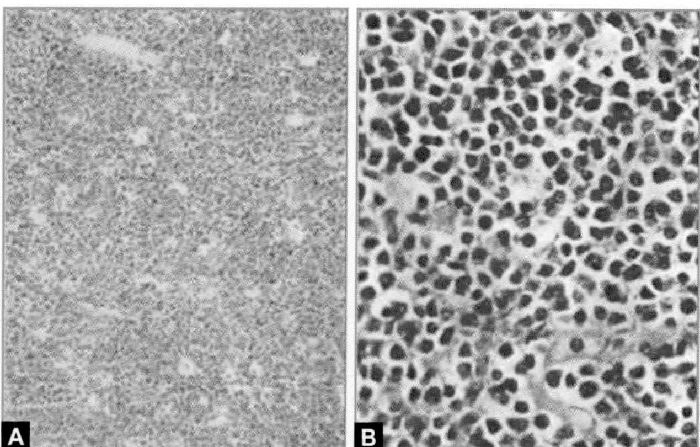

Figs 7A and B: Photomicrograph showing a tumor composed of monomorphic round cells arranged in diffuse sheets in Burkitt's lymphoma. (A) Characteristic starry sky pattern is evident (Hematoxylin and Eosin, ×100); (B) Photomicrograph showing small to intermediate sized cells having round nuclei with clumped chromatin (Hematoxylin and Eosin, ×400) *(Chapter 15)*

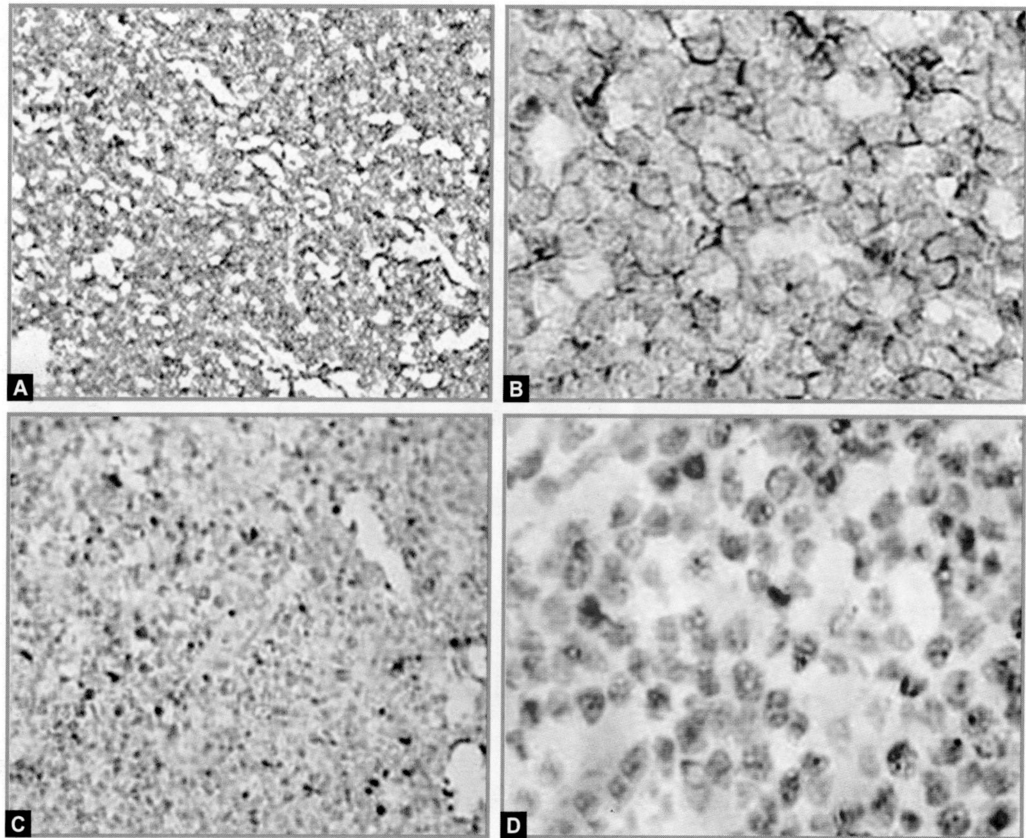

Figs 8A to D: (A) Tumor cells of Burkitt's lymphoma showing strong membrane positivity for leukocyte common antigen (LCA) [×100]; (B) Tumor cells showing strong membrane positivity for B-cell marker CD20 [×400]; (C) Tumor cells showing strong nuclear positivity for Ki-67 [×100]; (D) Tumor cells showing membrane negativity for T-cell marker CD3 [×400] *(Chapter 15)*

PLATE 7

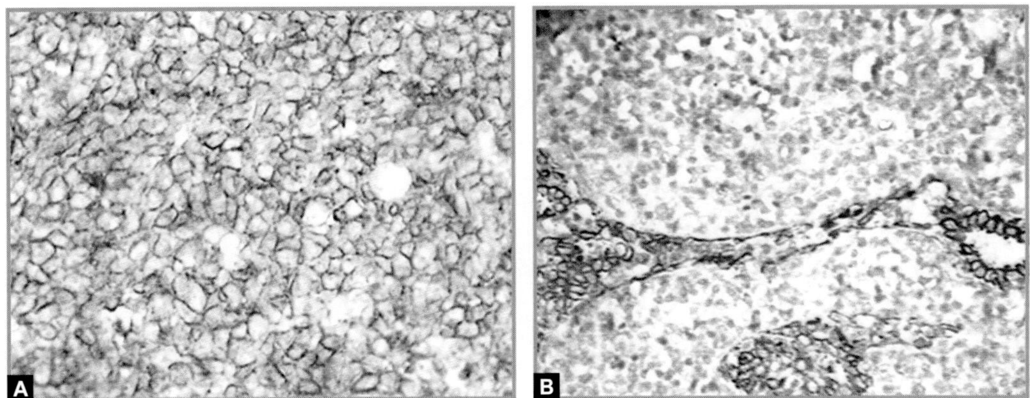

Figs 9A and B: (A) Immunohistochemistry showing diffuse cytoplasmic membrane staining of CD20 in the tumor cells of diffuse large B-cell lymphoma (DLBCL) in breast [×400]; (B) Immunohistochemistry showing negative expression of cytokeratin antigen by the tumor/lymphoma cells, while the entrapped ductal epithelial cells are positive for cytokeratin [×100] *(Chapter 15)*

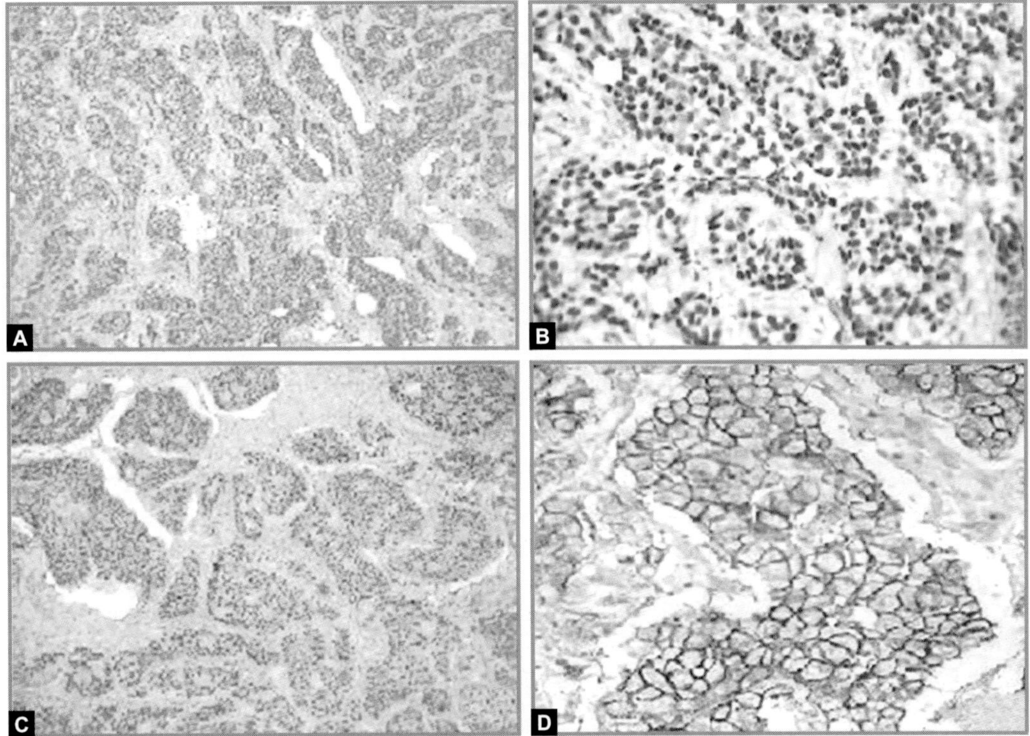

Figs 10A to D: (A) Microphotograph showing ER positivity (nuclear) in breast carcinoma (IHC, ×100); (B) Microphotograph showing strong ER positivity (nuclear) in breast carcinoma (IHC, ×400); (C) Microphotograph showing PR positivity (nuclear) in breast carcinoma (IHC, ×100); (D) Microphotograph showing Her-2/neu positivity (complete cytoplasmic membrane staining in >30% of tumor cells) in breast carcinoma (IHC, ×400) *(Chapter 15)*

PLATE 8

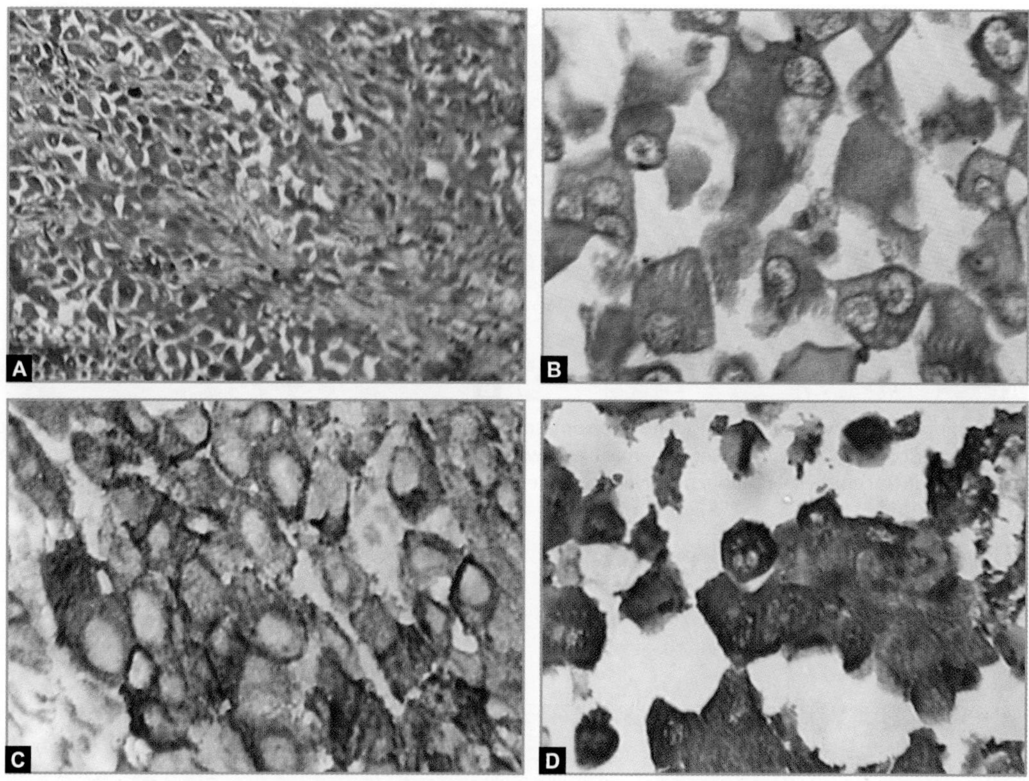

Figs 11A to D: Amelanotic melanoma (epithelioid type). (A) Microphotograph showing melanoma cells in paraffin section (H and E × 100); (B) High power view showing prominent nucleoli in melanoma cells and binucleated tumor cells (H and E × 400); (C) Immunocytochemistry on FNAC smears showing Melan A/Mart-1 positivity (cytoplasmic) in many melanoma cells; (D) Immunocytochemistry on FNAC smears showing S100 positivity (both nuclear and cytoplasmic) among tumor cells *(Chapter 15)*

PLATE 9

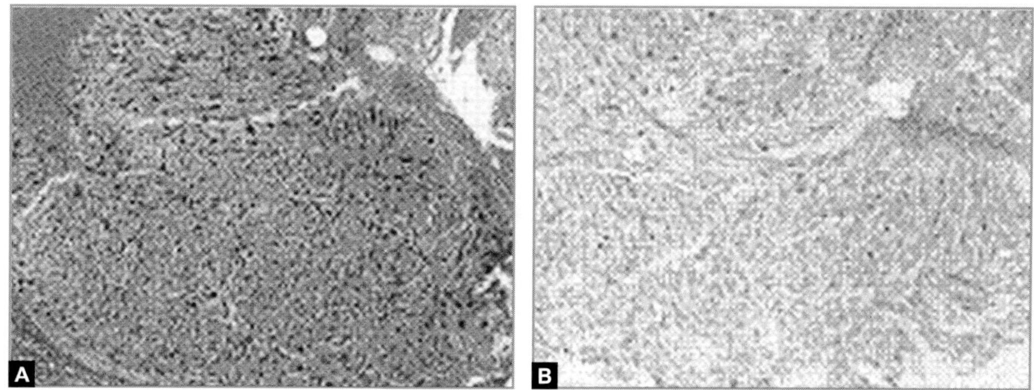

Figs 2A and B: (A) Cell block showing fascicles of spindle cell proliferation in GIST (hematoxylin and eosin stain, 100x magnification); (B) Immunohistochemistry of cell block demonstrating c-kit/CD117 positivity (100x magnification) *(Chapter 16)*

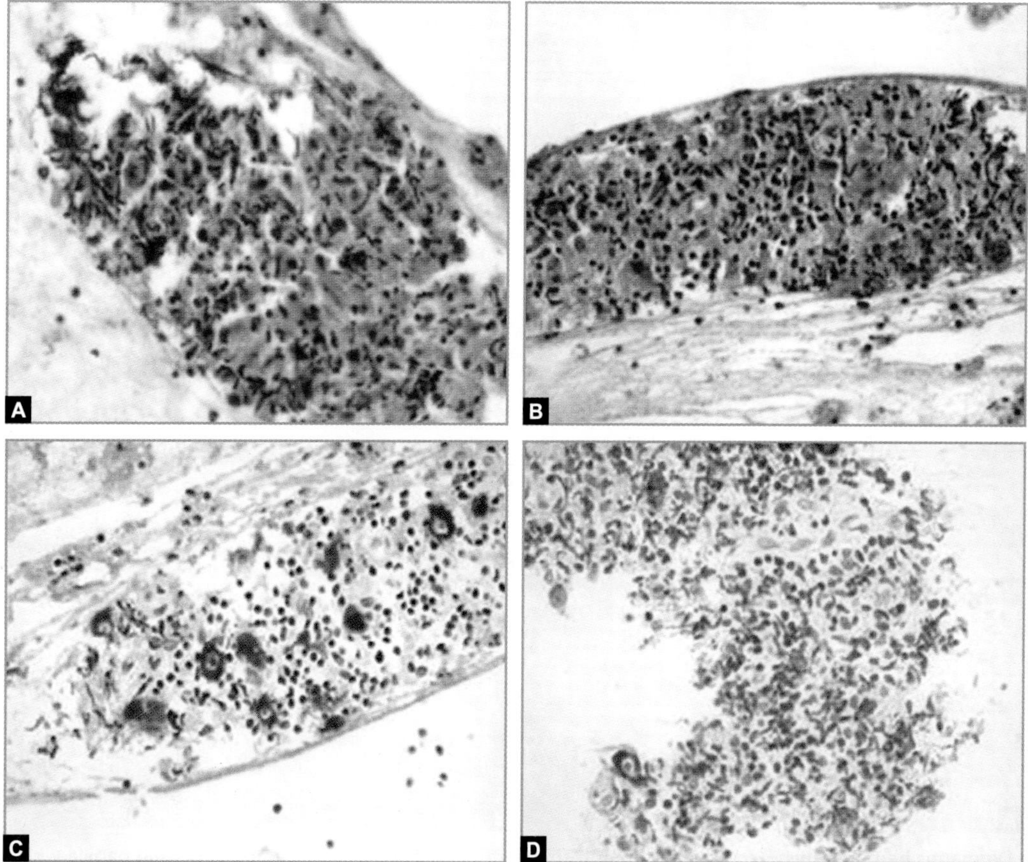

Figs 3A to D: A case of Hodgkin's lymphoma that was diagnosed by FNA. (A and B) showing the cell block of this case that contains few Reed-Sternberg (RS) cells. The cells were immunoreactive for CD 15 (C) and CD 30 (D) and were negative for CD 45 and CD 20, confirming the diagnosis *(Chapter 16)*

PLATE 10

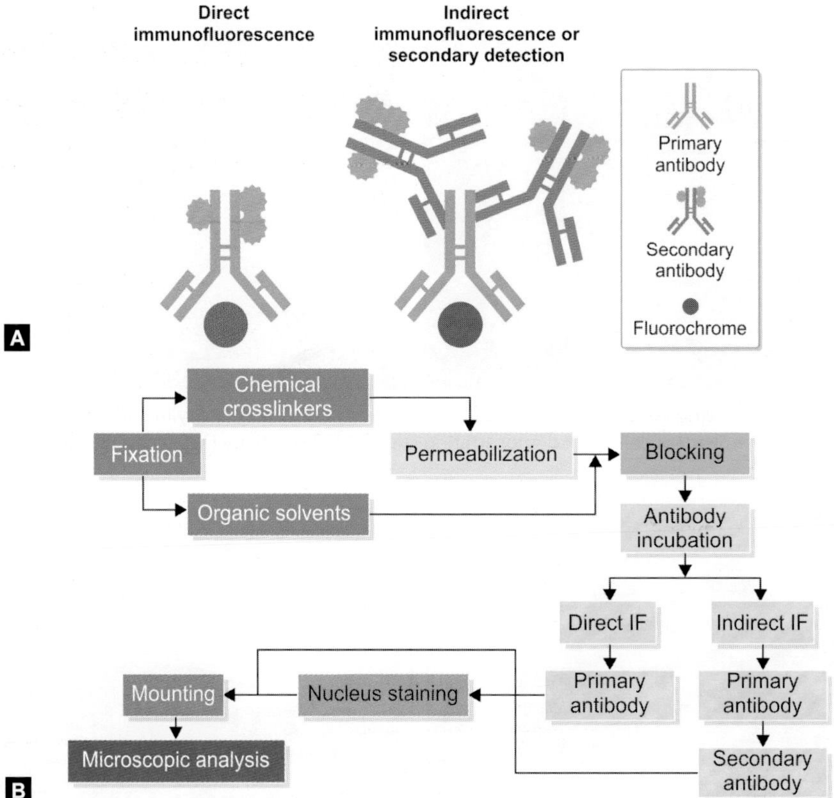

Figs 1A and B: Direct and indirect immunofluorescence *(Chapter 19)*

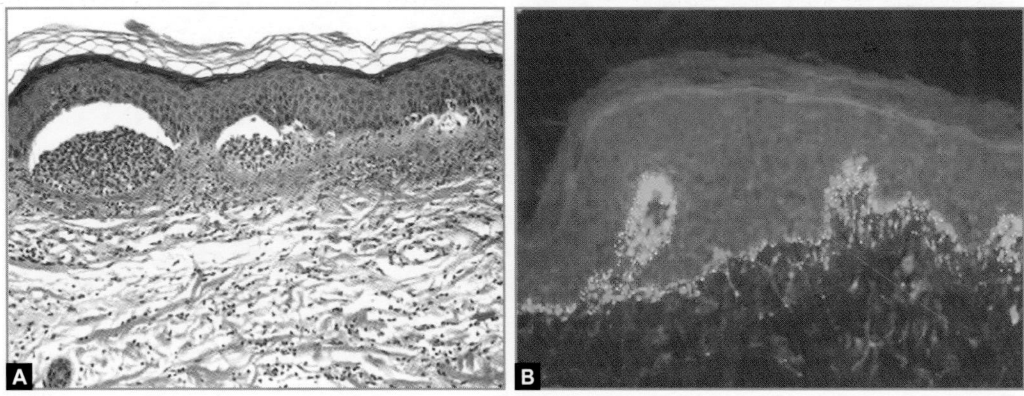

Figs 2A and B: Dermatitis herpetiformis. (A) Microphotograph showing microabscesses at the tips of dermal papilla which one forming a multilocular subepidermal bulla. Eosinophils are also present (H & E × 100). (B) Microphotograph showing immunofluorescence of granular and thready deposits of IgA at the epidermal basement membrane zone (EBMZ) *(Chapter 19)*

PLATE 11

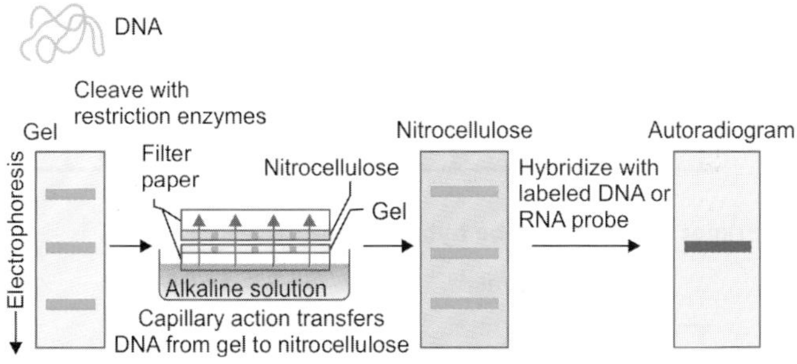

Fig. 2: Schematic diagram of Southern blot *(Chapter 22)*

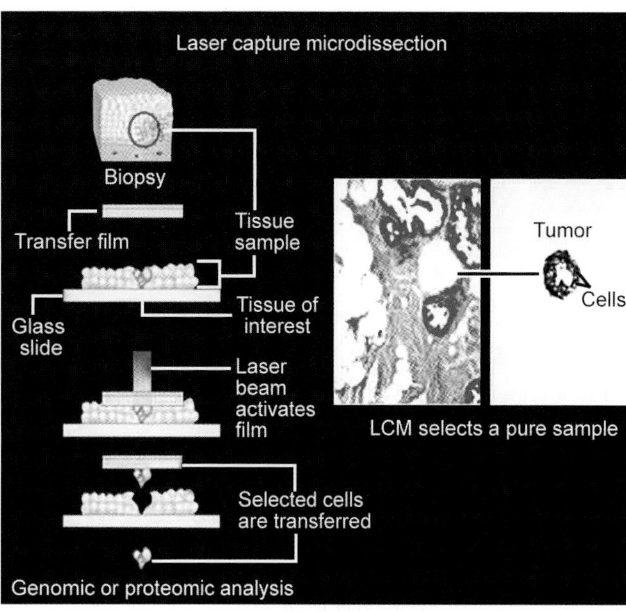

Fig. 7: Schematic diagram of laser capture microdissection technique *(Chapter 22)*

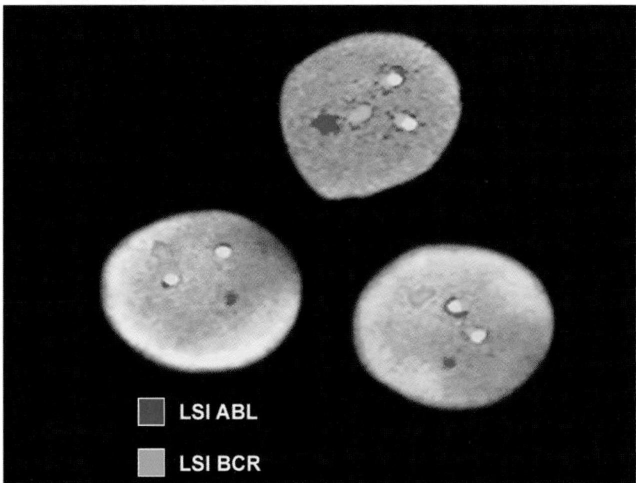

Fig. 6: Interphase cytogenetics, ABL-BCR transfusion in Philadelphia chromosome in chronic myeloid leukemia (CML). Normally, ABL gives red signal and BCR gives green signal. But when they are translocated and transfused to make a chimeric protein (in Philadelphia chromosome) they impart yellow signal *(Chapter 22)*

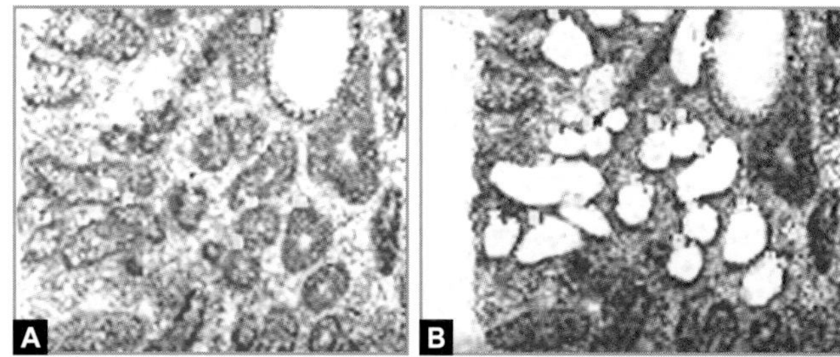

Figs 8A and B: (A) Before microdissection and (B) after microdissection. Note, areas marked in the left photographed have been taken out (microdissection) in the right photograph *(Chapter 22)*

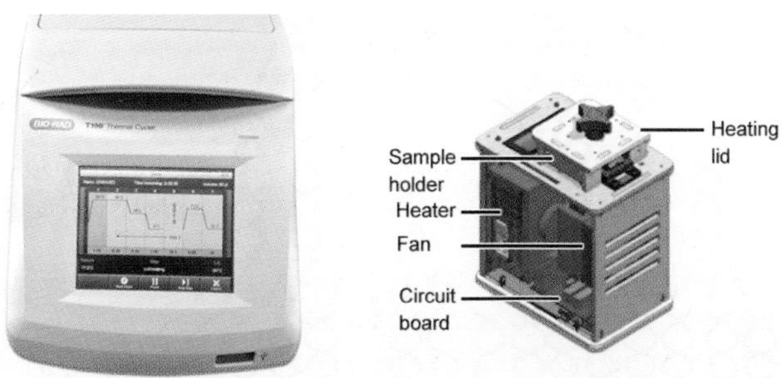

Fig. 9: PCR machine and its parts *(Chapter 22)*

PLATE 12

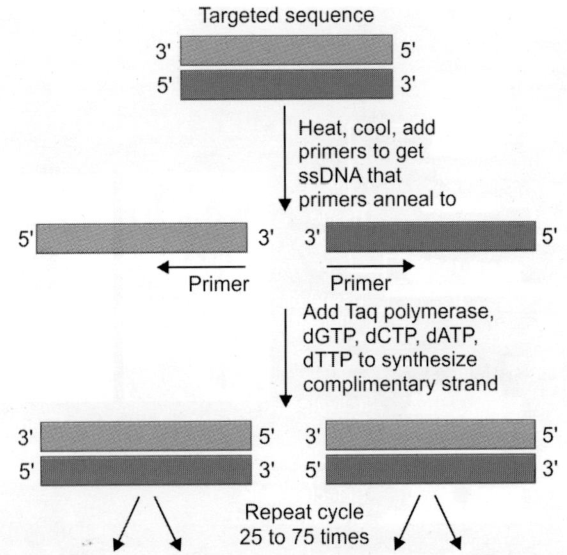

Fig. 11: Denaturation, annealing and extension; three important steps in PCR *(Chapter 22)*

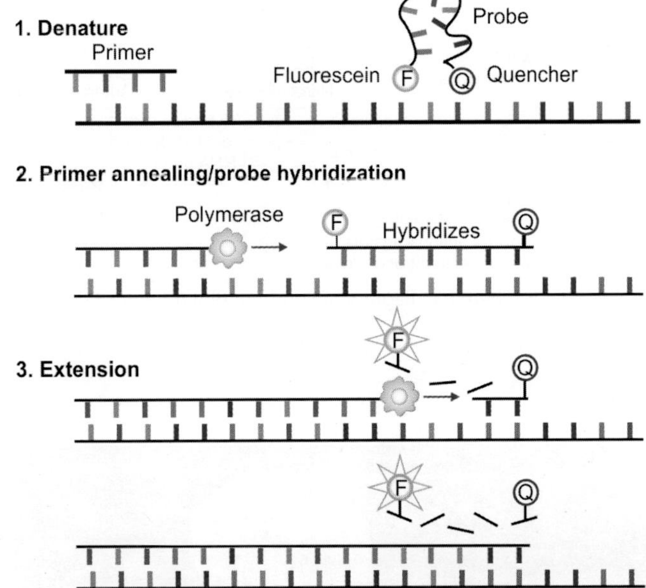

Fig. 14: Schematic diagram (TaqMan® probe method) of real-time PCR (RT-PCR) or quantitative PCR (Q-PCR) *(Chapter 22)*

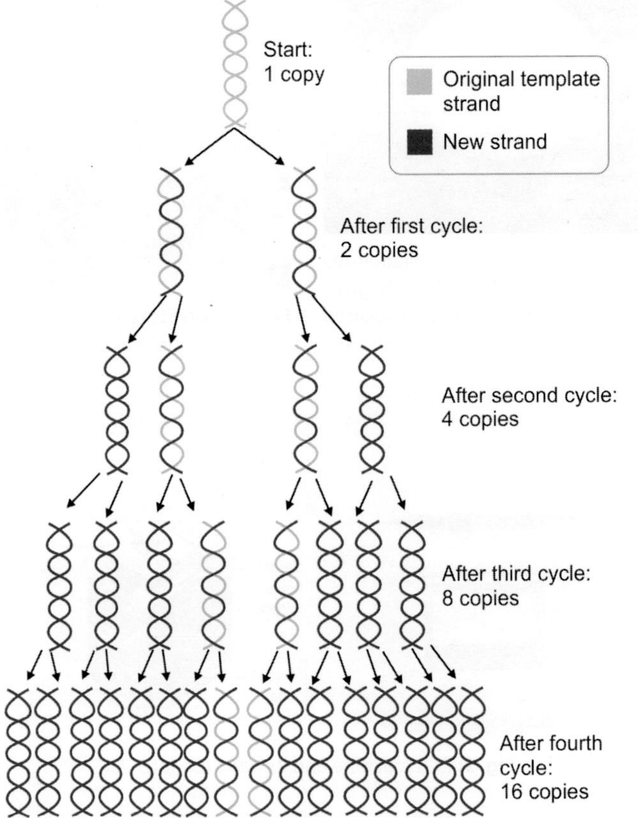

Fig. 12: Schematic diagram of different steps in a PCR *(Chapter 22)*

PLATE 13

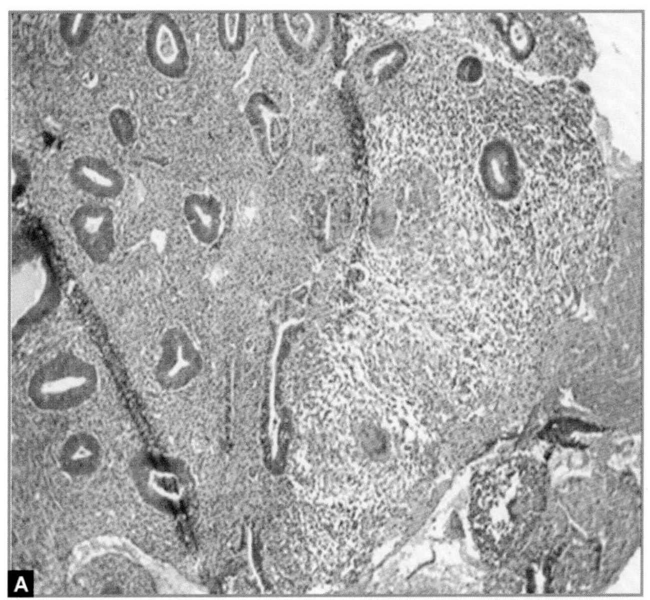

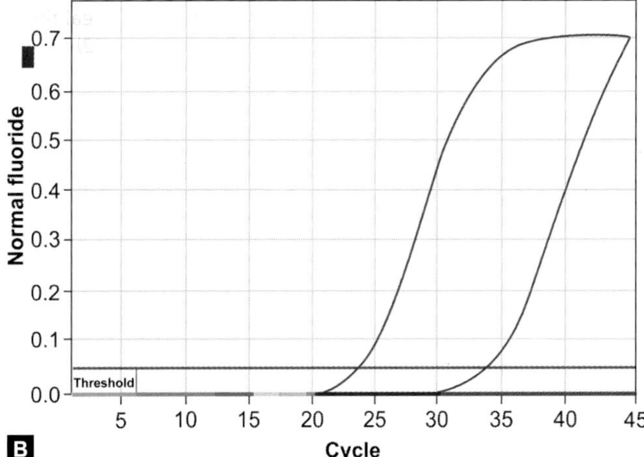

No.	Co-lor	Name	Type	Ct	Given Conc (copies)	Calc Conc (copies)	% Variation
1		C2	NTC				
2		C1	Standard	23.67	250,000	250,000	
3		Manibha Kumar	Unknown	33.89		Detected	

Legend: 1. C2 (NTC) – Negative control
2. C1 (Standard) – Positive control
3. Unkown – Patient sample

Figs 16A and B: (A) Photomicrograph showing few epithelioid granulomas of tuberculosis in the endometrium. The endometrium is in proliferative stage (H&E, × 100); (B) Real-time or RT-PCR detecting the *Mycobacterium tuberculosis* and its quantity/concentration *(Chapter 22)*

PLATE 14

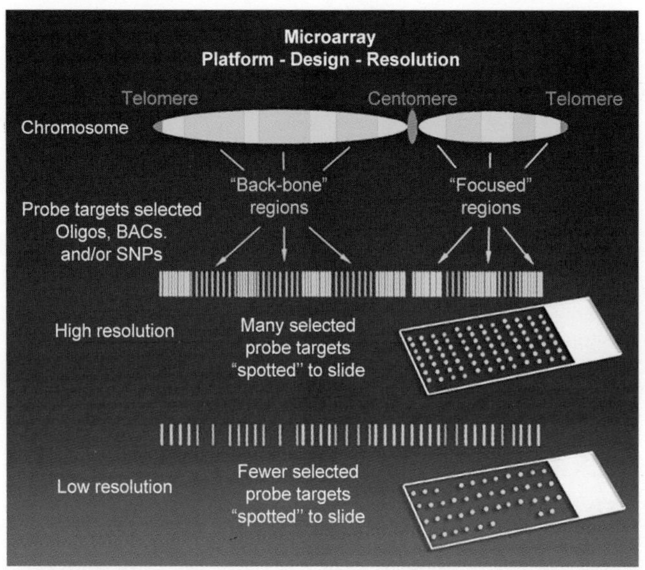

Fig. 17: Schematic diagram of DNA microarray *(Chapter 22)*

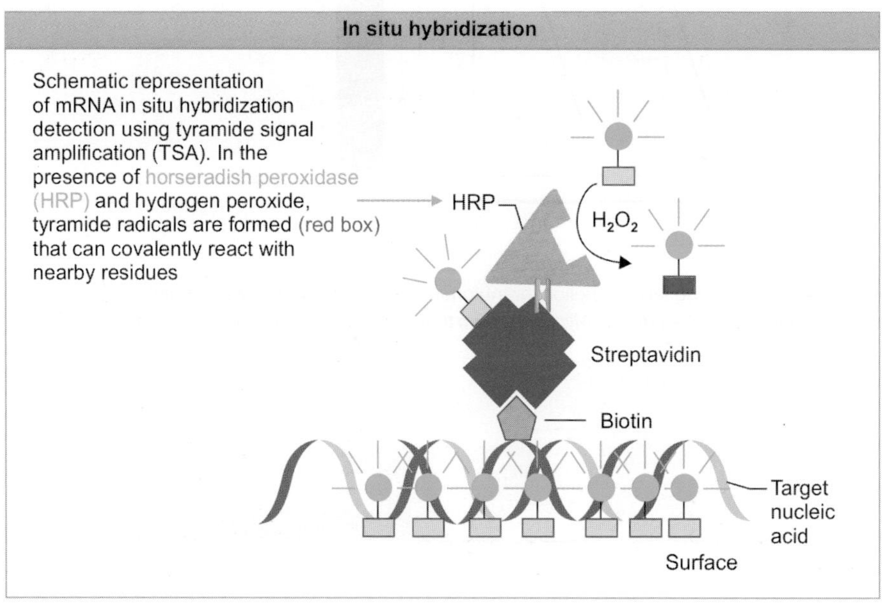

Fig. 1: Schematic diagram of mRNA in situ hybridization (ISH) *(Chapter 23)*

PLATE 15

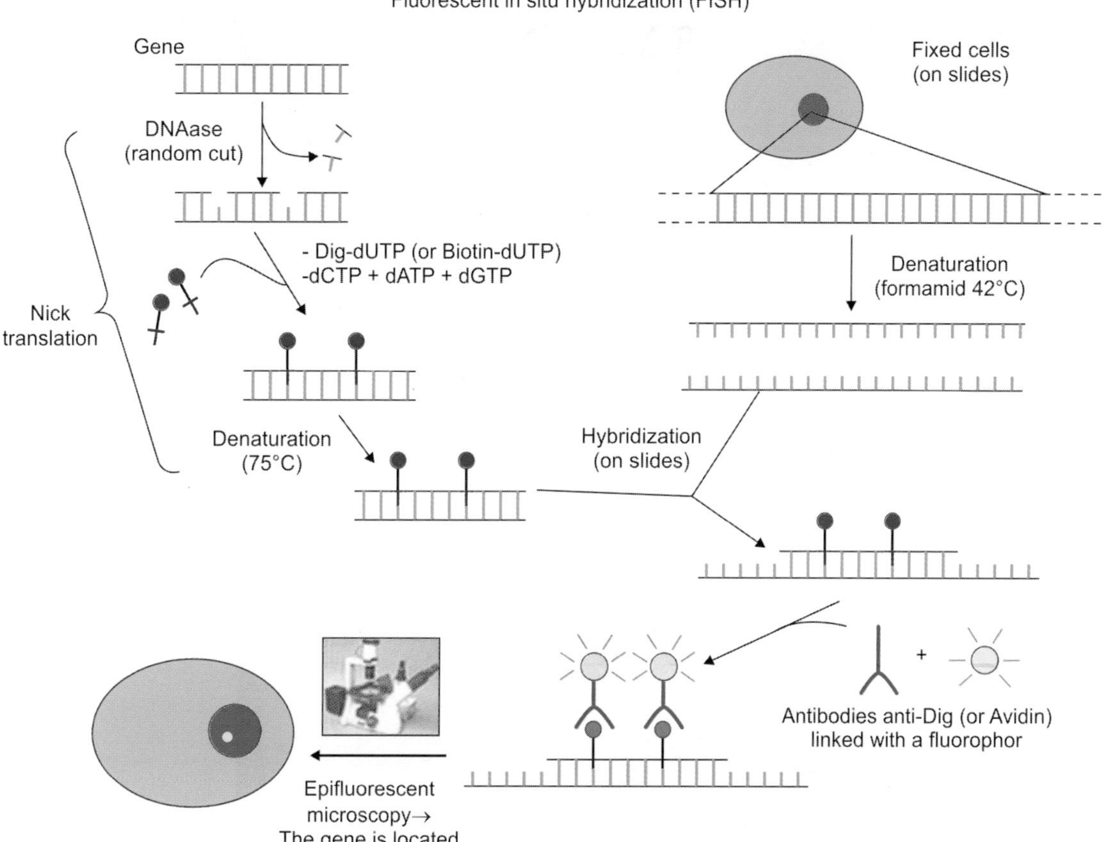

Fig. 2: Scheme of the principle of the FISH (fluorescent in situ hybridization). Experiment to localize a gene in the nucleus *(Chapter 23)*

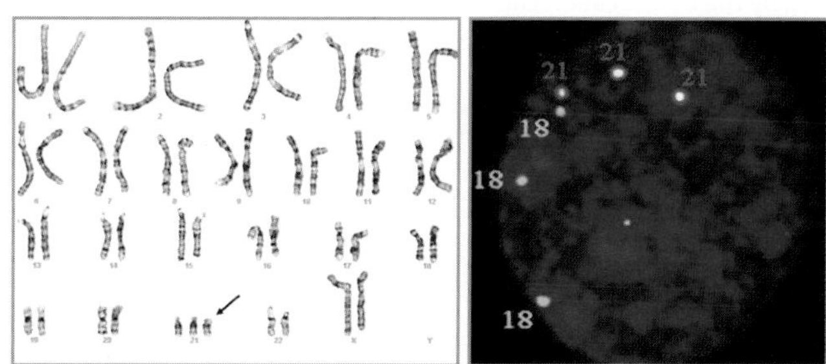

Fig. 3: Conventional cytogenetic G-banded karyotype demonstrating trisomy 21. The arrow indicates the third copy of chromosome 21. Trisomy 21 detected by FISH. An extra chromosome of 21, which gives red signal. Do not be confused about the chromosome 18 in the lower left corner which is part of a pairs of other chromosome 18 and is not part of chromosome 18 pair above it *(Chapter 23)*

PLATE 16

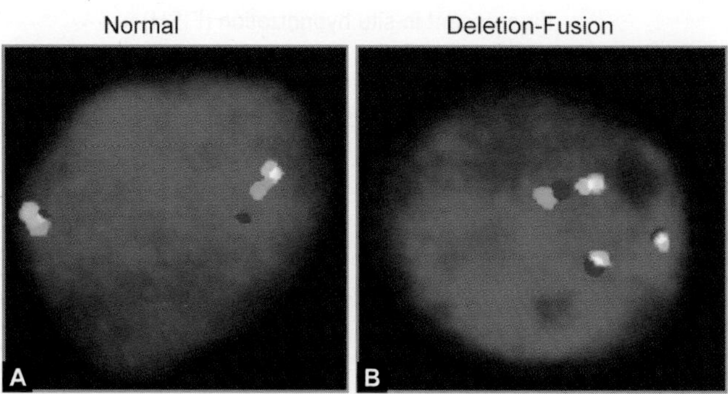

Figs 4A and B: Four-color FISH assay after probe hybridization in a normal (A) and prostate tumor cell (B). In the normal cell, all four of the probes (red, yellow, green, and blue) exist within close proximity to one another (in two four-colored foci corresponding to a diploid nucleus) since the probes recognize a distinct chromosomal locus containing two adjacent genes, TRMPRSS2 and ERG. The tumor cell on the right has had two deletion-fusion events at the TRMPRSS2 and ERG loci, as evidenced by two blue/red dimeric probe signals and the loss of the other two-colored signals (lower right side of nucleus) *(Chapter 23)*

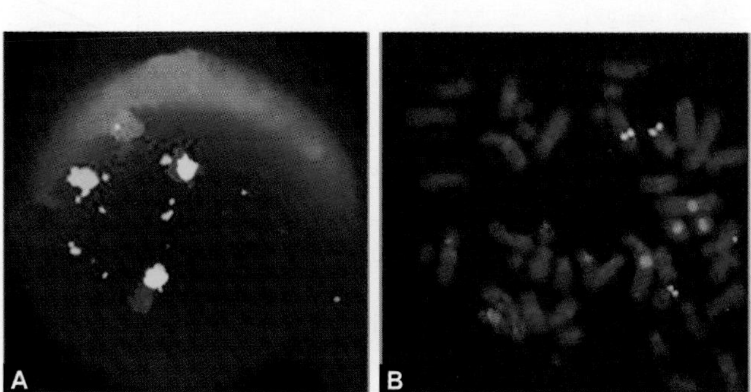

Figs 5A and B: Fluorescence in situ hybridization (FISH) analysis on interphase (A) and metaphase nuclei (B), using the ***LSI IGH/CCND1*** XT dual-color probes. Dual-fusion translocation DNA probe identifying the presence of the t (11;14) (q13;q32) chromosomal translocation. One orange (CCND1 on chromosome 11q13), one green (IGH on chromosome 14q32), and two fusion signal patterns [der (11) and (der14)], indicating the chromosomal rearrangements produced by the translocation can be observed *(Chapter 23)*

CHAPTER 1

Tissue Fixation and Fixatives

INTRODUCTION

Histological techniques are a series of processes by which the tissues are prepared for microscopic examination. It starts with fixation and continues with dehydration, clearing, embedding, cutting and staining.

When the tissues are removed from the body (e.g. surgical excision) or blood supply is cut off; tissues begin to decompose. This is due to lack of oxygen and other essential metabolites and also from the accumulation of carbon dioxide and other toxic metabolites in the cells and due to activation of different autolytic enzymes. Some tissues are decomposed rapidly whereas others are slow to decompose. The rapidity is proportional to the natural metabolic activity of the tissue. This is the basis of rapid decomposition in liver, pancreas, convoluted tubules in kidney.

To minimize the decomposition and to preserve as nearly as possible the natural activity of the cells; the tissues are put in a suitable fixative (usually 10–20 times of volume of surgical specimens). Fixation is defined as a complex series of chemical and physical events which prevents or at least minimizes tissue decomposition and it differs for the different groups of chemical substances found in the tissues. There are other reasons of fixation. In most of the cells, there is an outer complex membrane containing the fluid protoplasm. The protoplasm is a mixed, true and colloidal solution of carbohydrates, proteins, lipids, salts, organic acids and enzymes. Many of these substances would have been lost if tissues had not been fixed.

The aims of fixation are:

- Prevention of tissue autolysis and bacterial attack
- To maintain the shape and volume of the tissues during subsequent procedures (e.g. clearing, embedding, etc.)
- To keep tissues as close to their natural state and to minimize change of natural color and appearance
- To prevent loss of tissue substances or rearrangement of tissue ingredients.

To achieve the aims of fixation, an ideal fixative should:

- Prevent autolysis and bacterial decomposition
- To maintain the shape and volume, natural color and appearance of the tissues
- Make the cellular components 'fixed' after chemical and physical events of fixation and make cellular components insoluble to liquids during subsequent stages of processing
- It should be nontoxic, nonallergic and avoid excessive hardening of the tissues
- It allows enhanced staining of the tissues
- It should fix all the tissue components (carbohydrates, proteins, lipids) and prevents loss of any cellular components during next stages.

But, truly speaking, ideal fixative has not been found and search for it is still on. We commonly use fixatives which usually preserve protein (sacrificing carbohydrates, lipids) and conserve structures for routine purposes.

CLASSIFICATION OF FIXATIVES

- **Aldehydes**: Formaldehyde, glutraldehyde, acrolein.
- **Protein denaturating agents**: Acetic acid, methyl alcohol, ethyl alcohol.

- **Oxidizing agents**: Osmium tetroxide, potassium dichromate, potassium permanganate.
- **Physical agents**: Microwave, heat.
- **Other cross-linking agents**: Carbodiimides.
- **Miscellaneous**: Picric acid, mercuric chloride.

REACTIONS OF FIXATIVES WITH PROTEINS

The most important reaction in tissue fixation is probably the reaction which stabilizes the proteins. Most commonly used fixatives have the property to form cross-link between proteins leading to gel formation. Soluble proteins get fixed with structural proteins (insoluble) and make the soluble protein insoluble. This process also gives some mechanical strength which allows subsequent procedure to take place.

Most fixatives used in laboratory are liquids/aqueous solutions, although vapor may be rarely used.

GENERAL PRINCIPLES OF FIXATION

- **Amount of fixing fluid:** Approximately 10–20 times the volume of the specimen, except for osmium tetroxide.
- **Surgical specimens:** Should be placed in fixative as soon as possible after removal from body. Bacteriological study is possible if done immediately.
- **Autopsy specimen:** Autopsy examination should be done after death without delay, if not possible then it should be kept in mortuary refrigerator at 4°C or arterial embalming should be done. Bacteriological or toxicological study not advisable after these procedures.
- **Duration:** Usually for 8 hours at room temperature when tissues are fixed with 10–20 times volume of 10% buffered formalin. But duration of 4 hours is sufficient if fixation is done with agitation. If temperature is raised to 45°C then fixation time may be shortened to 25–40% of usual time.

Aldehyde (Formaldehyde/10% Formalin/Glutaraldehyde)

The reactions between fixative and tissue proteins are usually mild with a short reaction time. Cross-links between proteins are formed and the reaction starts with basic amino acid lysine. Lysine amino acids which are on the exterior aspect of the protein molecule can only react.

In case of formaldehyde the reaction is usually reversible within the first 24 hours by an excess of water but glutaraldehyde causes rapid and irreversible reaction.

Aldehyde fixation may denature proteins to some extent apart from their primary role in forming cross-links. As most of the proteins are not denatured, tissues fixed with aldehyde may be used for immunohistochemistry (IHC), enzyme histochemistry and high resolution electron microscopy. But glutaraldehyde may cause a loss of up to 30% of alpha helix structure of protein in contrast to formaldehyde.

Cross-linkages between proteins and aldehydes can be measured by changes in molecular size, mechanical strength and viscosity. When two proteins are cross-linked, their molecular weight (MW) become doubled and it keeps on increasing as the polymerization (cross-linking of proteins) proceeds (Table 1).

Table 1: Comparison of formaldehyde and glutaraldehyde as fixative

Formaldehyde	*Glutaraldehyde*
• Fixation reaction is slow and reversible (for first 24 hours)	• Fixation reaction is rapid and irreversible
• Protein denaturation is minimal	• Considerable (up to 30% loss of alpha helix structure of protein)
• Enzyme and immunological activity usually retained	• Usually lost
• Morphological picture is average	• Morphological picture is good
• In gel filtration little cross-link formation	• In gel filtration very good cross-linking of proteins
• Prolonged fixation (>24 hours) causes shrinkage and hardening of tissues	• Prolonged fixation longer than conventional period may be advantageous, e.g. electron microscopy
• Most commonly used fixative for light microscopy	• Used for special investigations as in electron microscopy

ROUTINE FORMALIN FIXATIVES

This is a fixative which is most commonly used in histological laboratories. The commercially available solution contains 30–40% formaldehyde gas by weight and is called formalin. So, a 10% formalin fixative gives 4% formaldehyde gas for tissue fixation. Most laboratories prefer 10% buffered formalin or 10% formal saline as fixative (Table 2).

Chemical Composition of Different Formaldehyde Containing Fixatives

Formal Saline (10%)

- Water (preferably distilled): 900 mL.
- Sodium chloride: 9 g.
- Formalin (40% formaldehyde): 100 mL.

10% Formalin (4% Formaldehyde)

- Formalin (40% formaldehyde): 100 mL.
- Distilled water or tap water: 900 mL.

Table 2: Advantages and disadvantages of formalin fixative

Advantages	*Disadvantages*
• It is cheap, relatively stable (when buffered) and easy to prepare • Tissue penetration is good • Does not make tissues very hard or brittle • Allows most routine stainings • Frozen section is possible with formalin fixed tissues • Natural color may be restored • Most commonly used fixative and is the best fixative for the nervous system (brain)	• It may cause dermatitis and asthma in allergic individuals • It is slow to act (less tissue penetration) • There may be formation of dark brown artefact granules especially in tissues containing much blood (e.g. spleen, liver) • Reagent grade formalin (contains 10% methanol in addition to formaldehyde) is unsuitable for electron microscopy as methanol denatures proteins. However, pure formalin is suitable • Gradual loss of basophilic staining of nucleus and cytoplasm. So, prolonged fixation is not advisable • Loss of myelin reactivity when Weigert iron hematoxylin stain is used

Neutral Buffered Formalin (10%)

- Water (preferably distilled): 900 mL
- Formalin: 100 mL
- Sodium dihydrogen phosphate monohydrate: 4 g ($NaH_2PO_4.H_2O$)
- Disodium hydrogen phosphate anhydrous: 6.5 g (Na_2HPO_4.).

REMOVAL OF FORMALIN PIGMENT

Kardasewitch's Method

- Put the histologic sections in water.
- Then place the sections in a mixture for 5 minutes to 3 hours (more the pigment, more the time required). The mixture contains:
  - 70% ethyl alcohol: 100 mL.
  - 28% ammonia water: 1–2 mL.
- After that take it out from the mixture and wash thoroughly in running tap water for 10–15 minutes.

Lillie's Method

- Keep the sections in water.
- Then place the sections in a mixture for 1–5 minutes. The mixture contains:
  - Acetone: 50 mL.
  - 3 volume hydrogen peroxide: 50 mL.
  - 28% ammonia water: 1 mL.
- Wash in 70% alcohol (ethyl) for 1–2 minutes.
- Wash in running tap water for 10–15 minutes.

Picric Acid Method

- Put the sections in water.
- Place the sections in a saturated solution of picric acid for 5 minutes to 2 hours (depending on the amount of artifactual formalin pigments) .
- Wash in running tap water for 10–15 minutes.

PROTEIN DENATURING AGENTS AS FIXATIVE

- **Alcohol:** This is used as 80–100% solution. It frequently shrinks and hardens the tissue. Does not preserve chromatin well but good for demonstrating glycogen, plasma cells, amyloid, iron and uric acid. Carnoy's fluid is generally used for specific purposes. Alcohol denatures and precipitates proteins probably by disrupting hydrogen bonds. Ethyl alcohol is used as a fixative for enzymes (Table 3).
- **Acetic acid:** It is used as 1–5% aqueous solution. It is good for nuclear fixation and has rapid penetration (so, fixation time is less) . Disadvantage of this fixative is that it forms pigments if used with formalin. Also it causes hemolysis of RBCs.

Carnoy's Fixative

- Absolute alcohol: 60 mL.
- Chloroform: 30 mL.
- Glacial acetic acid: 10 mL.

Oxidizing Agent as Fixative

Chromium salts in water (aqueous solution) form Cr-O-Cr complexes. This leads to breakage of internal salt linkages of proteins and increases the activity of basic groups leading to enhanced acidophilia. Oxidizing agents react with proteins and osmium tetroxide to form cross-links with proteins.

- **Osmic acid:** It is used as 1–2% solution. It is very powerful oxidizing agent and is very expensive. So it

Table 3: Advantages and disadvantages of alcohol fixative

Advantages	*Disadvantages*
• Methyl alcohol (80–100%) is excellent fixative for smears • Ethyl alcohol is used as a fixative for enzymes • Carnoy's fixative is used for urgent biopsy (paraffin processing within 5 hours) • Good fixative to demonstrate glycogen, alkaline phosphatise, etc.	• Should be used at 0°C or cooler, otherwise causes marked shrinkage • Distorts morphology and hardens the tissue • Contraindicated for lipid study • Although glycogen can be demonstrated it causes polarization (streaming of protoplasm to one pole of the cell) of glycogen granules

cannot be used with formalin or alcohol. It fixes and stains fat. It is sometimes used for special cytologic methods, e.g. demonstration of Golgi bodies.

- **Potassium dichromate:** This is used as 2–4% aqueous solution. Compared to osmic acid, this is a weak oxidizing agent. It is a poor nuclear fixative as it dissolves nuclear chromatin and causes moderate shrinkage. But it is a good cytoplasmic fixative.

Orth's Fluid

- 2.5% potassium dichromate, $K_2Cr_2O_7$ (aqueous): 100 mL.
- Sodium sulfate (optional): 1 g.
- Formalin (add just before using): 10 mL.

Regaud's (Moller's) Fluid

- 3% potassium dichromate: 80 mL.
- Formalin (add just before using): 20 mL.

Physical Agents as Fixatives

- **Microwave:** The optimum temperature for fixation is 45–55°C. Overheating (>65°C) may cause pyknotic nuclei, vacuolation and cytoplasmic over-staining whereas under-heating (<45°C) causes poor quality of tissue sections. It may be used for rapid fixation of tissues as required in urgent cardiac biopsies. Microwave fixed tissue may be used for electron microscopy aftert post-fixation in osmium tetroxide. Mode of action is through protein denaturation (no cross-linking of proteins as in formalin/aldehyde).
- **Heat:** Like the microwave controlled heat may be used as fixative.

Other Cross-linking Agents

They give alternative or improved fixation for electron microscopy or for gastrointestinal hormones demonstration. As for example, carbodiimides which were described as fixative by Hassel and Hand in 1974.

MERCURY FIXATIVES

Its tissue penetration is poor and cause tissue shrinkage. So, it is usually combined with other fixatives as a mixture. But tissue fixed with mercuric chloride usually results in black precipitates of mercury. This precipitates can be removed by keeping tissue sections in 0.5% iodine solution in 70% alcohol for 5-10 minutes. Then the sections are washed in water and decolorized in 5% sodium thiosulfate for 5 minutes. Again sections are washed in running water for 2-5 minutes (Table 4).

Table 4: Advantages and disadvantages of mercuric chloride fixative

Advantages	*Disadvantages*
• Better staining of nuclei and connective tissue. Recommended for fixing fetal brain • Gives best results for metachromatic staining (e.g. toluidne blue) • Cytoplasmic staining with acidic dyes is enhanced	• Solution rapidly deteriorates • Corrodes most metals except nickel alloy • Zenker's solution removes iron of hemosiderin and causes RBC lysis • Tissues become very hard and brittle if left for 1–2 days in fixation • Reduces the demonstrable glycogen in tissues • Not ideal for frozen sections

Zenker's Fluid

- Distilled water: 950 mL.
- Potassium dichromate: 25 g.
- Mercuric chloride: 50 g.
- Glacial acetic acid: 50 g.
- Fixation time: 4–24 hours followed by prolonged wash.

Helly's Fluid

- Mercuric chloride: 50 g
- Potassium dichromate: 25 g
- Sodium sulfate: 10 g
- Distilled water: 950 mL.
- Fixation time: Same as in Zenker's fluid but 50 mL of 40% formaldehyde is added to this fluid before use.

PICRIC ACID FIXATIVES

It is used as a mixture and common mixtures are Bouin's fluid, Rossman's fluid and Brasil's alcoholic picro-formol fixative. It reacts with histones and basic proteins to form crystalline picrates with amino acids. This is a very good preservative for glycogen (Table 5).

Bouin's Fluid

- Saturated aqueous picric acid solution: 75 mL.
- Formalin (40% formaldehyde): 25 mL.
- Glacial acetic acid: 5 mL.

Table 5: Advantages and disadvantages of Bouin's fluid

Advantages	*Disadvantages*
• It is a good fixative except mammalian kidney and penetrates rapidly. Shrinkage is minimal • Good fixative to demonstrate glycogen • Small fragments easily visualized because of yellowish color after fixation • Solution is stable	• Prolonged fixation (>24 hours) causes tissue hard and brittle • It lyses RBCs and reduces the iron content • Lipids are also decreased in amount and are altered

Brasil's Alcoholic Picro-formol Fixative

- Picric acid (50% water): 80 g
- Formalin: 2,040 mL
- Ethanol or isopropyl alcohol: 6,000 mL.
- Trichloroacetic acid: 65 g.

FIXATION OF TISSUES FOR ELECTRON MICROSCOPY

Fixation for electron microscopy should be done at 4°C in the refrigerator. The commonly used fixatives are glutaraldehyde and osmium tetroxide. Glutaraldehyde forms cross-linkages between molecules and preserves the cellular structure well. Whereas osmium tetroxide gels protein by formation of bridges between molecules. It rapidly fixes the tissue as well as stains the tissue structures.

FACTORS INVOLVED IN TISSUE FIXATION

- **Temperature:** Usually done at room temperature. For electron microscopy and some histochemistry low temperature (0–4°C) is preferred to slow down the autolysis. For fixation in bacteriology (e.g. leprosy, TB) and blood film heat may be used. For urgent biopsy, formalin may be heated up to 60°C. Fixation can be done within 5 hours at 40°C but higher temperature deteriorates some antigens, e.g. PCNA.
- **pH (hydrogen ion concentration):** Good fixation is achieved at a pH of 6–8. Outside this pH there may be damage to the ultrastructure. Storage granules of adrenaline and noradrenaline are most stable at pH 6.5 with formalin fixative. Gastric mucosa is best fixed at pH 5.5 .
- **Duration:** Primary fixation in buffered formalin for 2–8 hours (< 24 hours). Prolonged fixation causes hardening and shrinkage of tissue.
- **Tissue penetration:** This process is usually slow with usual fixatives. So, the blocks should be either thin or small (e.g. 1 mm^3 for electron microscopy). The depth of penetration is proportional to the square root of time (t) and can be expressed as $d = K\sqrt{t}$; where K (in tissue) is the constant and it is the coefficient of diffusibility of the fixative in tissues or gel. K value (tissue) is high (1.33) in potassium dichromate fixative whereas it is low (0.25) in chromium and glutaraldehyde fixative.
- **Concentration of fixative:** Ideal concentration should be used for good fixation, e.g. 10% buffered formalin, 3% glutaraldehyde or saturated solution of picric acid and mercuric chloride. The concentration may be changed with change of pH or addition of buffer to a fixative. Like glutaraldehyde can be used at 0.25% if the pH of the vehicle is correct and can be used for immuno-electron microscopy.
- **Osmolality:** The preferred osmolality is slightly hypertonic solution or isotonic solution.
- **Substances added as vehicles:** Sodium chloride added to mercuric chloride fixative to increase the binding of it to amino groups of proteins. Likewise, tannic acid enhances fixation of protein, lipid and complex carbohydrates especially for electron microscopy.
- **Volume changes:** Volume of tissue may be changed during fixation. Nucleuses in frozen sections are usually bigger whereas prolonged fixation in formalin causes shrinkage. Some intercellular material like collagen swells when they are fixed.

SECONDARY FIXATION (POST-FIXATION/ POST-CHROMATIN)

It is the use of two fixatives in succession. The first one is the primary fixative and the second one is the secondary fixative. As for example, after primary fixation in buffered formalin, tissues are kept in secondary fixative of mercuric chloride-formaldehyde solution. Advantage of this sublimate post-fixation is that tissues are more easily cut and flatten better, also they give better staining quality. Likewise, tissues fixed with glutaraldehyde may be post-fixed with osmium tetroxide which makes the membranes relatively permeable and better stained (Table 6).

Table 6: Choice of fixatives for different cellular component or surgical specimens

Surgical specimens/tissues	*Choice of fixative*
Routine specimen/general surgical specimen	10% buffered formalin
Glycogen	Bouin's fluid (picric acid fixatives), alcohol fixatives (absolute alcohol)
Fat/lipid	Osmic acid
Golgi bodies	Osmic acid
Enzymes	Ethyl alcohol
Smears (blood or cytologic)	Methyl alcohol
Urgent biopsies	Carnoy's (alcohol) fixative
Electron microscopy	3% glutaraldehyde, osmium tetroxide
Nuclei	Mercury fixative (Zenker), acetic acid
Cytoplasm	Potassium dichromate
Gastrointestinal hormones	Carbodiimide
Metachromasia	Mercury fixative (Zenker's)
Testis	Bouin's fluid, buffered formalin
Nucleic acid (DNA and RNA)	Carnoy's fluid
Mucoprotein	Glutaraldehyde
Neuroendocrine granules	Ethanol, methanol, acetone
Cholesterol and its esters	Bouin's fluid, Zenker's fluid
Glycoproteins	Chromates
Gouty crystals (monosodium urate)	Absolute alcohol
Intermediate filaments	Carnoy's fluid, Methacarn
Trephine/bone marrow biopsy	Zenker or Zenker's formalin (previously B5)

CHAPTER 2

Tissue Processing, Microtomy and Paraffin Sections

TISSUE PROCESSING, MICROTOMY AND PARAFFIN SECTIONS

Tissue contains intracellular as well as extracellular water which should be removed as paraffin wax (commonly used as embedding medium) is not miscible with water. Also most fixatives are water based (like formalin) so there must be some processes which remove this water and allow paraffin wax impregnation. The whole process is called tissue processing.

The steps in tissue processing are:

- **Dehydration:** Common agents are ethyl alcohol/ethanol/acetone, methyl alcohol, isopropyl alcohol and dioxane.
- **Clearing:** Common agents are xylene (xylol) toluene (toluol), chloroform, citrus fruits oils, paraffin and Histoclear.
- **Impregnation:** Common agents are paraffin wax, other waxes (like ester wax, polyester wax), resins (acrylic, epoxy), agar, gelatin and celloidin.
- **Embedding:** Final stage with paraffin blocks.

DEHYDRATION

This step removes water and fixative from the tissue and replaces then with dehydrating fluid. Naturally dehydrating fluid should mix with and has water affinity so that so that it can easily penetrate the tissue cells. The best reagent is ethanol or ethyl alcohol.

A. Ethyl alcohol (ethanol): It is a clear colorless flammable liquid. It is used as graded alcohol beginning with 70% then to higher grades, e.g. 85% or 95%. But for delicate tissues like embryo, animal tissues or brain it should be more gradual (begins with 50%). As it is hydrophilic, it is miscible with water and many other organic solvents.

B. Acetone: This is also a clear and volatile, colorless, flammable fluid which is miscible with water, ethanol and many organic solvents. Though it has rapid action, it has poor tissue penetration and prolonged used may cause tissue brittleness. It is cheaper than ethanol but more amounts (at least 10 times the volume of tissue) is needed.

C. Methanol: It is highly toxic but can substitute ethanol, rarely used now a day.

D. Isopropyl alcohol: Becoming very popular as it is cheaper and no excise duty is required as in alcohol. It is miscible with water, ethanol and most organic solvent. It is recommended for microwave oven processing method.

E. Dioxane (diethyl dioxide): It has the advantage of being miscible with water, alcohol, xylene, balsam and paraffin wax. The dioxane can be reused after removing the water from dehydrating fluid with calcium chloride or quicklime (CaO). But it is toxic and is not recommended for routine use.

CLEARING

This step replaces the dehydrating fluid and embedding medium (paraffin wax). So, this stage acts as a bridge between dehydration and subsequent embedding. When the dehydrating fluid is totally replaced by these agents, the tissue looks translucent, hence the name clearing agent came.

- **Xylene (xylol):** This is an excelling clearing agent but immersion must not be prolonged (>3 hours) as it makes tissue hard and brittle. It is cheap and can be used with celloidin section. This is not suitable for lymph nodes and brain, as it makes them very brittle.
- **Toluene (toluol):** It has almost similar properties to xylene but has the advantage of not making the tissues hard and brittle.
- **Chloroform:** It is slower in action than xylene. It causes little brittleness and is recommended for nervous tissue, eye, granulation tissue, lymph nodes and larger tissue blocks (up to 1 cm) can be processed. It is non-inflammable but highly toxic. Unlike other clearing agents it does not make tissues translucent.
- **Citrus fruit oils:** It is extracted from orange and lemon rinds. It is nontoxic and miscible with water. But it has the disadvantage of dissolving out small mineral deposits in tissues (copper, calcium).
- **Paraffin wax:** Recently introduced as a cleaning agent because of its cheapness. Time of immersion is similar to chloroform.
- **Histoclear:** It has been recently introduced. This nontoxic agent is derivative of food-grade material and has much promise.

IMPREGNATION

This step involves replacement and clearing agent with the embedding medium. This impregnating medium fills all natural cavities, interstices and spaces of the tissues. It makes the tissues sufficiently firm to allow thin section cutting but without alteration of the spatial relationship of the tissues and cellular components and also not to distort the tissues. Subsequently, making of blocks is done with embedding medium. Usual duration is 1–3 hours.

Vacuum Impregnation

This process fasten impregnation step and remove excess air bubbles from tissues which has undergone clearing step. This process benefit tissues like lunge, spleen, muscle, skin, central nervous system and decalcified bone. As for example, lung tissue after clearing to a heated paraffin wax bath can be transferred to vacuum impregnation with a degree of vacuum <500 mm Hg. This way excess residual air can be removed from the tissue and the impregnation time is also reduced by half (Fig. 1).

Apparatus

The apparatus may be of two types; gas and electric. Both of these two types work on same principle and consist of thermostatically controlled vacuum embedding bath. The lid or door of the bath is fitted with a well-fitting rubber washer and, when evacuated by either a mechanical and water pump, must be able to maintain a vacuum. The degree of vacuum is controlled by the use of a mercury manometer or by a gauge on the newer electric model. There is a trap between manometer and water evacuation pump to prevent backflow of water directly into the oven, in case the water supply inadvertently turned off before the exhaust trap on the oven has been closed.

Procedure

Firstly, close the lid or door and put slight pressure on it during initial part of evacuation. Now, close air intake valve, open exhaust valve and start the evacuation pump.

Reduce the pressure slowly and stop when a pressure of 400–500 mm Hg is obtained. Close the exhaust valve and switch off the evacuation pump.

To enter air in the oven, slowly open the air intake valve until the pressure within the oven equals that of the atmosphere.

EMBEDDING

Tissues which have been impregnated in paraffin wax is put in freshly melted paraffin wax and allowed to solidify. This can be done by using metal containers like Tissue

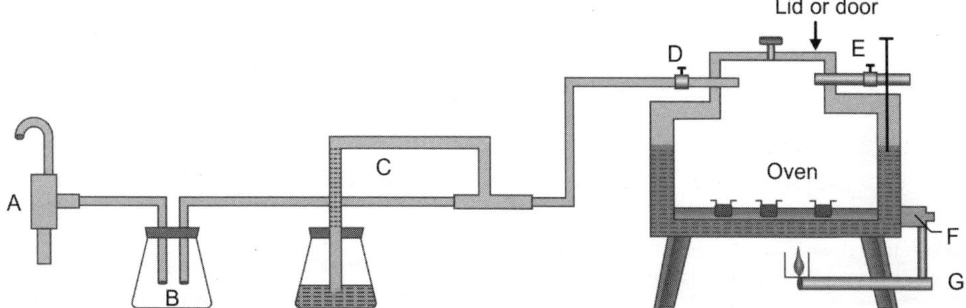

Fig. 1: Vacuum embedding and impregnation. A, water vacuum pump; B, trap; C, mercury manometer; D, exhaust outlet; E, air inlet; F, evacuation pump

Tek, Leukhart's L or paper boats, etc. The tissue should be carefully oriented so that the surface to be cut is placed downwards. Commonly two methods are used in histology namely paraffin wax, resins and celloidin method.

- **Paraffin wax**: It is probably the most popular embedding medium as it is chip, easily handled and section cutting is easier. Melting point ranging between 40–70°C. Wax with higher melting point has higher hardness. Wax with a melting point off 54–58°C is preferred for routine use. Sometimes, substances like bee wax, rubber, ceresin, dental wax, diethylene glycol are added as additives to increase the hardness of paraffin wax hence, more thin sections can be cut (Fig. 2).
- **Resins**: This is particular used for thin sections for high resolution, for lection microscopy and for undecalcified bone.
- **Celloidin**: Celloidin or its variant low viscosity nitrocellulose (LVN) was popular for large tissue blocks and for nervous tissue (like eye). Sections are cut by base sledge or a sliding microtone.
- **Agar**: It does not have sufficient support for sectioning of tissue alone. Its main use is to adhere small friable tissue pieces after fixation. After solidification in motten ager, tissues are embedded in paraffin wax.
- **Gelatin**: Its main use is in frozen sectioning.
- **Paraplast**: It is a mixture of purified paraffin wax and synthetic plastic polymers whose melting point is 56–57°C. Sections can be cut without cooling the block face by ice. Ribbon like sections are more easy to cut and does not tend to crack. Larger blocks and bone blocks may be cut easily as it is more resilient than paraffin wax.
- **Carbowax**: Alcohols with more carbon atoms (≥12) are solid at room temperature and may be used in tissue embedding. Alcohols with 18–12 carbon atoms are suitable for this purpose. Carbowax (polyethylene glycols) is good for this purpose. Carbowax is soluble in and miscible with water, hence embedding may be done directly from the formalin fixation bypassing the first dehydration and second clearing steps of normal tissue processing. Normally, four changes of carbowax (70%, 90% and two changes of 100%) are used at 56°C for 30 minutes, 45 minutes and 1 hour respectively with agitation (Table 1).

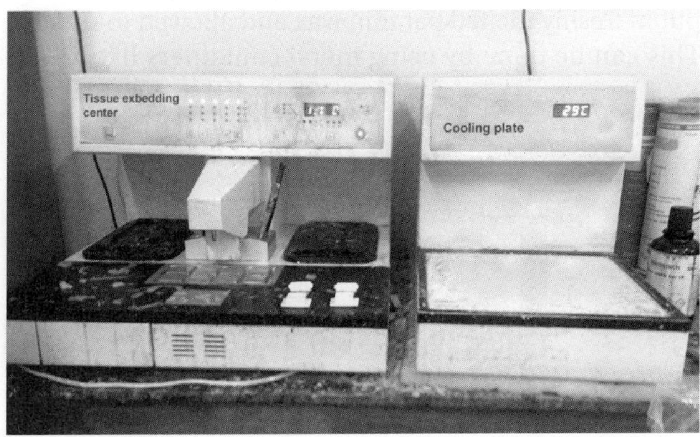

Fig. 2: Automated paraffin embedding

Table 1: Advantages and disadvantages of Carbowax

Advantages	*Disadvantages*
• Dehydration and clearing steps may be bypassed • As it does not undergo those two steps, lipids and neutral fats are not removed. So, these may be demonstrated in these sections • The processing time is short compared to the routine tissue processing • It reduces tissue shrinkage and distortion • It is also good for many enzyme histochemistry studies	• Carbowax sections have a tendency to crumble, so obtaining good sections may be difficult. Softer grade may be used to overcome this problem • If carbowax is overheated, various polymers with high molecular weight are formed and the blocks become more crumbly during section cutting • As it is water soluble, sections cannot be floated on water bath. For this diethylene glycol or gelatin mixture is used

The specimens are then put in fresh carbowax at 50°C for blocking and the blocks are immediately cooled in the refrigerator.

As carbowax is very hygroscopic, blocks and sustained sections must not come in contact with water or ice and are stored in dry, airtight containers.

Manual Processing (2 Days)

Container	*Fluid*	*Time*
1	70% alcohol	1 h (9.00 am–10.00 am)
2	95% alcohol	1 h (10.00 am–11.00 am)
3	95% alcohol	2 h (11.00 am–1.00 pm)
4	100% alcohol	1.5 h (1.00 pm–2.30 pm)
5	100% alcohol	1.5 h (2.30 pm–4.00 pm)
6	100% alcohol	1.5 h (4.00 pm–5.30 pm)
7	100% alcohol	Overnight
8	Xylene	1 h (9.00 am–10.00 am)
9	Xylene	1.5 h (10.00 am–11.30 am)
10	Paraffin wax	1.5 h (11.30 am–1.00 pm)
11	Paraffin wax	1.5 h (1.00 pm–2.30 pm)
12	Paraffin wax	2.5 h (2.30 pm–5.00 pm)

In case of large blocks the schedule can be modified by extending the time in each container to all days in container 1, overnight in container 2, all day in container 3 and so on.

Rapid Processing for Small Biopsies or for Urgent Work

Rapid processing within 2–5 hours is done using heat (37°C or 47°C) or vacuum which speed up tissue processing. Usually fixation is done by ethyl alcohol, so immunohistochemistry is difficult with this processed tissue. Formalin is not used as it takes more time for fixation; urgency is the main reason for rapid processing. Biopsy should be trimmed to <2 mm in thickness.

Short Processing Schedule for Urgent Work and Small Biopsies

Container	Fluid	Vacuum (<500 mm Hg)	Heat, °C	Time
1	10% formalin	Yes	45	20 minutes
2	95% ethyl alcohol	Yes	45	5 minutes
3	95% ethyl alcohol	Yes	45	5 minutes
4	100% ethyl alcohol	Yes	45	5 minutes
5	100% ethyl alcohol	Yes	45	5 minutes
6	100% ethyl alcohol	Yes	45	5 minutes
7	100% ethyl alcohol	Yes	45	5 minutes
8	Absolute alcohol	Yes	45	5 minutes
9	Xylene	Yes	45	5 minutes
10	Xylene	Yes	45	5 minutes
11	Paraffin wax	Yes	45	5 minutes
12	Paraffin wax	Yes	45	5 minutes
Total time				75 minutes

Draining time is 5 minutes after each stage. So there will be 11 × 5 = 55 minutes draining time for the above schedule with 12 stages. Hence, total time for the above schedule will be (75 + 55) minutes = 130 minutes or 2 hours 10 minutes.

AUTOMATED TISSUE PROCESSING

Many histopathology laboratories now a days use automatic tissue processors to process tissues. These machines have reduced the processing time compared to manual time (at least 24 hours). Other advantage is superior quality of tissue processing due to constant agitation.

Two types of processing machines are used: Carosel type and enclosed pump fluid type. But the older carousel type is currently being replaced by newer enclosed pump fluid type. Enclosed tissue processor is advantageous over carousel type, as in case of any electric fault, these machine sounds and alarm and automatically stops (Fig. 3). Other advantages of enclosed tissue processors are:

- More rapid schedule

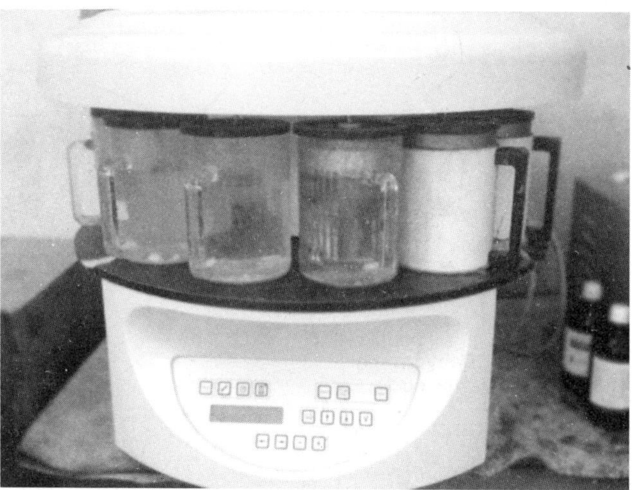

Fig. 3: Automated tissue processor

- Vacuum and heat application at any stage to speed up processing
- Fluid spillage containment
- Less toxic fumes emitted
- If required longer delay schedule permitted.

Most laboratories use an overnight schedule of approximately 16–18 hours. In case of weekend and holidays, when delay is required, then the tissues are kept in first container with 10% formalin. Some delicate tissues require special treatment, as for example, enucleated eyes. The eye must be thoroughly fixed dissected before processing. To soften hard tissue like lens and sclera, phenol is added to the lower percentage of alcohol. Chloroform is chosen as a clearing agent as it is less harsh than xylene and causes less shrinkage, thus keeping the retina attached (Fig. 4).

Overnight Schedule (Automation Technique)

Container	Fluid	Time (hours)
1	10% formalin	0
2	70% alcohol	1/2
3	95% alcohol	1/2
4	100% alcohol	1/2
5	100% alcohol	1/2
6	100% alcohol	1/2
7	100% alcohol	1/2
8	100% alcohol/xylene	1/2
9	Xylene	1
10	Xylene	2
11	Paraffin wax	2 and 1/2
12	Paraffin wax	4
Total time		14 and 1/2 hours

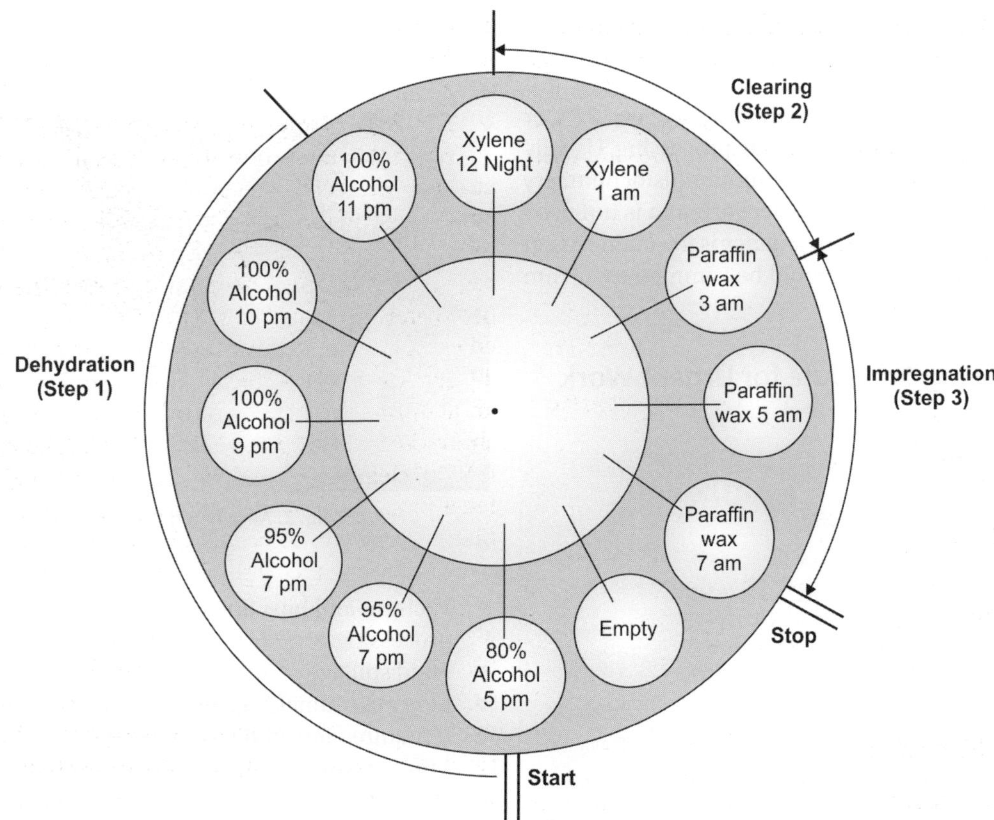

Fig. 4: Automatic tissue processing in different timer discs. Step 1: Dehydration; Step 2: Clearing; Step 3: Impregnation in paraffin wax

MICROTOMY

Microtomy is the process by which tissues are sectioned by microtomes and these sections are attach to a surface for visualization by microscopes. A microtome (from Greek micros, meaning 'small' and temmein, meaning 'to cut' is a tool used to cut extremely thin slices of material, known in histology as sections.

Microtomes are basic instrument for microtomy and are designed for accurate cutting of sections (thin slices). Generally there are several types of microtome:

- Rotary microtome
- Rocking microtome
- Sliding microtome
- Freezing microtome
- Ultrathin microtome
- Rotary rocking microtome
- Base sledge microtome
- Vibrotome.

ROTARY MICROTOME

This microtome was invented by Minot in 1885–1886. Probably this is the most popular microtome for routine paraffin wax embedded tissues (Fig. 5). Serial sections can

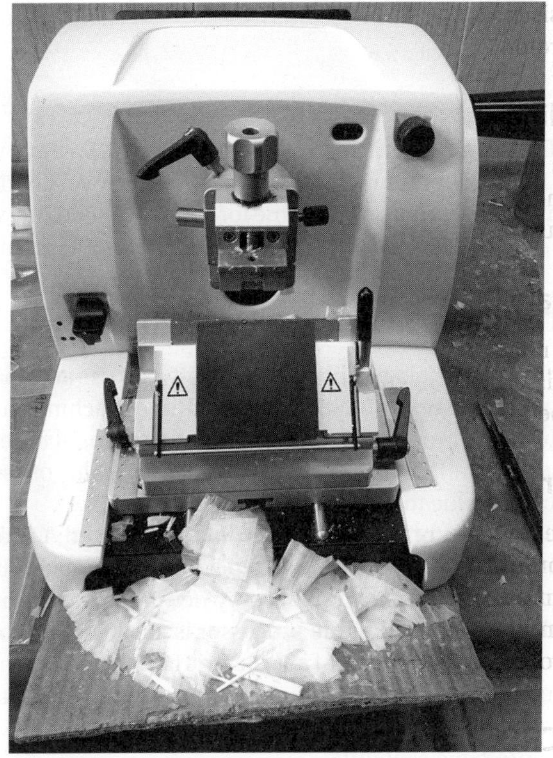

Fig. 5: Rotary microtome

be cut conveniently. A large number of paraffin blocks can be cut. Electrically driven rotary microtomes are costlier compared to manual microtomes and are used when the control is necessary to produce ribbons for serial sections. Electrically driven or manual rotary microtomes are used in cryostats for frozen sections.

Disadvantages

- Only a small length of knife is available for cutting, so large blocks cannot be cut (cutting facet base sledge microtome)
- Cellodin embedded blocks cannot be cut (cutting facet sliding microtome)
- Relatively costlier.

Rocking Microtome

It was used in the past and Cambridge rocking microtome was most commonly used. It is cheap and was also used in cryostats first. But hard tissues cannot be cut and size of blocks should be small.

Base Sledge Microtome

This mirotome is favored when large blocks and very hard tissues should be sectioned. In neuropathology, this microtome is preferred as large blocks of brain are made. It is also good for resin embedded undecalcified bone. But consistent thin sections are difficult to cut unlike in rotary microtome.

Sliding Microtome

This machine is dangerous as knife is taken along with runners to the block and knife guards cannot be attached. It was used in the past for celloidin embedded blocks cutting.

Rotary Rocking Microtome

This microtome has the advantage of making flat surface to the tissue block. It is usually used in cryostat though paraffin embedded blocks can also be cut.

Vibratome

Here a vibrating knife is used which oscillates variably according to the voltage supplied through a transformer when passed through a tissue during section cutting. Its main use in some enzyme demonstration in unfixed, unfrozen sections.

MICROTOME KNIVES

There are many types of microtome knives. The common types are:

- Wedge shaped
- Plano concave
- Biconcave
- Tool edge.

We should know how to set these microtome knives to cut sections from paraffin embedded blocks. The actual cutting part of the knife forms a very small area, the sides of which (cutting facets) are more acutely inclined towards each other than the sides of knife proper. The angle formed between the cutting facets where they meet at the cutting edges is known as the 'Bevel angle' which is normally is 27–32°. The angle of these facets is kept constant for each knife during the process of honing and stropping. Knives should be inclined relative to the cutting plane, so that there is 5–10° clearance or 'Clearance angle' between the cutting facet presenting to the block and the surface of paraffin block. If there is no proper clearance angle, then missed sections or alternately thick and thin sections may result.

In rotary microtome, the axis (plane) of knife edge is kept at right angles to the plane of cutting (line of movement of block). But in case of hard tissue blocks, large tissue blocks or celloidin embedded blocks, the axis of knife edge is inclined to 30–45°, so that it is oblique rather than right angle (90°), this gives a slicing cut with less wedging (Figs 6 to 8).

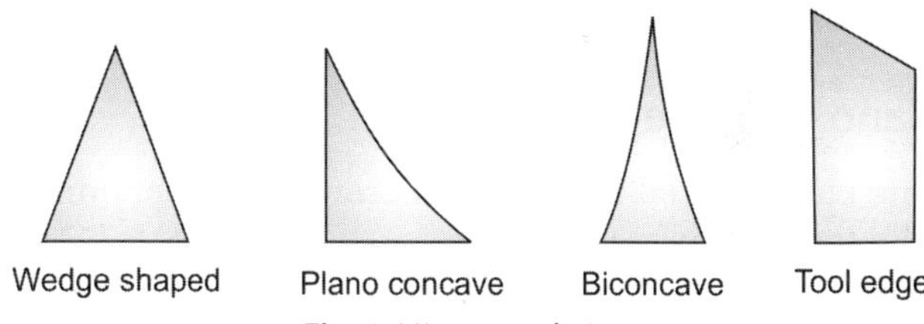

Fig. 6: Microtome knives

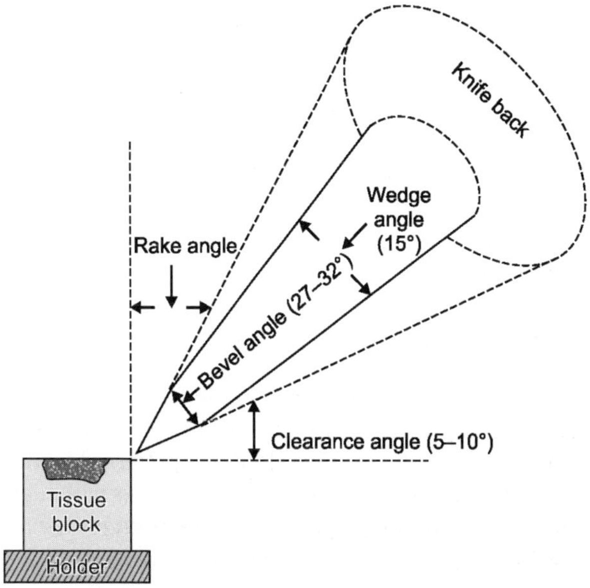

Fig. 7: Setting the microtome knife

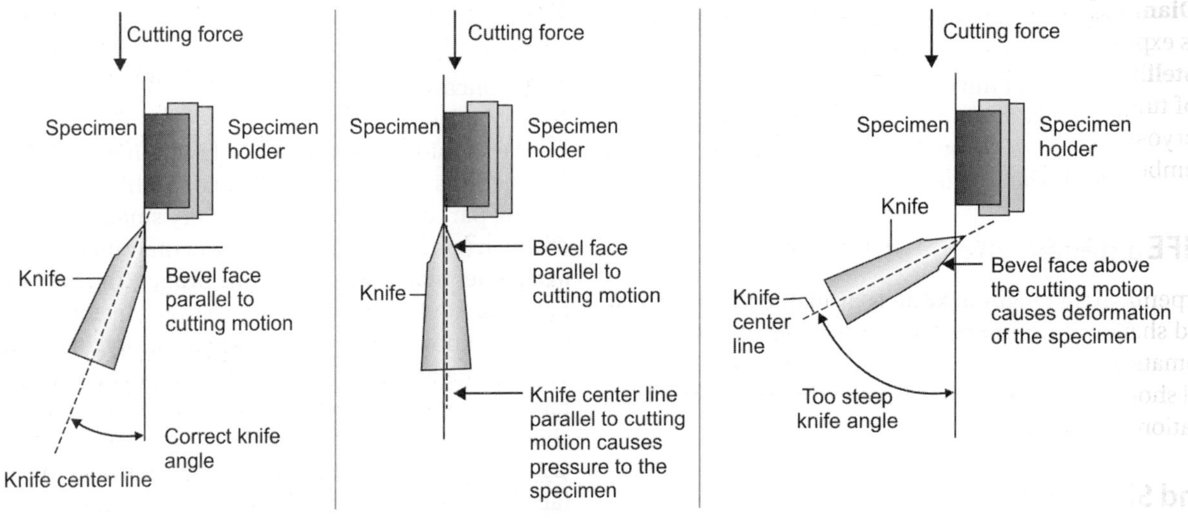

Fig. 8: Knife angle in microtomy

Wedge-shaped Knife

This is the most common knife used nowadays for section cutting. The sides of the wedge knives are inclined at an angle of approximately 15° (wedge angle). Surfaces of these knives are highly polished so that sections will move on surface and will not adhere to surface. This minimizes chances of folding, distortion and facilitates ribbon formation.

Plano Concave

This knife is used in sliding microtome for sectioning cellodin embedded material.

Biconcave

This is not recommended for normal routine work as rigidity is sacrificed because of its shape. But a very keen edge can be produced.

Tool Edge

This kind of knife is rigid and is recommended for use in hardest of tissues and embedding media. So, it is preferred for resin embedded undecalcified bone. This type is used in Jung K microtome.

KNIFE MATERIALS

Knives used for microtomy are made from good quality tool steel or high carbon, tempered from the tip inwards for one-third of the width of knife. Hardness preferred for these knives is about 700 on Vickers hardness. Knives with higher hardness are difficult to sharpen and knife edges become brittle. There are several types of knives:

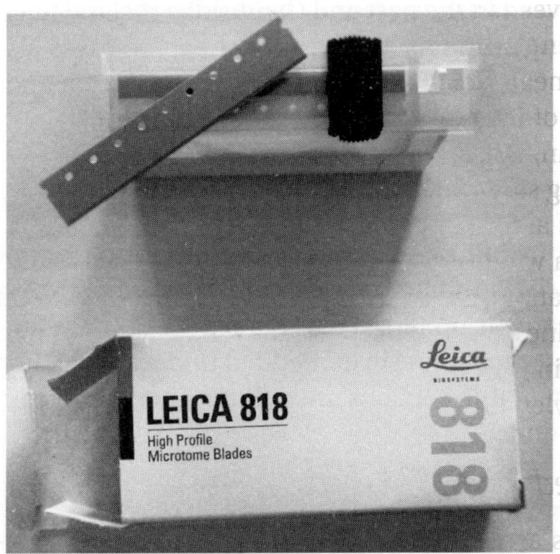

Fig. 9: Disposable blade for rotary microtome

- **Disposable blades**: Nowadays, this is the most commonly used for routine paraffin embedded sectioning. Modern blades are usually coated with a special PTFE which allows ribbons to be sectioned easily. Recently discovered magnetic disposable blades are attached to blade holders and may be used in cryostat. Disposable blades have some advantages, as they are cheap and flawless and 3–4 µm sections can be cut from paraffin blocks when compared to conventional steel knife (Fig. 9).
- **Glass knives:** These are used in ultra-thin microtomy. 'Ralph' type glass knives were used for sectioning glycol methacrylate resin embedded tissues.
- **Tungsten carbide tipped knives:** These are used in lather tools. The sintered tungsten carbide blades are brittle and are mixed with a steel body to make a composite knife which is more stable and harder.

- **Diamond knives**: It is used in electron microscopy and is expensive.
- **Stellite-tipped knives:** Stellite is an alloy which is made of tungsten, cobalt and chromium. It may be used in cryostat but not recommended for routine paraffin embedded sectioning.

KNIFE SHARPENING

Sharpening can be done either by hand or by a machine. Hand sharpening was used in the past and is replaced by automatic knife sharpening. The final sharpening materials used should have a grain size smaller than the permissible serrations remaining the edge.

Hand Sharpening

It can be done by two ways: (1) By hones and (2) By abrasives and plate glass. A hone is a natural stone or hard grinding surface for sharpening a cutting tool or knife. The finer the grain, the harder the hone. There are many types of hones—Carborundum, Arkansas stone, yellow Belgian, Belgian black vein (blue-green). Amongst these honing stones Belgian stones are finest whereas Arkansas hones are of the medium fineness. Carborundum hones have a wide variety of fineness. Oil is commonly used as lubricating agent, so hones are also called a oilstones. Light machine oil is probably the best, other lubricants are liquid paraffin (mineral oil), vegetable oil, neutral soap solution and xylene.

Procedure of Honing

Hones are wiped with a soft cloth to clean it. Then it is covered with a thin film of lubricant. Now the knife is filled with its own back and laid obliquely on the stone, edge forward. Gentle even pressure is made on knife with thumbs and forefingers. Knife is now drawn obliquely forward on the honing stone in a steady movement. First heel end (handle end), then toe end. When the knife reached the other end of hone, knife is rotated on its back, so that the other cutting facet lies on the stone. Now the knife is drawn toward the operator, again from heel to toe. This forward-backward movement of knife over the hones is called double stroke. Usually 20-30 double strokes are required for sharpening. After honing knife edges are wiped clean with a rag moistened in xylene.

Plate Glass Honing

Here, a piece of plate glass which is about 14 inches long, 1-2 inches wider than the length of the knife blade and 1/4 to 3/8 inch thick is used. Abrasive powder (Corundum 303 or 304) is used for removing nicks and for grinding in conjunction with plate glass. As the plate glass is wider (1-2 inches) than length of knife, there is no need to place the knife obliquely as in honing stones. The knife is pushed and pulled (forward and backward movement) at right angles to the transverse axis of the plate.

Automatic Hones

These are usually flat plate glass hone and may be of two types. One is a large circular glass plate and the other is a smaller rectangular frosted glass plate. The smaller hone is preferred as it has precision, greater fitness, economical and case of dressing (Fig. 10A).

Stropping

Though perfectly honed knife does not require stropping theoretically, but in practice stropping is still required. Strops should be made from best quality shell horse leather (rump or thick part of horse hide). The strop or leather should be 18 inches wide, mounted on a solid wooden block. For stropping, the knife is first fitted with knife back, and then placed obliquely on the strop. Then it is pushed backward and pushed forward (toe to heel) and its back edge always leading which is opposite to honing. Usually 40-120 double strokes are required for stropping. Before and after use, the strop should be wiped with a soft cloth to remove particles. Sometimes, xylene moistened cloth is used for cleaning. But care must be given as xylene may remove the oil (like castrol oil), used to impregnate the strop (Fig. 10B).

Using two types of stropes mounted on the same block is advantageous. One of the pure fine leather, while the other impregnated with a fine abrasive (fine carborundum paste

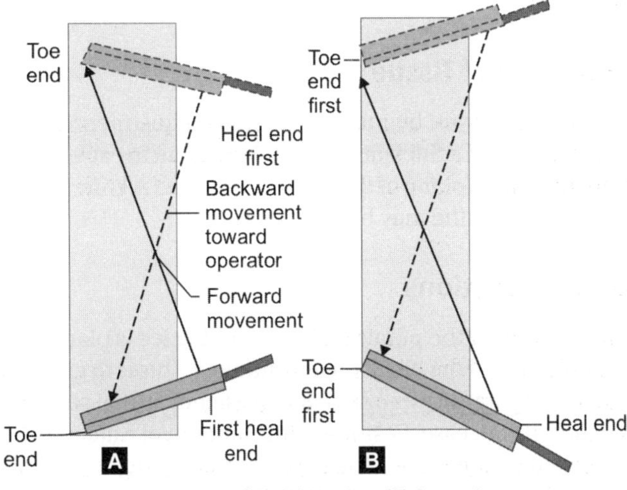

Figs 10A and B: (A) Honing; (B) Stropping

or diamond dust). This second or coarser strop may be used to touch up knife when there is no time for honing.

Automatic knife sharpeners: With the advent of disposal blades, the steel knives are becoming obsolete. But some microtomists still prefer the older steel knives for section cutting from paraffin blocks. Few types of automatic knife sharpening machines are available:

- The rotating buffing wheel type (made by Temtool)
- Glass plate type (made by Shandon)
- Large circular glass plate type.

Fanz sharpener was very popular until the recently developed Shandon-Elliot Autosharp III.

Manual knife sharpening device: Best device was developed by Bell which is also most scientific. The advice includes a large circular bronze lapping plate with parallel grooves to prevent accumulation of debris on the honing surface.

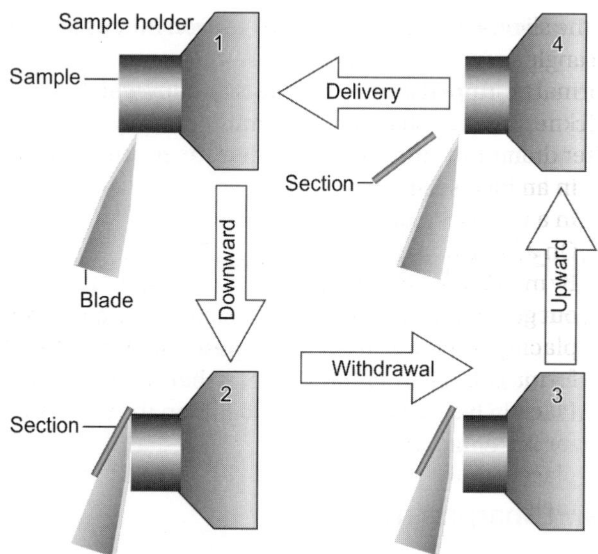

Fig. 11: Tissue cutting by microtome

PARAFFIN SECTION CUTTING

Setting of the Microtome

Here we will follow the steps in a rotary microtome, although basic steps are same for other microtomes. The numbered paraffin block is secured in place in the microtome object clamp. Special microtome clamps are available for specific embedding systems, e.g. Tissue Tek, TIMS, for those mounted on fiber blocks and for unmounted (e.g. Peel-A-Way) blocks.

The object holders are adjusted so that top of the paraffin block just touches the knife edge. If the tissue has varied consistency, e.g. skin it is performed to have the soft part of the tissue strikes the knife edge first. After placing the knife in position, both the clearance angle and angle of slope should be adjusted. A clearance angle of 3–4° and angle of slope of 40° are found to be satisfactory.

Trimming of Tissue Blocks

Trimming is done by means of course adjustment of the microtome and a thickness of 10–15 µm is cut in each stroke until the whole plane of the tissue is reached. A knife which is awaiting honing may be used for this.

Cutting Sections

After trimming the paraffin block; melting ice is placed on suitable area of the block for few minutes. This is to give the tissue and paraffin wax a similar consistency so that sections can be cut with ease. Besides, a little amount of water will be absorbed by the tissue. The tissue will swell slightly which will make section easier. For routing purpose sections are cut at 4–5 µm thickness. Some tissues are cut at 3 µm (e.g. kidney, bone marrow, trephine and lymph node biopsies) and other thicker at 5–6 µm (e.g. bone and brain). Ribbon sections are very good for handling cut sections. After cutting a ribbon (6–8 sections) the first section is hold by forceps while the last section is taken away by a small brush from the knife edge, the brush itself will be attached to the last section. An experienced technician or microtomist may cut a ribbon of 9–10 inches long. But for mounting, the ribbons are cut into suitable length (2 inches) (Fig. 11).

Floating Out Sections

Now, the ribbon sections are taken out and placed in floating out bath. Usually water-bath is used and temperature of water should be 10°C below the melting point of paraffin wax. Small amount of detergent or alcohol may be added to the water which will reduce the surface tension and will make sections flatten easily. The trailing end of the ribbon should be in contact with the water first. The shining side of sections should be down on water bath.

In case there are folds, they may be adjusted by gentle teasing with forceps. Usually 0.5–2 minutes time is good for a section to be flattened.The water should be cleaned by dragging a tissue paper across the surface. It should be done after each block cutting.

Placing of Slides and Drying

The surface of the slide coated with adhesive is then approximated to whole length of the section (ribbon) gently. Now,the slide is raised in an even motion. As the slide touches the edge of section, the section will adhere to the slide as it is drawn upward. Then the slides are stood an angle of 60–85° for 2–5 minutes for draining of water. For normal routine work, 75 × 25 mm slides are used. Preferred thickness of the slides is 1–1.2 mm.

After draining, the sections may be dries in several ways;

- In an incubator at 37°C overnight.
- In a wax oven at 56–60°C for 2 hours.
- On a hot plate at 45–55°C for 30–45 minutes.
- By mounting the sections in 0.1–0.25% aqueous floating-out gelatin or albumenized slides draining excess fluid, placing them in a Coplin jar containing 2–3 mL 40% formaldehyde in the incubator at 37°C for 4–18 hours.
- Placing in a blower type electric slide dryer at 50–55°C for 20–30 minutes. For urgent works the slides may be placed above the Bunsen flame until the paraffin wax melt.

SECTION ADHESIVES

If the slides are grease free and sections are adequately dried, then sections do not float during staining and there is no need of adhesives. But there are some circumstances when sections will float:

- Significant exposure of acid alkalis during staining.
- Cryostat sections for immunofluorescence, immunohistochemistry and urgent diagnosis.
- Decalcified tissues, tissue containing blood clot, CNS tissues.
- Sections submitted to high temperature.

Protein adhesives such as gelatin, albumin and starch are prone to contaminate due to bacterial or fungal overgrowth which may cause confusion in PAS and gram stain. Use of a glass rod applicator fixed in the stopper of the container and use of thymol will help prevent this.

Mayer's Egg Albumen-Glycerol

- Whites of fresh egg: 50 mL
- Glycerol: 50 mL.

Mix well and filter the solution by using several layers of gauze. Add about 100 mg thymol to prevent mould growth.

Gelatin in Floating Out Bath

Adding 15–30 mL of 1% aqueous gelatin to the water of floating bath and mixing well is an alternative to direct coating of slides.

But nowadays two new adhesives are being used, replacing the previous one due to chances of contamination.

- **Poly-L-lysine:** This is readily available as 0.1 solution and is further diluted for use, 1 in 10, with distilled water. The coated slides should be used within few days as poly-L-lysine loosely attaches the section to the slide and tends to dissociate after few days.
- **3-Aminopropyltriethoxysilane (APES):** Probably this is the best section adhesive. Slides are dipped in 2% APES in acetone, drained and again dipped into acetone. After that, slides are drained again and dipped into distilled water. Then the slides are dried. These APES coated slides are particularly useful for cytospin preparation of blood or proteinaceous material.

CUTTING HARD TISSUES

Due to advent of disposable blades and introduction of automatic knife sharpener, cutting hard tissue is now less difficult. Poor fixation or processing is main reason for difficult section cutting. If difficulty is faced, then the blocks may be placed in running tap water for 30 minutes or it may be treated with melted ice for prolonged tine. This will soften the tissue. By reducing knife slant slightly, good result may also be obtained.

If the above procedures fail, then softening fluid like Mollifex, saturated in a cotton wool may be applied on the block surface. This Mollifex will penetrate the block up to 15–20 μm thickness (Fig. 12).

BLOCKING OUT MOLDS (SHAPES, CUPS)

There are several types:

- **Leuckhart's embedding irons:** These consist of two L-shaped pieces of heavy brass or similar metal. Advantages are adjustability to give wide variety of block sizes, even blocks with parallel sides. But it is cumbersome and too slow for a busy laboratory (Figs 13 and 14).

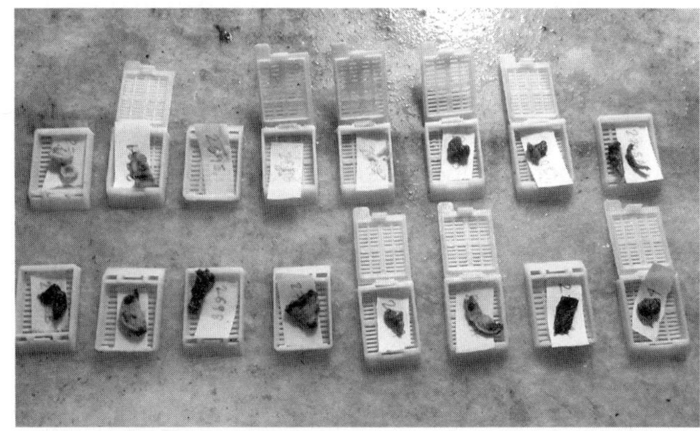

Fig. 12: Surgical specimens after grossing in tissue cassettes

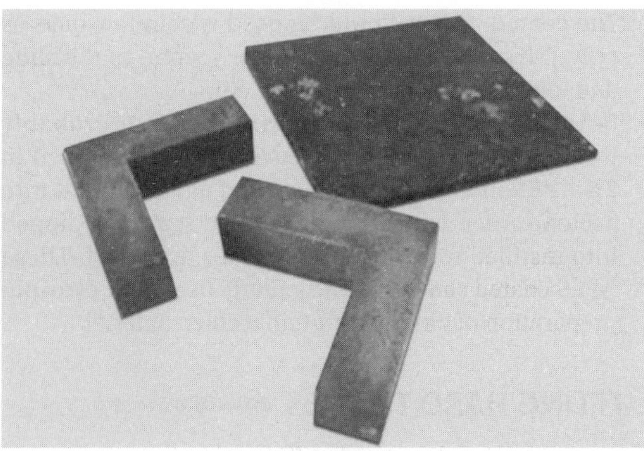

Fig. 13: Leuckhart's embedding iron without paraffin

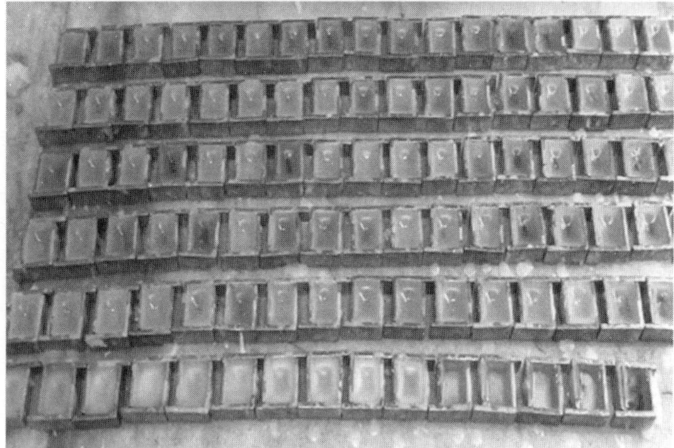

Fig. 14: Leuckhart's embedding iron with paraffin

- **Tissue-Tek system:** This system has stainless steel base molds in which the tissue block is embedded. A plastic mold is then placed on top and filled with wax. There are two types. Mark I and Mark II. Mark II uses about one-third less wax than Mark I system. Also they occupy much less storage space.
- **Peel-A-Way:** These are disposable thin plastic embedding molds. When paraffin wax has solidified, the plastic walls are simply peeled off, hens the name. It gives perfect blocks and requires no trimming. These blocks may be placed directly to the chuck of the microtome.
- **Tray of cups:** Made of different types of papers (waxed, thin or stout) were used in the past.
- **TIMS tissue processing and embedding system:** These are made of molded plastic capsules or 'bottoms'. These capsules consist of three pieces: a bottom, a frame center piece and a perforated lid. The tissue block may be fixed, dehydrated, cleared and embedded, i.e. all the steps of tissue processing may be done using this. When cooled and ready for section cutting, the bottom

Table 2: Problems and their solutions in paraffin wax sectioning

Problems	*Solutions*
1. Thick and thin zones parallel to knife edge (chatters)	
a. Tissue or wax too hard for sectioning	Use heavy duty knife and microtome. Reduce slant type angle of knife. Use softening fluid or melting ice on tissue
b. Knife or block loose in holder	Tighten it
c. Very steep knife angle	Reduce knife angle but still leave clearance
2. Ribbons and sections are curved	
a. Consistency of tissue is varying	Reorientation of the block by turning to 90 degree. Apply melting ice on block
b. Loading and trailing edges not parallel	Use sharp scalpel to trim the block
3. Alternate sections thick and thin	
a. Wax is too soft for tissue sectioning	Cool block with melting ice for prolonged time or re-embed the tissue in wax with higher melting point (54–58°C)
b. Low clearance angle	Increase the clearance angle slightly
c. Knife or block loose	Tighten knife or block
4. Sections do not join to form ribbons	
a. Knife angle either steep or shallow	Adjust to optional angle
b. Wax very hard for section cutting	Re-embed in wax with lower melting point
c. Debris on knife edge	Clean it with a cloth moistened with xylene
5. Spitting or scoring at right angles to knife edge	
a. Hard particles in tissues	If mineral or other particles, remove it with fine sharp pointed scalpel. If it is calcium, then decalcify
b. Nick in knife edge	Resharpen the knife or use different part of knife
c. Hand particles in wax	Re-embed in fresh wax which is filtered to remove hard particles
6. Sections become attached to block on return stroke	
a. Debris on block edge	Trim the block with sharp scalpel
b. Insufficient clearance angle	Increase and adjust clearance angle
c. Wax debris on knife edge	Clean it with xylene

Table 3: Different types of mounting media used in histology

Mounting Media	*Properties/use of the media*	*Formula/Preparation*
1. Resinous mounting media a. Canada balsam (RI 1.5)	i. Hardens slowly ii. Prussian blue stain is bleached slowly iii. Becomes yellow after long time	Dry powder is dissolved in xylol to 55–70% by weight Calcium carbonate is added to reduce acidity. Ready made mount is also available commercially
b. DPX (RI 1.52)	i. Hardens fast	Distrene 10 g Dibutylpthalate 5 mL Xylol 35 mL
2. Aqueous mounting media a. Glycerine jelly (RI 1.47)	i. Used for frozen sections ii. To demonstrate fat	Gelatin 10 g Distilled water 60 mL Glycerine 70 mL Phenol 0.25 g Dissolve gelatin with gentle heat in distilled water. Add other ingredients. As the solution solidifies, warm it to liquidify before use
b. Apathy's medium (RI 1.52)	i. To mount sections from distilled water ii. To mount sections for fluorescent microscope iii. To demonstrate fat	Gum arabic 50g Sucrose 50 g Distilled water 50 mL Thymol - One crystal Dissolve the ingredients
c. Farrant's medium (RI 1.43)	i. More convenient than glycerine jelly as it is liquid ii. Air bubbles may form	Gum Arabic 50g Distilled water 50 mL Glycerine 50 mL Arsenic trioxide 1g Dissolve the gum arabic in distilled water with mild heat. Add other ingredients. Instead of arsenic, sodium methiolate may be added
d. Highman's modification of Apathy's medium (RI 1.52)	i. Recommended for use with metachromatic stains	Gum Arabic 20 g Potassium acetate 20 g Cane sugar 20 g Sodium methiolate 10 mL Distilled water 40 mL Dissolve the ingredients by applying mild heat

is removed and opened surface of the block is cut. Microtome clamp or chuck grips the center frame piece. After section cutting, the bottom piece is replaced so that the block surface is protected for storage. Problems and their solutions in paraffin wax sectioning are given in Table 2.

MOUNTING OF SECTIONS

Mounting is the placing of mounting media on the stained tissue section and covering it with coverslips.

Functions of Mounting Media

- To fill the tissue and tissue cavities.
- To prevent damage to the section, easy handling and storage.
- To release entrapped air bubbles.
- To be visible on microscope and therefore it should have refractory index (RI) close to the glass (RI 1.5) as light passes through glass slides and coveslips. Different types of mounting media being used in histology are depicted in Table 3.

CHAPTER 3

Cryostat and Frozen Section

The basic principle in frozen section is to freeze the tissue so that the water within the tissue transforms into ice. The tissue becomes firms. This ice acts as the embedding medium. We can adjust the consistency of the frozen block by adjusting the temperature of the tissue. Raising the temperature the tissue becomes softer while reducing the temperature will make harder block.

Majority of unfixed nonfatty tissues sectioned well at around –25°C depending upon the tissue type. But fixed tissues section well at around –10°C or warmer temperature. Because in fixed block of tissue there is more water compared to unfixed block of tissue and the fixed tissue will have a harder consistency. Hence a higher or warmer temperature is required to make the fixed block of tissue soften and get good sections.

ADVANTAGE OF FROZEN AND CRYOSTAT SECTIONS

- They are indispensable for rapid diagnosis during operations (to know the tumor type, margin involvement, etc.), i.e. 'on-table' diagnosis of malignancy.
- For certain staining procedures these are essential, e.g. fat staining by Oil Red O method, some methods in CNS and silver impregnation method. Lipid and some carbohydrates can also be demonstrated.
- Most of enzymes are destroyed at temperature >56°C; so cannot be demonstrated in paraffin section excepting a few like phosphatases. Frozen section is ideal to demonstrate the enzymes in tissues.
- They are also used in immunofluorescent method and in immunocytochemical method.

THE CRYOSTAT (MACHINE)

The cryostat was introduced in 1954 and there have been improvements in the instrument which facilitated both safety and section cutting. The cryostat is a refrigerated cabinet and microtome is placed inside. Presently, rotary microtome is the type of choice. This microtome is controlled from outside the cabinet.

Modern cryostats are caster mounted cabinet models of the open-top type which permits easy access and visibility through the double thickness, hinged plastic cover. The rust proof microtome is usually mounted at 45° angles in the stainless steel cabinet. This cabinet is equipped with an antifogging air circulating system, a drain for defrosting and sterilization and a shelf with spaces for 4–6 metal block carriers.

Unfixed tissues should be fresh and freezing should be rapid. The common freezing techniques are:

- Liquefied nitrogen (–190°C)
- Isopentane cooled by liquid nitrogen (–150°C)
- Carbon dioxide gas (–70°C)
- Carbon dioxide 'cardice' (–70°C)
- Aerosol sprays (–50°C)

Liquefied nitrogen is commonly used. It is the most rapid freezing agent.

Operating Temperature and Type of Tissue

Because there are differences in composition, cellularity, connective tissue and fat content, the optimum temperature varies as per the nature of tissue. Human and animal tissues may be classified in three groups in accordance to optimum temperature:

- **Optimum temperature –5 to –15°C:** Brain, kidney, liver, lymph nodes, thyroid, testis, soft cellular tumor, uterine curetting.
- **Optimum temperature –15 to –25°C:** Muscle, connective tissue, uterus, cervix, pancreas, skin without fat, prostate, ovary, gut, nonfatty breast tissue.
- **Optimum temperature –25 to –35°C:** Fatty tissue (omentum, breast, skin with fatty subcutis).

Most unfixed tissues will section well between –15 to –23°C. The tissue containing more amount of water section well at warmer temperature while harder tissue (containing less amount of water) require cool temperature. Practically the optimum working temperature for cryostat is –18 to –20°C. But most fixed tissue will be cut well at a temperature of –7 to –12°C.

Fixed Tissue and the Cryostat

Occasionally fixed tissues are required to avoid diffusion of labile substances and enzymes (e.g. acid and alkaline phosphatases) in unfixed tissues. Cold formol-calcium is usually used for fixation. The tissue must be absolutely fresh and placed in formol-calcium at 4°C (cool temperature) for 18 hours. For sectioning fixed tissues blocks are prepared in this technique using gum sucrose a solution (Fig. 1).

Gum Sucrose

- Gum acacia: 2 g
- Sucrose: 60 g
- Distilled water: 200 mL
- Store the solution at 4°C.

Method of Cryostat Sectioning of Fixed Tissues

- Fix fresh tissue at 4°C for 18 hours in formol-calcium
- Rinse in running tap water
- Dry it by blotting
- Place the tissue in gum sucrose solution for 18 hours at 4°C. Small segments like jejunal biopsies may be kept for shorter intervals
- Blot dry
- Freeze tissue onto block holder moderately slowly to optimum cryostat temperature (–7 to –12°C).

Cryostat Mounting Media for Section Cutting

In the ascending order of merit these are: water, bovine albumin (20–30%) and von Apathy's gum syrup. But probably the best is mixture of synthetic water soluble glycols and resins. Lab Tek's optimum cutting temperature (OCT) compound is very good and is recommended.

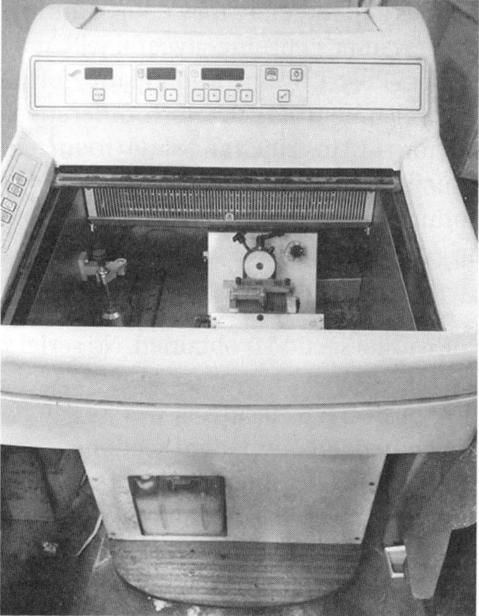

Fig. 1: Frozen section instrument and inner cabinet

Cryostat Sectioning Procedure

A suitable block of fresh tissue is selected and trimmed with a sharp scalpel to make slides parallel. The blocks are then covered with cryostat mounting media (like OCT compound) and placed in the quick freeze shell of the cryostat. The tissue will be cooled and frozen in 1–3 minutes.

After the tissue is adequately frozen, the object disc is inserted into microtome clamp, the tilt and angle being so oriented that the face of the block and of the object disc is in the plane of sectioning and the block edge is parallel to that of the knife. All clamps are tightened. Trim the block using quick or manual advance until the desired full section is obtained. Now, set the automatic advance mechanism and section thickness control.

Edge and undersurface of antiroll plate and surface of knife should be absolutely clean. Now, make the edges of antiroll plate parallel to and even with the knife edge. Close the cabinet for 1–2 minutes, so that temperature equilibrates.

It should be kept in mind that cryostat cuts individual section and not ribbons. For cryostat sections, the tissues are cut with a slow and even motion. Firm and fast strokes are applied for cutting harder tissues. The cut section will glide smoothly and flat beneath the antiroll plate.

The sections may be picked up on clean slide with the help of a knife, on coverglass which may be held by hand or by forceps.

Fixing Cryostat Sections to Slides

Fresh, unfixed tissue usually does not require adhesive on slides. But formation or otherwise fixed tissue may not adhere to slides and therefore may detach during staining. Albumen or Zwemer's chrome-glycerol jelly may be used in these cases. Poly-L-lysine and gelatin-formaldehyde mixture may also be used. The 40°C difference between cryostat section (–18 to –20°C) and slide (room temperature 37°C) is usually sufficient to attach the section to slide as well as producing some heat fixation.

Disadvantages of Frozen Section

- Only individual section is obtained. No serial section or ribbons possible.
- Staining of unfixed tissues is not as satisfactory as paraffin embedded permanent sections.
- Structural details are somewhat distorted during section cutting as no embedding medium (like paraffin) is used.
- Sometimes freezing artifacts are produced due to improper techniques. These include presence of ice crystals in tissues, separation of mucosal and other epithelial surfaces, nuclear vacuolization and ballooning.

Staining of Cryostat Sections

There are many methods of which two are very popular (1) Rapid hematoxylin and eosin (H and E) stain; (2) Polychrome methylene blue or crystal violet staining.

Rapid H and E Staining Method

- Fix cryostat sections in formol-acetic acid alcohol for 20–30 seconds.
- Rinse in water 10–15 seconds.
- Stain in Harris hematoxylin for 1.5–2 minutes.
- Rinse in lithium carbonate, Scott's tap water or alkaline tap water.
- Rinse in water (5–10 seconds)
- Stain in eosin (1% alcoholic eosin) for 10–25 seconds.
- Rinse in tap water (10–30 seconds)
- Dehydrate through graded alcohols.
- Clear in xylene.
- Mount in DPX/Canada balsam/Clarite/Permount or HSR.

Polychrome Methylene Blue/Crystal Violet Staining

Usually the zinc free chloride form of methylene blue is used and it contains some azures or methylene violet. The polychroming involves the oxidation of the methylene blue resulting in loss of methyl group which leaves lower homologues of the dye (azures) and deaminized oxidation products (thiazoles). The resulting mixture of methylene blue, azures, and thiazoles are known as polychrome methylene blue which has a violet color. This stains nuclei blue and mast cell granules, cartilage matrix, mucin, connective tissue reddish violet.

Methods

Slides are stained with polychrome methylene blue for 0.5–1 minutes. Then rinsed and mounted in an aqueous mountant or blotted dry, cleared in xylene and mounted in DPX/Canada balsam.

Accuracy of Frozen Section

Studies have shown that accurate diagnoses are made overall in >95% of cases whereas discordance with the final diagnosis (permanent paraffin section) occurs in 1–2% of cases. Deferral of the availability of permanent section diagnosis occurs in 1–4% of cases.

Indications of Frozen Sections

- To establish a tissue diagnosis (to detect any malignancy that will guide intraoperative patient management and extent of surgery).
- To determine the nature of lesion which will require other ancillary testing like flow cytometry or electron microscopy.
- For tissue identification, as for example to confirm the presence of parathyroid tissue in parathyroidectomy.
- To identify metastatic disease.
- To obtain sufficient diagnostic tissue, as for example, immunohistochemistry in frozen sections.
- To assess surgical margins (whether the margins are free of tumor or involved) and extent of the tumor, pathological or TNM staging.

FREEZE DRYING

This is a method for rapid-freezing ('quenching') of fresh tissue at –160°C, and subsequent removal of water molecules from tissue in the form of ice by the process of sublimation in a vacuum at a higher temperature, e.g. –40°C. Then these freeze-dried blocks are raised to room temperature (37°C) and either fixed in vapor fixative or embedded in paper medium. Freeze drying has three stages:

- Initial rapid freezing, known as 'quenching'

Table 1: Differences between frozen tissue and paraffin-embedded tissue

	Frozen tissue	*Paraffin embedded tissue*
1. Fixation	Pre/Post-sectioning	Pre-embedding
2. Sectioning	Cryostat	Microtome
3. Storage	Usually up to one year at –80°C (longer at –190°C)	Several years at room temperature (antigenicity may decrease)
4. Advantage	Preserves certain enzymes and antigen functions	Preserves tissue morphology
5. Limitations	Formation of ice crystals may adversely affect tissue structure	Over fixation can mask the epitopes
6. Precautions	Tissue should not be frozen slowly to prevent ice-crystal formation. Tissues should be allowed to warm to cutting temperature (-20 to –22°C) in cryostat to avoid shattering	Duration and intensity of tissue heating should be kept to a minimum as melting temperature of paraffin wax (50–60°C) may be deleterious to staining of some antigens
7. Routine use	• Rapid diagnosis and status of margins (involved or not) during operation • Fat stain, enzyme demonstration and some other special stains need cryostat sections	• Histologic sections, subsequent staining (H and E and others) and microscopical examination for confirmatory diagnosis of tumors, infections and other pathologic lesions • Also useful to demonstrate normal histology and to make control sections

- Drying of frozen tissue
- Fixation and embedding.

Quenching

Small pieces of tissue (≤1 mm thickness) are placed on a thin strip of folded aluminum foil or copper foil and plunged into isopentane cooled to a temperature of -160°C to -180°C with liquid nitrogen. Now, the frozen tissue is taken from the foil and the isopentane poured of. Initial rapid freezing with low temperature is very important, otherwise large crystals of ice will be formed which will disrupt cell structure.

Drying

The freezing tissue is quickly transferred to the drying apparatus, wherein a high vacuum is established and ice in tissue transferred by sublimation to vapor trap. Drying of tissue takes place when heat is supplied to the frozen tissue in a vacuum of 133 mPa or better.

Fixation and Embedding

Vapor fixatives which may be used are formaldehyde, glutaraldehyde and osmium tetroxide. Among these, formaldehyde is best as it gives excellent tissue preservation and also tissues can be used for all histochemistry excepting enzymes.

Tissues can be embedded in paraffin wax following fixation or straight from the freeze dryer unfixed (Table 1).

Use of Freeze Drying

- Initially it was used to demonstrate fine structure detail
- Scanning electron microscopy
- Fluorescent antibody studies, formaldehyde-induced fluorescence
- Mucosubstances, proteins
- Microspectroflrometry of autofluorescent substances
- Autoradiography.

CHAPTER 4 Staining of Tissues—Basic Concept

The staining of different tissue elements and pathological products depends upon a number of factors which are mostly chemical or physical in nature. The following steps are essential before staining cut sections after paraffin embedded tissues.

- The slides are placed in xylol to remove paraffin.
- Xylol is removed by placing the tissue in several changes of alcohol.
- The sections are then washed in water and are ready for staining.

The tissues fixed in Zenker's fluid or any fixative containing mercuric chloride have to be treated with weak solution of iodine in 0.5% alcohol for 5–10 minutes to remove mercuric deposits .The iodine stain is then removed by treating the sections with 0.5% aqueous solution of sodium thiosulfate for 5 minutes.

Most of the time dye used in stain is taken up by the tissues during staining. This uptake is due to dye-tissue or reagent tissue affinities. Affinity is used to describe the attractive forces which bind dye to tissues. So if a tissue has affinity for a dye, it is intensely stained. The magnitude of affinity depends on dye-solvent, solvent-solvent, dye-dye and dye-tissue interactions.

FACTORS CONTRIBUTING TO AFFINITIES BETWEEN DYE AND TISSUES

	Factors	*Example*
1.	**Solvent**-solvent interactions (Hydropic bonding)	Using aqueous solutions of dyes or other organic reagents, e.g. enzyme substrates
2.	**Reagent-reagent interactions**	Using basic dyes in metachromatic staining, e.g. silver impregnation, Gomori type enzyme histochemistry
3.	**Reagent-tissue interactions**	
	a. Van der Waal's forces	These forces act when large molecules such as elastic fibers stains and final product such as bis-formazans in enzyme histochemistry
	b. Covalent bonding	PAS stain, Feulgen nuclei, mercury orange
	c. Columbic attractions	Ionic reagents including inorganic salts, acid and basic dyes
	d. Hydrogen bonding	Glycogen (polysaccharides) staining by carminic acid from nonaqueous solutions

Hydrophobic Bonding

This describes the bonds between hydrophobic groupings like phenylalanine and tryptophan side chains of proteins, although they are dispersed in aqueous environment initially. In water, many molecules are held together by hydrogen bonding and hydrophobic bonds stabilize these clusters.

Metachromasia and Metachromatic Stains

If a dye absorbs light at different wavelengths depending upon its concentration and surroundings, then metachromasia occurs. As for example, toluidine blue when used at low concentrations, absorbed onto nuclear chromatin and transmits in the blue (orthochromatic staining). But when toluidine blue is used at high concentrations and is absorbed into substrates like mast cells, basophils or cartilage matrix, it transmits in the purple (metachromatic staining).

This metachromatic staining is due to dye-dye interactions. When two or more dyes come close proximity, their electronic energy levels interact. This interaction gives a new wavelength of absorption which is responsible for metachromatic color.

Van der Waal's force: These forces act between all reagents and tissue substrate. These forces are strong as they are short range. The substrate groupings which fall into this category are tyrosine and tryptophan residues of proteins, large aromatic regent molecules such as bis-azo dyes and tetrazolium salts, the heterocyclic bases of nucleic acids, enzyme substrate based on naphthyl and indoxyl systems and halogenated dyes such as rose bengal.

Covalent Bonding

It is responsible for many reactive stains between metal ions and mordant dyes facilitate dye-tissue binding (mordanting).

Columbic Attractions

They are also known as salt links or electrostatic bonds. These arise when interactions between two unlike ions occur. As for example, interactions between the colored cations of basic dyes and tissue structure rich in anions such as phosphated DNA and RNA or sulfated and carboxylated mucosubstances.

Hydrogen Bonding

This is a localized bond and is formed when a hydrogen atom lies between two electronegative atoms (e.g. nitrogen or oxygen). Hydrogen bonds are not important for reagent tissue affinity when aqueous solvents are used. But in aqueous solvents it plays a major role like in Best's carmine stain for glycogen.

Sometimes dyes are not taken up by the tissues during staining. In negative staining, some structures are not stained while other structures are stained. The shape of these unstained structures can be visualized as they are surrounded by stained structures, e.g. demonstration of the canaliculi of bone matrix, individual macromolecules for electron microscopy, etc.

In vital or supravital staining, reagents can be taken up by live cells unlike dead tissues in normal histological staining. For example, supravital staining of reticulocytes by brilliant cresyl blue, new methylene blue or azure blue. Reticulocytes contain remnants of ribosomes and RNA which are present in the cytoplasm of their precursors, i.e. normoblast which interact with supravital dye to form a blue precipitate. Here the reticulocytes are not fixed and are still alive. Recent use of supravital staining is in the use of fluorescent probes.

Now, we will discuss some queries which come up into our minds.

- Why tissues retain dyes after its removal from staining bath?
- Why stains are selectively taken up by some parts while not taken by others?
- Why are dyes colored during staining?

Why Tissues Retain Dyes After its Removal from Staining Bath?

The processing fluid and mounting media have low affinity for the stain. Also the stain dissolves very slowly into these substances, so that the stained tissue fades slowly. For example, prussian blue used in Perls' method for demonstrating iron which is virtually insoluble in alcohol or xylene (used for tissue processing).

A cationic or basic dye like crystal violet or methylene blue dissolves in the lower alcohol rapidly and freely. So sections stained in basic dyes are dehydrated in alcohol quickly, with the use of nonalcoholic solvents or by air drying. Anionic or acid dyes such as orange G or eosin Y are less soluble in alcohol unlike basic dyes. In case of nonionic dyes (neither basic or acidic) like Sudan stain which is used in fat staining, are soluble in common dehydrating agents as well as clearing solvents. Hence, nonionic dyes should be mounted in aqueous media.

Why Stains are Selectively Taken up by Some Parts While not Taken by Others?

This selectivity of stain depends on various factors like: (1) Numbers and affinity of binding sites, (2) Rates of reagent uptake, (3) Rate of reaction, (4) Rate of reagent loss. Reagent-tissue affinity and number of binding sites are variable. As for example, both acid and basic dyes are used in most commonly used hematoxylin and eosin stain during routine histological staining. Here, negative charged acidic dyes have high affinity for tissue structures carrying cationic or positive charges like protein in the nucleus. But acidic dyes have low affinity for structures containing negative charges like phosphate nucleic acids and sulfated glycosaminoglycans which are formed in cytoplasm. These particles are stained by basic dyes due to high affinity to basic dyes, so acid dyes stain the nuclear part whereas basic dyes stain the cytoplasmic part in H and E staining.

Progressive staining is the rate-controlled and also is time based, as for example, mucin staining by alcian blue method. When staining is done for shorter period, selectivity occurs and only mucin containing structures are stained. If it is stained for a prolonged time (more than stipulated time for mucin staining) it also stains other basophilic materials like RNA-rich cytoplasm and nuclei.

Sometimes three or more acid dyes are used in analogous methods. Here, staining rates are variable in different acidophilic substances—for instance, collagen fibers stain rapidly, whereas RBC stain slowly and muscle fibers are intermediate.

The selective staining also depend on selective rates of reaction. As for example, in enzyme histochemistry, rate of reaction varies as the pH varies. At low pH, hydrolysis of an organic phosphate will be rapid in tissues which contain acid phosphatases. But tissue containing alkaline phosphatases,the hydrolysis will be slow as pH optima is higher for these substances, another example is periodic oxidation in PAS staining, periodic acid-Schiff (PAS) can oxidize many chemical structures but optimum oxidation time is chosen. It only selectively oxidizes fast reacting 1, 2-diol groupings, which are abundant in polysaccharides like glycogen.

Why are Dyes Colored During Staining?

Dyes appear colored as they absorb radiation in the visible region of the electromagnetic spectrum, i.e. light, between wavelengths of about 400–650 nm. Acid-fuchsin absorbs blue-green light strongly from the middle of visible spectrum and transmits red light. On the other hand, picric acid absorbs predominantly blue-violet light from short wavelength end of visible spectrum and yellow light is transmitted.

POLYCHROMASIA

Stains may sometimes give selective color; even it is not bound selectively. Such polychromasia can occur with dyes as well as reactive stains. For example, toluidine blue or methylene blue (basic dyes) are absorbed by tissue basophils or mast cells. The chromatin is stained blue (orthochromatic staining) but granules in basophils/mast cells and cartilage matrix become reddish purple (metachromatic staining). This is different coloration of different structures using the same stain is called polychromasia.

THEORY OF STAINING

The theory of staining is not simple and many theories have been put forward to explain it. However, it can be explained by physical theories and chemical theories.

Physical Theories

These theories depend on two things: (1) Simple solubility and (2) Adsorption.

- **Solubility:** A good example of solubility of stains is fat stains like Oil Red O, Sudan black, etc. Here, the fat stains are more soluble in fat rather than in 70% alcohol or other solvents which are used for conventional hematoxylin and eosin stain.
- **Adsorption:** It is the action of a substance in attracting and holding other materials or particles on its surface. This action may be selective under certain circumstances (e.g. adsorption may be affected by both substances). Usually, in adsorption one large body attracts minute particles over its surface. Bayliss in 1906, had proposed this theory and named it as electrical theory of staining.

Chemical Theories

Previously, it was thought that during staining, an actual chemical combination of dye and tissue take place. It is generally agreed, that basic dyes stain acidophilic materials (nucleus) whereas acid dyes stain basic elements (cytoplasm).

But till date, most popular theory of staining is perhaps combination of the adsorption (physical theory) and chemical theory.

STAINS AND DYES

In 1714, Leeuwenhoek was probably the first scientist to use a dye as biological stain. He used saffron (crocus in wine) to muscles as biological stain. Later on, carmine was applied by Goppert and Cohn in 1849, and hematoxylin in 1863 by Waldeyer. It was in the year 1856, when aniline dyes were introduced. But the major advancement was in 1891, when Heidenhain discovered the iron hematoxylin technique which is still very common used as stain.

Biological stains are used in biology unlike commercial stains which are used for processed tissues. But, property wise both are similar (Fig. 1).

Acidic dyes	Basic dyes
Eosin	Hematoxylin/Methylene blue
Carry net negative charge	
React/bind with cationic components of the cell/tissue	Carry net positive charge with anionic components of cell/tissue
Less specific (as compared with basic dyes)	Highly pH specific
Acidophilic/eosinophilic (cytoplasmic filaments, intracellular membranous components, extracellular fibers)	Basophilic substances (PO_4 of nucleic acids, SO_4 of MPS, CO proteins)

Fig. 1: Basis of staining

Classification of Dyes

Dyes may be classified into following groups:
- The nitro group
- The nitroso group
- The thiazol group
- The azo group
- The anthraquinone group
- The phenyl-methane group
- The quinine-imine group
- The xanthene group.

Natural Dyes

Though most of the dyes used nowadays in laboratory are synthetic, some natural dyes are still in use. Some of the natural dyes which are used presently are—hematoxylin, cochineal (carmine), orcein and litmus.

Hematoxylin

The hematoxylin stain is probably the most widely used histological stain. It is extracted from the heartwood (logwood) of the tree *Hematoxylin campechianum* which grows in Campeche, Mexico.

Hematoxylin as supplied cannot be used as a stain unless it is 'ripened' by oxidation into hematin. This ripening or oxidation can be done by two ways. It can be natural oxidation by exposure of prepared solutions to the light and air for 6–8 weeks. It can also be done by chemical oxidation by adding an oxidizing agent such as mercuric oxide (e.g. Harris's hematoxylin), sodium iodate (e.g. Mayer's hematoxylin) or potassium permanganate.

After ripening (oxidation) into hematin, the stain cannot be used as the hematin has poor affinity for the tissues as it is anionic. So, a mordant is used with it. The mordant/metal cation gives a net positive charge to the dye-mordant complex (here it is hematin dye). This change of charge from anionic to cationic (positive charge) enables them to bind to anionic tissue sites such as nuclear chromatin. The commonly used mordants are salts of iron, aluminium or tungsten, i.e. salts of a metal. Occasionally, lead is also used as a mordant to demonstrate argyrophilic cells.

Carmine

It is produced from cochineal after treatment with alum. The cochineal is extracted from the female cochineal insect (*Coccus cacti).* It should be used along with a mordant.

Orcein and litmus: This is extracted from lichens. Litmus is used as an indicator (to demonstrate acid or alkaline pH), whereas orcein is used to stain elastic tissues.

Mordants

The term mordant is only strictly applicable to salts and hydroxides of divalent and trivalent metals. The mordants most commonly used in histological technique are salts, usually sulfates of aluminium, iron and chromium. Generally, double sulfates or alums are used (Fig. 2).

The mordants form a link between the tissue and the stain. The combination of the dye and the mordant forms a compound which is capable of attracting itself to the tissue firmly. This compound is sometimes called 'lake'. Some lakes are not stable and should be used immediately. As for example, Heidenhain's iron hematoxylin stain and Gram's stain.

Accentuators and Accelerators

They are a group of substances which increase the selectivity or staining power of the dyes which are already capable of staining without the accelerators. Unlike the mordants, the accentuators and accelerators do not form lakes with the dyes, or make any chemical union. Examples of accentuators are phenol in carbol thionin and carbol fuchsin, and potassium hydroxide in Loffler's methylene blue.

Accentuators when used with metallic salt and is applied during impregnation of nervous system are called accelerators. Practically these accelerators are hypnotics. Examples of accelerators are chloral hydrate in Cajal's method for motor and plate and vernal in Cajal's method for axis cylinders.

Direct Staining

If tissue sections are kept into alcoholic or simple aqueous solutions of certain dyes, tissues are stained. Such staining without the help of a mordant or accentuators/accelerators is called 'direct' or simple staining. These stains even after washing in water or alcohol, may be selective. As for example, methylene blue will stain the nucleus and cytoplasm of a cell in different shades of blue.

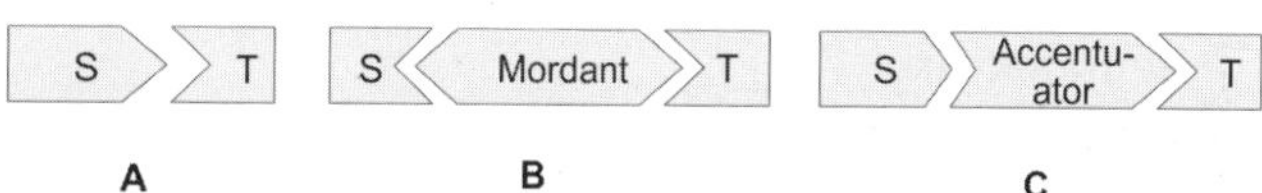

Figs 2A to C: Diagrammatic representation of different types of staining. (A) Direct or simple staining: direct union of stain or dye with tissue; (B) Mordant staining: Mordants firmly attach both the stain and tissues forming a compound union; (C) Accentuators or accelerators: These increase the affinity of tissues but without this help, staining is still possible (which will have lesser staining power or affinity)
Abbreviations: S, stain; T, tissue

CHAPTER 5

Routine Hematoxylin and Eosin Stain

A good routine histologic stain must be able to stain nuclei and cytoplasm but also connective tissue. A properly stained histologic section by hematoxylin and eosin differentiates and distinguishes the nuclei, the cytoplasm and connective tissue. The nuclei appear blue, whereas the cytoplasm and connective tissue fibers will have shades of pink. As it can stain and differentiate well all these structures, so it is the most popular routine stain.

Hematoxylin is used in conjunction with eosin as routine stain. Usually 0.5–1% aqueous solution of eosin is used as a counter stain, though some prefer phloxine (0.5–1%) as a counter stain. Phloxine gives a brighter and vivid red stain but eosin is more informative as it differentiates better. Some other counter stains are orange G, Bordeaux red and Biebrich scarlet.

Hematin (oxidation product of hematoxylin) is inadequate as a nuclear stain without the presence of a mordant. So, hematoxylin solutions are classified according to which mordant is used.

- **Alum hematoxylin**: Ehrlich's hematoxylin, Harris's hematoxylin, Mayer's hematoxylin, Cole's hematoxylin, Gill's hematoxylin and Carazzi's hematoxylin.
- **Iron hematoxylin**: Weigert's hematoxylin, Verhoeff's hematoxylin, Loyez's hematoxylin, Heidenhain hematoxylin.
- **Tungsten hematoxylin**: Phosphotungstic acid hematoxylin (PTAH)
- **Lead hematoxylin**.
- **Molybdenum hematoxylin**.
- **Hematoxylin without mordant**.

PRINCIPLE OF ALUM HEMATOXYLIN STAINING

The mordant used in alum hematoxylin is aluminium either potash alum (aluminium potash sulfate) or ammonium alum (aluminium ammonium sulfate).

Initially, the nuclei become red after staining, which turn blue or blue black when stained sections are washed in weak alkali. Practically, tap water can be used for washing as it is alkaline enough to produce desired color change. Sometimes, alkaline solutions like Scott's tap water, saturated lithium carbonate or 0.05% ammonia in distilled water is used for this color change. This process of changing color from red to blue is called 'blueing'.

Progressive staining: Here, the sections are stained for a predetermined time, so that the nuclei become well stained but the background is relatively under stained.

Regressive staining: In this procedure, the sections are first over stained, and then excess stain is selectively removed in acid alcohol. Advantage of this staining procedure is that the degree of staining is controlled (some tissue elements retain more stain/dye compared with others). Hence, the nuclei take good staining whereas the cytoplasm and background are perfectly clear.

Ehrlich's Alum Hematoxylin

Composition of solution:

- Hematoxylin: 2 g
- Absolute alcohol: 100 mL
- Distilled water: 100 mL

- Glycerine: 100 mL
- Glacial acetic acid: 10 mL
- Potassium alum: 15–20 g (approximately).

Preparation: The hematoxylin should be dissolved in absolute alcohol. Other components are added in the order given. Lastly, potassium alum (mordant) is added and solution is shaken. Keep on adding this mordant unless there is alum crystal on the bottom of the solution (i.e. addition of excess mordant). Role of glycerin is to stabilize the stain against over-oxidation, even and precise staining and to prevent rapid evaporation.

Ehrlich's alum hematoxylin lasts for months in a Coplin jar whereas it can retain its staining power for years. Filter before use.

Ripening: After freshly prepared solution, the stain is kept in an unstoppered or loosely plugged bottle in a warm, light place. This is done for natural oxidation of hematoxylin to hematin (this process is called ripening). This natural ripening usually takes 2 months time. It can be shortened by placing the bottle in sunny place. So, time is shorter in summer than in winter.

Advantage: Nuclei are stained intensely and crisply. Stained sections fade slowly compared to other alum hematoxylin stains. It also stains mucin and mucopolysaccharides of cartilage. So, staining of bone and cartilages are recommended by this method.

Disadvantage: Not suitable for frozen sections.

Staining time: 20-45 minutes (progressive method).

Harris's Alum Hematoxylin

Composition of solution:

- Hematoxylin: 2.5 g
- Absolute alcohol: 50 mL
- Ammonium or potassium alum: 50 g
- Distilled water: 500 mL
- Mercuric oxide: 1.5 g
  Or
  Sodium iodate: 0.5 g
- Glacial acetic acid: 20 mL.

Preparation: The hematoxylin is dissolved in the absolute alcohol and it is then added to previously prepared alum solution (alum in distilled water). The two solutions are mixed well. The mixture is now heated to boiling point and mercuric oxide or sodium iodide is added. Then the mixture is rapidly cooled by plunging the flask in cold water or into a sink containing ice pieces. The solution is ready for staining.

Addition of glacial acetic acid is optional but is preferred, because this gives more precise and selective nuclear staining. Filter before use when previously made solutions are used.

Advantages: It is a good nuclear stain and is used for general purpose. As the nuclear staining is very clear, it is also used in exfoliative cytology. In routine histologic sections, Harris's hematoxylin used regressively but in exfoliative cytology it is used progressively.

Disadvantages: Nuclear stain fades after a few months which is also seen in other chemically ripened alum hematoxylin (of natural ripening of Ehrlich's alum hematoxylin). In stored solution, there is formation of a precipitate after few months and the solution is not good for staining. At this stage, the stain can be used by filtering the precipitate and increasing the staining time. But best thing is to use freshly prepared stain.

Staining time

- Progressive in cytology: 4–30 seconds
- Regressive method: 5–15 minutes.

Mayer's Hematoxylin

Composition of solution:

- Hematoxylin: 1 g
- Distilled water: 1000 mL
- Ammonium or potassium alum: 50 g
- Citric acid: 1 g
- Chloral hydrate (SLR): 50 g
  Or
  Chloral hydrate (AR): 30 g.

Preparation: The hematoxylin, alum and sodium iodate are dissolved in the distilled water either by warming and stirring, or by keeping at room temperature overnight. Then citric acid and chloral hydrate are added, and the mixture is boiled for 5 minutes. The mixture is now cooled and filtered. The stain should be used immediately and should be filtered before use.

Advantage: It is very precise for nuclei and the stain is used progressively (usually as counter stain, for example, after glycogen or mucicarmine staining) but can be used regressively as well. The stain is very good to demonstrate amoebae in histologic sections.

Disadvantage: Prepared solution should be used immediately and cannot be kept for future use.

Staining time:

- Progressive: 10–20 minutes
- Regressive: 5–10 minutes.

Carazzi's Hematoxylin

Composition of solution:

- Hematoxylin: 5 g

- Glycerol: 100 mL
- Potassium alum: 25 g
- Distilled water: 400 mL
- Potassium iodate: 0.1 g.

Preparation: Dissolve the hematoxylin in glycerol and alum in most of the water (say 350 mL) overnight. After overnight stay, the alum solution is added to the hematoxylin solution slowly. Now, potassium iodate is dissolved in rest of the water (say 50 mL) with gentle warming. This, potassium iodate solution is added to the hematoxylin-glycerol-alum solution. The final solution is shaken to mix well and can be used immediately. The solution is stable for 6 months and can be used (filter before use). It may be used as progressive stain (1–2 min) but also as regressive stain (45 sec).

Advantage: It can be used for urgent reporting as in frozen section. More clear staining of the nuclei is possible if double or triple strength hematoxylin solution (10 g or 15 g) is used instead of conventional 5 g hematoxylin.

Disadvantage: It stains nuclei well but does not stain cytoplasmic component.

Staining time:
- Progressive: 1–2 minutes
- Regressive: 45 seconds.

Staining Procedure Using Alum Hematoxylin with Eosin

- Dewax histologic sections.
- Hydrate through graded alcohol first, then to water.
- Stain the nuclei with preferred alum hematoxylin for required time.
- Wash the stained sections for 5 minutes in tap water till the blueing of the nuclei.
- Differentiate the sections, in 1% acid alcohol (1% HCl in 70% ethyl alcohol). For 5–10 seconds.
- Wash again in tap water until the sections are 'blue' for 5 minutes or less.
- Stain in 1% eosin (eosin Y is preferred) for 10 minutes.
- Wash in tap water for 1–5 minutes.
- Dehydrate through graded alcohol (70%, 95% and then 100%).
- Clearing in xylene, then mount it.

Results of Alum Hematoxylin-Eosin Stain

- Nuclei: Blue/black
- Cytoplasm: Varying shades of pink
- Fibrin: Deep pink
- Red blood cells: Orange/red
- Muscle fiber: Deep pink/red
- Fungal hyphae: Faintly blue
- Calcium deports: Deep blue-black

Rapid Staining Using Carazzi's Hematoxylin for Urgent Frozen Section

- Place the tissue block onto a chuck in the cabinet of cryostat for freezing.
- After the tissue is frozen, cut cryostat section at 3–4 μm thickness.
- Cut sections are placed onto glass slides.
- Fix the section in 10% natural buffered formalin for 20 seconds at room temperature.
- Rinse in tap water (5–10 seconds).
- Stain in double or triple strength of Carazzi's hematoxylin for 1 minute.
- Wash in tap water (10–20 seconds).
- Stain in 1% aqueous solution of eosin Y for 10 seconds.
- Rinse in tap water (5–10 seconds).
- Dehydrate in graded alcohol, clear and mount.

Result:
- Nuclei: Blue/black
- Cytoplasm: No/poor stain (pink).

Iron Hematoxylin

Here iron salts are used both as oxidizing agent and as mordant in the hematoxylin solutions. Ferric chloride and ferric ammonium sulfate are commonly used as iron salts. Common iron-hematoxylins are:
- **Weigert's hematoxylin:** Nuclei becomes black
- **Verhoff's hematoxylin:** For elastic fibers
- **Loyez hematoxylin:** For myelin
- **Heidenhain hematoxylin:** Mitochondria, myelin, muscle stations, chromatin (nuclear), etc. become gray black.

In comparison to alum hematoxylin, iron hematoxylin can demonstrate wider range of tissue structures but staining technique is time consuming and also it needs microscope evaluation during differentiation stage.

Weigert's Iron Hematoxylin

Composition of staining solutions:
- Hematoxylin solutions
  - Hematoxylin: 1 g
  - Absolute alcohol: 100 mL
- Iron solution
  - 30% aqueous ferric chloride solution (anhydrous): 4 mL
  - Hydrochloric acid (concentrated): 1 mL
  - Distilled water: 95 mL

Preparation: First the solution (i) or Hematoxylin solutions must be allowed to ripen. For natural ripening, it takes 4–5 weeks time. It may also be prepared from a stock solution of 5% hematoxylin in absolute alcohol (previously ripened solution). Now, mix equal parts of solution (i) and solution (ii) immediately before use. When mixing is done in a test tube, it is advisable to pour solution (i) in the tube first, and then add solution (ii) as it contains conc HCl. The staining solution/mixture ideally should be violet-black in color. If the color became brown, then the mixture should be discarded.

Advantage: Main use is as a nuclear stain in techniques where acid is used subsequently (e.g. picric acid in van Gieson stain). It resists removal of counter stain containing differentiating agent like picric acid. It stains nuclei black unlike blue/blue-black in alum-hematoxylin. The stained nuclei won't be decolorized by light. So, it is a more permanent stain than alum-hematoxylin.

Disadvantage: More time consuming and needs microscopic control for accuracy. It has been replaced by more convenient Celestine blue-alum hematoxylin. Still it is in use for CNS tissues.

Staining time: 20–30 minutes.

Heidenhain Hematoxylin

Composition of staining solutions:

- Iron alum solutions
  - Ferric ammonium sulfate (violet crystals): 5 g
  - Distilled water: 100 mL
- Hematoxylin solutions
  - Hematoxylin: 0.5 g
  - Absolute alcohol: 10 mL
  - Distilled water: 90 mL
- This solution must be kept ready for 4–5 weeks for natural ripening.
  or
  5% stock solution (ripened) alcoholic hematoxylin: 10 mL
- Distilled water: 90 mL
- This solution is ready for immediate use.

Staining Method

1. Dewax histologic sections (either putting it into xylol for 1–2 minutes or by heating).
2. Hydrate through graded alcohol to water.
3. Mordant in 5% iron alum/iron alum solution for 1 hour.
4. Rinse in distilled water (10–20 seconds).
5. Stain in Heidenhain hematoxylin solution for 1 hour.
6. Wash in running water until the sections are blue (usually takes 10 minutes in tap water of pH 8). Lithium carbonate may be added to water if it is not sufficiently alkaline.
7. Differentiate in 5% iron alum until the desired structured is clearly demonstrated under microscope.
8. Wash in running tap water for 8–10 minutes.
9. Dehydrate in graded alcohol (70%, 95% and then 100%)
10. Clear and mount in DPX or Canada balsam.

Advantage: It can be used to demonstrate many structures as per degree of differentiation. Mitochondria, muscle striations, myelin, nuclear membrane, chromatin, chromosomes, nucleoli, centrioles, yolk and ground cytoplasm can be demonstrated which become jet black or grey black. Good for photography. The stain is permanent, if the alum is properly removed. It is applicable after use of any fixative.

Disadvantage: It is used only regressively and experience is required for good staining quality. For beginners use half-strength iron alum is advisable until they gain experience.

Verhoeff's Hematoxylin

This stain is used to demonstrate elastic fibers. In this staining procedure, ferric chloride is included in the iron-alum staining solution along with Lugol's iodine and 2% aqueous ferric chloride is used as the differentiator (CF 5% iron alum in Heidenhain hematoxylin).

Coarse elastic fibers become black after staining, Verhoeff' stain is ideal for photography of stained elastic fibers as it gives intense black color which produces good contrast required for photography (unlike other elastin staining methods which stain fined fibers and give weak coloration).

Tungsten Hematoxylin

The original technique was described by Mallory who combined hematoxylin with 1% aqueous phosphotungstic acid (which acts as mordant). Later on Shun and Hon in 1969 prepared a staining solution which contains hematin instead of hematoxylin. The advantage of using hematin is that it does not require oxidation for ripening and can be used immediately. On the contrary hematoxylin needs ripening either by oxidation with chemicals like potassium permanganate (takes 1 day) or by natural way in light and air (takes several months). Though natural ripening is time consuming, it may be used for several years whereas chemically ripened solution can be used for 24 hours.

Mallory's Phosphotungstic Acid Hematoxylin (PTAH)

Natural ripening	*Chemical ripening*
Composition of staining solution: Hematoxylin: 1 g Phosphotungastic acid: 10 g Distilled water: 1000 mL	**Composition staining solution:** Hematoxylin: 1 g Phosphotungastic acid: 20 g Distilled water: 1000 mL Aqueous potassium permanganate (0.25%): 50 mL
Preparation: The solids are dissolved in separate containers having distilled water, then it is mixed as per above formula. The solution is kept in loosely stopped bottle for several months for natural ripening	**Preparation:** The hematoxylin (1 g) is dissolved in 200 mL of distilled water, and the phosphotungstic acid in the rest 800 mL. The two solutions are mixed. Then potassium permanganate solution is added. Though the stain can be used next day, best staining is obtained after 7 days

Mallory's hematoxylin is good routine stain for CNS tissues. The first few steps (described below in steps 4–7) are for bleaching which helps differential staining and are known as the Mallory bleach (Figs 1 and 2).

Staining Method

1. Dewax histologic sections.
2. Hydrate through graded alcohol to water.
3. Treat them with Lugol's iodine or alcohol (0.5% in 80% alcohol) and sodium thiosulfate (3%) (Refer to removal of deposits in mercury fixed tissues).
4. Place in 0.25% aqueous potassium permanganate for 5 minutes.
5. Wash in water for 2 minutes.
6. Rinse in distilled water.
7. Place in 5% oxalic acid for 10 minutes.
8. Rinse in distilled water.
9. Wash in water for 5 minutes, then rinse in distilled water.
10. Stain with staining solution of PTAH for12–24 hours.
11. Dehydrate in graded alcohol (just dip and remove, otherwise red color will be removed by alcohol).
12. Clear in xylol and mount in DPX or Canada balsam.

Results of PTAH Staining

- **Blue color**: Nuclei, neuroglial fibers, myoglia, fibroglia, cross-section of muscle fibers, fibrin and centoles.
- **Yellow or brick red**: Reticulin, collagen, cartilage, osteoid and ground substance of bone.
- **Dark blue**: Amoebae.
- **Pale pinkish-brown**: Cytoplasm.

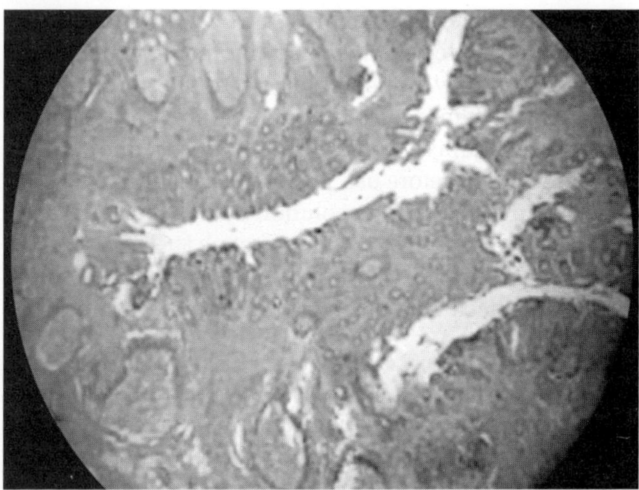

Fig. 1: Photomicrograph showing mucosal glands of appendix and lymphoid aggregates forming lymphoid follicles (H and E, low power view,100×) *(For color version, see Plate 1)*

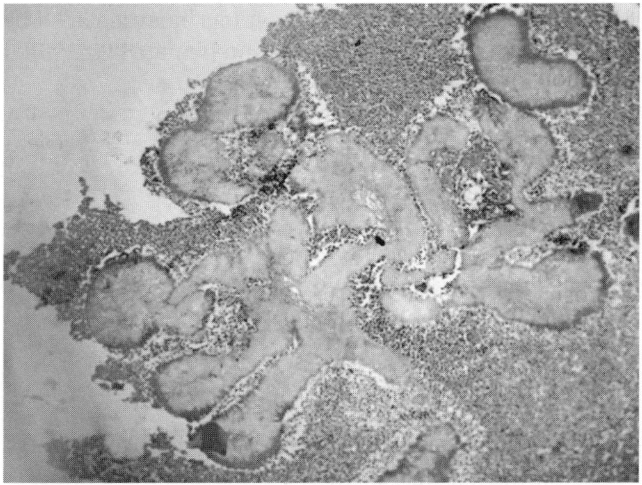

Fig. 2: Microphotograph showing fungal mycetoma (eumycetoma) or 'madura foot'. Multiple aggregates of fungal hyphae and sulfur granules, surrounded by neutrophils/microabscess (H and E, low power view,100×) *(For color version, see Plate 1)*

Counterstains Routinely Used with Hematoxylin Nuclear Stain

Most commonly, eosin is used as counterstain. Other counterstains which may be used are orange G, phloxine, Bordeaux red and Biebrich scarlet. But these substitutes give undesirable intense red color to the tissue and fail to achieve subtle differentiation as in eosin.

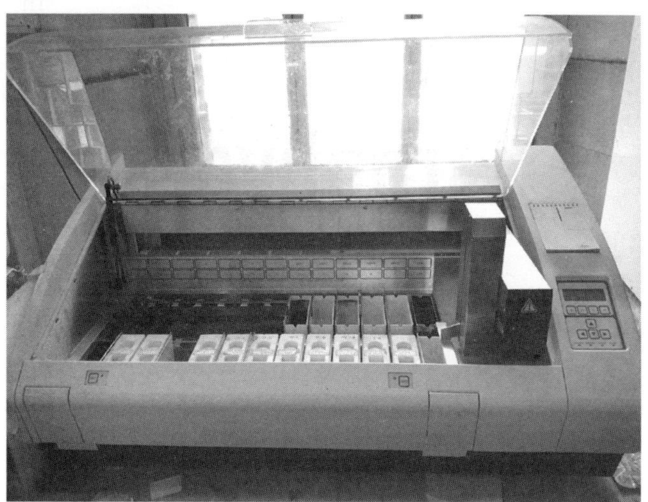

Fig. 3: Automatic tissue stainer machine (Autostainer)

Automatic staining

- In this procedure an automatic stainer is required
- It has a timer, which controls the time
- It has a mechanical device which shifts the slides from one container to next after the specified time

Advantages of automated stainer are:

- It reduces the man power
- It controls the timing of staining accurately
- Large number of slides can be stained simultaneously
- Less reagents are used

Note:

Slides stained either manually or by automatic stainer, pass through same sequences

Fig. 4: Automatic staining summary

The eosins are xanthene dyes are common types are eosin Y, ethyl eosin and eosin B. Of these three types eosin Y is most widely used. The Y stands for yellowish as reagent is yellowish in color. Eosin Y is both water and alcohol soluble. Commonly, eosin Y is used as 0.5–1% solution in distilled water. Glacial acetic acid may be added which augments staining. Also, few crystal of thymol may be added to prevent fungal growth (Figs 3 and 4).

Composition of Staining Solution of Eosin

- Eosin Y (water soluble): 1 g
- Distilled water: 80 mL
- 95% ethyl alcohol: 320 mL
- Glacial acetic acid: 0.4 mL.

Preparation: Dissolve 1 g eosin Y in 80 mL of distilled water, and then add 320 mL of 95% ethyl alcohol. To this mixture add few drops (0.4 mL) of glacial acetic acid. This acetic acid increases the staining intensity of eosin. The ideal solution should be cloudy, if it looks clear then add few more drops of acetic acid.

Uses of eosin

- Its ability with proper differentiation, to distinguish between the cytoplasm of different types of cells, and between the different types of connective tissue and matrix. Eosin stains then with different shades of red and pink.
- As counterstain to hematoxylin in H and E staining: Cytoplasm stains pink-orange and nuclei stained darkly blue-purple.
- It stains RBC intensely red.

CHAPTER 6

Carbohydrates

INTRODUCTION

Carbohydrates are compounds of carbon, hydrogen and oxygen, the latter two usually in the proportion of water. The most important carbohydrates are sugar, starches, cellulose and gums. These are classified as mono-, di-, tri- and heterosaccharide.The word "carbohydrate" actually is descriptive of the 1: 1 ratio of carbon molecules to water (hydrate).

In order to understand different types of carbohydrates and their location in different parts of the body, let us know the classification of carbohydrates based on chemical nature:

- **Group I: Polysaccharides**, e.g. glycogen.
- **Group II: Mucopolysaccharides**:
  - Simple or sulfate free, e.g. hyaluronic acid in synovial fluid or umbilical cord.
  - Complex or sulfate containing, e.g. chondroitin sulfate, mucoitin sulfate of gastric mucin, corpora amylacea, and mast cell granules.
- **Group III: Mucoproteins and glycoproteins**: These are protein-carbohydrate compounds having high protein or peptide within it.
  - Mucoprotein without sialic acid, e.g. serum mucoprotein, submaxillary and Brunner's gland mucin, beta granules of anterior pituitary.
  - Mucoprotein containing sialic acid (N-acylneuraminic acid), e.g. sialomucin or carboxylated mucin.
- **Group IV: Glycolipids**: These are carbohydrate lipid compounds and have fat residue within it, e.g. cerebrosides.
- **Group V: Phosphatides: or Phospholipids**, e.g. lecithin, cephalin and sphingomyelin.

Mucins are hexosamine containing polysaccharides covalently bound to varying amounts of proteins. The original term of "mucin" was coined by an American worker named Carpenter in 1846. Subsequently different names of mucin follow, i.e. mucosubstances, mucopolysaccharides and glycosaminoglycans. Later on, Reid and Clamp in 1978 suggested a general term "glycoconjugates", which again subdivided into proteoglycans or glycoaminoglycans and glycoproteins. To avoid confusion of terminologies we prefer to use the term mucin. The synthesis of mucin starts in the rough endoplasmic recticulum in the synthesizing cells and complete in the Golgi apparatus. For staining different types of staining techniques are employed. These are PAS (periodic acid-Schiff), Alcian blue, mucicarmine, aldehyde fuchsin, high iron diamine, etc.

- Mucins are high molecular weight glycoproteins and are commonly found in epithelium of gastrointestinal tract, respiratory tract and reproductive tract. Mucins are composed of a central protein core with multiple chains of carbohydrates (polysaccharide) attached. Carbohydrate component of mucin accounts for 60–80% of total molecular weight. The protein core of mucin contains high contents of two amino acids—**serine and threonine**.
- But there are other glycoproteins which share structural similarities with mucin (which is a high molecular weight glycoprotein) and are often confused with mucins. Proteoglycans are high molecular weight glycoconjugate complexes. These are found in abundance in connective tissues and in extracellular matrix. In the past proteoglycans were frequently referred to as connective tissue mucins. However,

protein core of proteoglycon is different and distinct from that of mucins.

- Histochemical reactivity is largely dependent upon the carbohydrate component of mucin. Some carbohydrate molecules do not carry electric charge as they do not have ionizable groups under normal conditions (e.g. glucose, mannose and galactose). In contrast to these monosaccharides, other monosaccharides may contain acidic groups or ions such as **carboxyl (COOH) and sulfonic (SO_3H) groups** which are capable of ionization to confer an overall negative charge on the molecule. The carboxylated monosaccharide N-acetyneuraminic acid is commonly known as sialic acid. The presence of these ionizable groups determine the chemical reaction with dyes of the stains.
- From histochemical perspective, mucins can be grouped into acid mucins and neutral mucins based on the presence of ions in their carbohydrate components. The charged or so called "acid" mucins contain **carboxylate (COO-) or sulfonate (SO_3-) ions (anions).** Both of these ionizable groups are ionized (acid groups/anions) at a physiologic pH to produce an overall negative charge on these mucins. But carbohydrate component of neutral mucins lack acidic groups, and hence they do not carry no net charge (neutral). The acid mucins are found widely in the epithelium of gastrointestinal tract and respiratory tract. The neutral mucins can be found in the gastric glands, Brunner's glands of duodenum and prostatic epithelium.
- The special stains of acid mucin usually contain catonic dyes molecules (positively charged) at a specific pH. This applies to stains like alcian blue, mucicarmine and metachromatic dyes (Azure A or toluidine blue). The cationic dye molecules bind via electrostatic forces to the anionic caboxylated or sulfated polysaccharide chains of the mucin molecules.

Mucins have some common characteristics:

- They are soluble in alkaline solutions.
- They stain intensely with basic dyes.
- They are precipitated by acetic acid excepting gastric mucin.
- They are metachromatic in many of the cases, so they turn into red to reddish blue when stained with toluidine blue or thionin.

From histochemical standpoint, mucins can be subdivided into following groups:

Acidic Mucin

Strongly Sulfated Mucin

- Epithelial mucin: Seen in bronchial serous glands, lesser extent in intestinal goblet cells.
- Connective tissue mucin or proteoglycans: Chondroitin sulfate A, chondroitin sulfate B, chondroitin sulfate C, heparin/heparin sulfate, keratan sulfate.

Weakly Sulfated Mucin or Sulfomucin

- Epithelial mucin: Colonic goblet cells
- Atypical mucin: They are not stained by usual mucin stains (e.g. PAS) but stained by alcian blue, e.g. tracheobronchial mucous glands.

Carboxylated Sialomucin

- Enzyme-labile: They are digested by enzyme sialidase, hence called labile. Examples are submandibular salivary glands, bronchial submucous glands, and goblet cells of small intestine.
- Enzyme resistant: These are resistant to denaturation by the enzyme sialidase. Also, they are PAS-negative unlike enzyme labile mucins. Examples are mucosal glands of large intestine, lesser extent in stomach and bronchus.

Carboxylated Nonsulfated Uronic Acid Mucin

Hyaluronic acid: Composed of N-acetyl-D-glucosamine and D-glucuronic acid. These are widely distributed connective tissue mucin and are also found in synovial fluid, synovial membrane, umbilical cord and early placenta (surface of placental syncytiotrophoblasts).

Sulfated Sialomucin

These mucins are a mixture of sulfomucins and sialomucins. Found in synovial sarcoma and prostatic carcinoma.

Neutral Mucin

As there is no acidic group or ion (carboxyl or sulfonic group), they are neutral. They are composed of different hexosamines. Mostly they are epithelial in origin, e.g. stomach, prostate, and Brunner's gland of duodenum.

There are many types of carbohydrates (as we see in the above classification) of which glycogen and mucins are most important. Now let us know about different types of carbohydrates which may be present in our body. This will enable us to understand role of different types of carbohydrates in many diseases including cancer (Table 1).

FIXATIVE FOR MUCINS

To demonstrate mucins in tissues, neutral or acid, formalin fixatives are good in most of the cases. Alkaline formalin

Table 1: Different types of carbohydrates in normal and abnormal conditions of body

Sl. No.	*Type of carbohydrate*	*Location in the body*
1.	Glycogen	Liver, hair follicles, voluntary muscles, endometrial glands, mesothelial cells, megakaryocyte and umbilical cord
2.	Neutral mucin	Stomach, prostate, Brunner's gland and duodenum
3.	Sialomucin (enzyme-labile)	Submandibular salivary glands, bronchial submucoral glands, goblet cells of small intestine
4.	Sialomucin (enzyme-resistant)	Large intestine, lesser extent in stomach and bronchus
5.	Strongly sulfated epithelial mucin	Bronchial serous glands, lesser extent in intestinal goblet cells
6.	Weakly sulfated epithelial mucin (sulphomucin)	Colonic goblet cells
7.	Sulfated sialomucin	Prostatic adenocarcinoma
8.	Hyaluronic acid	Synovial fluid/synovium, skin, umbilical cord and early placenta
9.	Keratan sulfate	Intervertebral disc and hyaline cartilage
10.	Heparin/Heparan sulfate	Mast cells and aorta respectively
11.	Chondroitin sulfate A	Hyaline cartilage
12.	Chondroitin sulfate B	Heart valves, skin
13.	Chondroitin sulfate C	Umbilical cord, skin
14.	Cellulose	May be present abnormally in gastro-intestinal tract and skin
15.	Chitin	Hydatid cyst of liver, lung and brain

should not be used as they are soluble in alkaline solutions. For metachromatic staining ideal fixative is mercuric chloride. In case formalin or alcohol fixed tissues are to be used, then tissues should be pre-mordanted in 5% mercuric chloride for 5 miutes, followed by treatment with iodine and sodium thiosulfate.

CHOICE OF STAINING METHOD

Mucin can be demonstrated in paraffin, frozen and celloidin sections. Though there are so many stains, Southgate's mucicarmine was most popular in the past. Metachromatic stains are also very good as they also stain many types of carbohydrates.

Recently PAS is getting popularity which also stains most of the carbohydrates/mucin excepting sialomucin and strongly sulfated mucin. Alcian blue and aldehyde fuchsin are sometimes preferred because of ease in staining

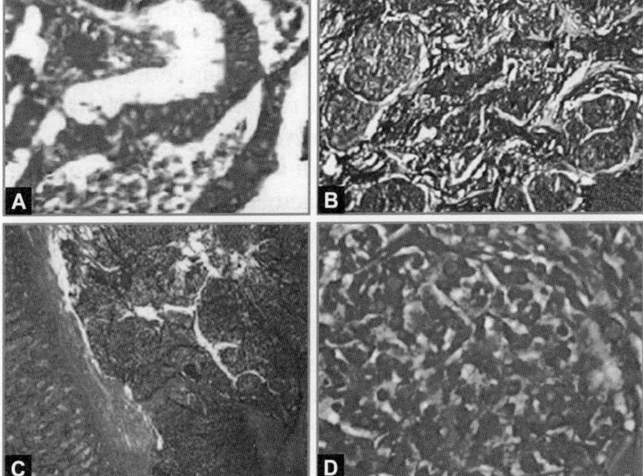

Figs 1A to D: (A) Adenocarcinoma of colon showing malignant cells with neutral mucins (PAS,400×); (B) Mucinous carcinoma showing pools of acidic mucin (Alcian blue,400×); (C) Mucinous carcinoma showing acidic and neutral mucins (Combined Alcian blue and PAS,100×); (D) Signet ring cell carcinoma showing neutral mucin (Combined Alcian blue and PAS, 400×) *(For color version, see Plate 1)*

technique. High iron diamine staining is not used nowadays (Figs 1A to D and Table 2).

- **PAS stain**: Stains glycogen, neutral mucin and carbohydrate portions of glycoproteins and glycolipids. This technique is perhaps the most versatile and widely used mucin stain.
- **PAS stain with diastase pretreatment**: Glycogen is digested, not stained by PAS but stains glycoproteins, glycolipids and glycomucins.
- **Alcian blue (pH 2.5)**: Best stain for acid mucins (strongly sulfated) which is produced by mesenchymal cells.
- **Combined Alcian blue-PAS stains**: best general mucin stain and considered as "pan" mucin stain. This combination is also useful for studying inflammatory and metaplastic conditions of gastrointestinal tract. For example, intestinal metaplasia in stomach (differentiates goblet cells of intestine and gastric mucosa).
- **Mucicarmine stain**: It stains strongly sulfated or acid mucin, other acidic mucin, hyaluronic acid. But neutral mucins are negative or weakly positive. Mucicarmine is commonly used but relatively insensitive stain for epithelial mucin. Mucicarmine is one of the oldest techniques and is replaced by other sensitive techniques.

METACHROMASIA AND MUCIN

Ranvier, Cornil, Jurgens and several other scientists discovered metachromasia in 1875 by using several different dyes like dahlia and cyanine. But the term

Table 2: Different types of carbohydrates and their staining pattern

Sl. No.	*Type of carbohydrate*	*PAS*	*AB at pH 2.5*	*AB at pH 0.2*	*Aldehyde Fuchsin*	*High iron diamine*	*Diastase digestion*	*Sialidase digestion*	*Metachromasia*	*Grocott–hexamine silver*
1.	Glycogen	+	–	–	–	–	+	–	–	+
2.	Neutral mucin	+	–	–	–	–	–	–	–	+
3.	Sialomucine (enzyme labile)	+	+	–	–	–	–	+	+	+
4.	Sialomucin (enzyme resistant)	–	+	–	–	–	–	–	+	–
5.	Strongly sulfated mucin (epithelial)	–	V	+	+	+	–	–	+	–
6.	Weakly sulfated mucin (epithelial)	V	+	–	+	+	–	–	+	+
7.	Sulfated sialomucin	+	+	–	+	+	–	+	+	+
8.	Chitin	+	–	–	–	–	–	–	–	+
9.	Cellulose	+	–	–	–	–	–	–	–	+

Abbreviations: PAS, periodic acid-Schiff, AB, alcian blue; "+", positive; "–", negative; V, variable

'metachromasia' was first used by Ackroyd in 1876. The dyes which show metachromasia exist in orthochromatic form (normal form). When they bind to certain substances (chromotropes), these dyes are converted to polymeric (metachromatic) form. This is because the negative charges of certain chromotropes attract many positively-charged polar groups on the metachromatic dyes to polymerise and polymeric (metachromatic) form is found.

Due to this polymerization, there is a shift of absorption towards the shorter wavelength of light. Normally, toluidine blue dye exists in the blue monomeric form and when they stain nonchromatropes, they polymerize and give purple to red color. Other metachromatic stains are thionin, Azure A, methylene blue, and few fluorochromes like acridine orange, etc.

The carbohydrates or mucins which contain acidic groups or negative charges (both sulfated and carboxylated mucins) show metachromasia with metachromatic stains/dyes. The neutral mucins, as they do not have acidic groups (caboxylate or sulfonate), do not show this property (Table 3).

GLYCOGEN

It is a simple polysaccharide which contains D-glucose units in branched or straight chains. Glycogen has two main forms—alpha and beta. It, in colloidal solution, is found in the cytoplasm of certain cells. Glycogen is derived from sugar and it breaks down into sugar within one hour of death. So tissue containing glycogen either should be fixed in fixatives or it should freeze as death of tissue results in breakdown into sugar.

Choice of Fixative

Fixatives containing picric acid or alcohol are preferred for demonstration of glycogen, e.g. Bouin's fluid or Rossman's solution and 80% alcohol, the original method was done by Best in 1906 in celloidin embedding after alcohol fixation. It was thought that celloidin is essential to prevent diffusion of glycogen from the tissues. But later on Lillie (1947) and Vallance-Owen (1948) proved that glycogen is not lost in running water, at least for 24 hours if tissues are properly fixed.

Table 3: Mucin expression in different malignancies/tumors

S.No.	*Type of malignancy*	*Neutral mucin*	*Acid mucin (strongly sulfated)*	*Glycogen (PAS positive)*
1.	Gastrointestinal carcinoma	+	+	–
2.	Ovarian carcinoma	+/–	+/–	+/–
3.	Renal cell carcinoma	–/+	–	–
4.	Endometrial carcinoma	+	+	–/+
5.	Mucoepidermoid carcinoma	+	+	–
6.	Liposarcoma	–	+	–
7.	Rhabdomyosarcoma	–	+	+
8.	Osteogenic sarcoma	–	+	–
9.	Smooth muscle tumors	–	+	–/+
10.	Neurogenic tumors	–	+	–
11.	Colloid carcinoma	+	+	–
12.	Seminoma	–	–	+
13.	Ewing's sarcoma	–	–	+

In routine practice, formol saline or other aqueous fixatives (e.g. formalin) give adequate result. But freeze drying should be used for histochemical studies. This freeze drying technique is superior to other methods in glycogen preservation and it almost preserves 100% glycogen. This method also prevents streaming of the intracytoplasmic glycogen to one pole of the cells (polarization).

Embedding Medium

Although celloidin was used as embedding medium in the original method by Best, paraffin wax is also equally good. But frozen sections are not suitable for glycogen demonstration.

USE OF ENZYMES

- **Diastase:** This is most commonly used enzyme for glycogen digestion, as it is cheap, stable and easy to use. It may be obtained from malt or saliva. Malt diastase is available commercially and is more reliable than saliva, but salivary diastase is routine as it is easily available. Disatase removes some other things (e.g. ribonucleic acid) besides glycogen, but as these things are not PAS positive, this does not pose a threat.
- **Amylase:** This can be alpha amylase or beta amylase. Alpha amylase is extracted from hog pancreas (also available in some organisms like *B.sublitis* and *Aspergillus oryzae*). Alpha amylase digests both branched and straight chains of glycogen. Beta amylase is derived from sweet potato or barley. It digests only straight chains of glycogen.

PERIODIC ACID-SCHIFF REACTION AND STAIN

Periodic acid is a very strong oxidizing agent and under the controlled condition of the staining reaction, it reacts with the aldehyde group of the carbohydrates. This periodic acid cleaves the carbon-carbon bond in amino or alkyl amino derivatives or 1.2-glycols to form aldehydes. These aldehydes will react with fuchsin-sulfurous acid and this product combines the basic pararo-saniline to give a positive result (magenta colored compound). This compound is chemically alkyl sulfate (Figs 2A and B).

Any substance that fulfills the following criteria will give a positive result during PAS reaction (Hotchkiss, 1948).

- The substance must not diffuse away during fixation
- It must produce an oxidation product which is not diffusible
- The substance must have the 1.2-glycol grouping or the equivalent amino or alkyl-amino derivative or the oxidation product CHOH-CO
- Sufficient concentration of the substance must be present in the tissue to give a positive reaction (magenta color).

PAS Technique

- **Periodic acid solution (0.5%)**
  Periodic acid: 1 g
  Distilled water: 200 mL
- **Schiff's reagent:** Dissolve 1 g basic fuchsin in 200 mL of boiling distilled water. When dissolved; cool it to 50–60°C. Add 2 g of potassium metabisulfite and mix

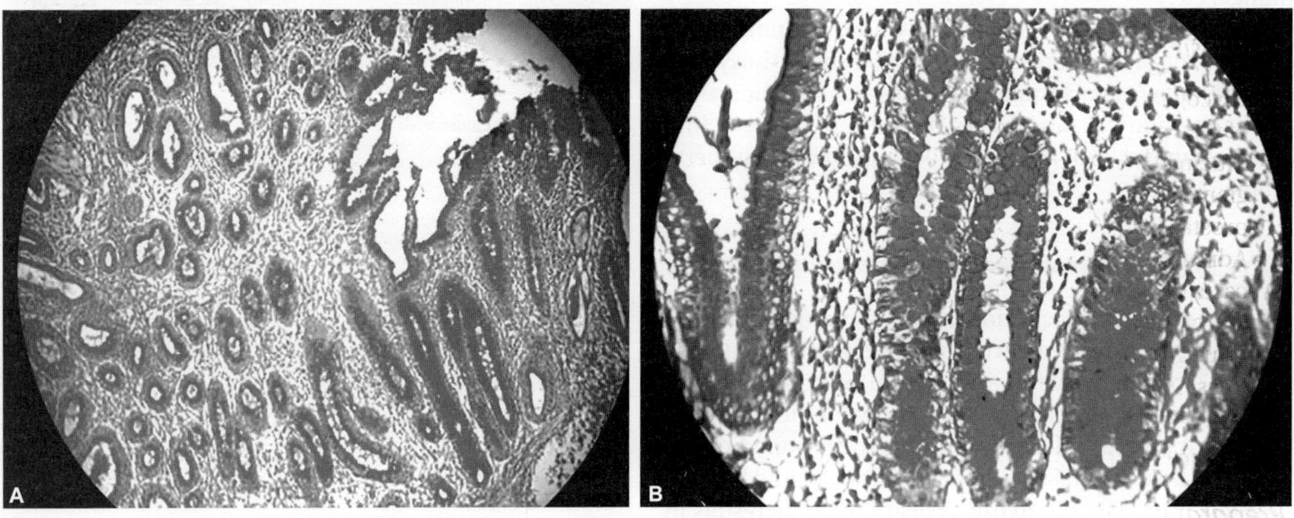

Figs 2A and B: PAS positive materials (mucin) are stained as magenta/bright red: (A) PAS: Appendix, low power; (B) PAS: Appendix, high power *(For color version, see Plate 2)*

it. Bring the mixture to room temperature and then add 2 mL of hydrochloric acid and mix it. Also add 2 g of activated charcoal and this chemical solution is kept at room temperature in a dark place overnight. Next morning, filter it (Whatman paper no. 1).The ideal solution after filtration should be pale yellow or clear. Store this solution at 4°C in dark container.

Staining Method

1. Deparaffinize histologic sections and bring the section to water. If Zenker's fluid is used as a fixative, remove mercury precipitate in iodine. Wash in water and decolorize in hypo solution.
2. Rinse in distilled water.
3. Oxidize in 0.5% periodic acid for 5–10 minutes.
4. Wash in running water for 5 minutes and rinse in distilled water.
5. Treat with Schiff reagent for 10–30 minutes.
6. Wash in running tap water for 5–10 minutes.
7. Counterstain (optional) with Harris's hematoxylin for 1–3 minutes to stain the nuclei. Differentiate in 1% acid alcohol (3–5 dips). Blueing the sections in running tap water.
8. Wash in water.
9. Rinse in absolute alcohol.
10. Clear it xylene and mount in DPX or Canada balsam.

Results

- Glycogen and other PAS positive substances: Magenta/ bright red
- Nuclei: Blue
- Other tissue constituents: Yellow.

PAS Positive Substances

- Glycogen, most basement membrane, amyloid, fibrin of thrombi, colloid of thyroid.
- Mucins: Intestinal glands, gastric glands, endocervical glands, salivary glands, bronchial glands, conjunctiva, prostatic gland secretion, corpora amylacea.
- Adrenal lipofuscin, actinomycosis (clubs only), hyaline casts of kidney, cartilage matrix, ocular lens capsule, starch, zymogen granules of pancreas, beta cell of pituitary.
- Russel bodies of plasma cells, megakaryocyte granules.

Glycogen Extraction by Enzymes

Preparation of Solution

- Diastase: 1 g
- Distilled water: 100 mL
- Mix them well.

Staining Method

1. Deparaffinize two test sections and two positive control section.
2. Treat one test section and one positive control section in diastase solution for 1 hour at 37°C.
3. Wash the sections in running tap water for 5–10 minutes.
4. Now stain all the sections with the desired staining technique for glycogen (e.g. PAS, alcian blue, mucicarmine, etc.).

Result

Presence of glycogen will be confirmed by loss of staining of glycogen after enzyme treatment, but the untreated sections will give positive staining reaction.

Alcian Blue Staining

Alcian blue is a water soluble copper thalocyanin. Although the exact staining mechanism is not known, it is presumed that alcian blue stains by salt linkage to acidic groups. Common alcian dyes are alcian blue 8GX, alcian yellow and a mixture of these two known as alcian green 2 GX (staining an emerald green color) and alcian green 3 BX (staining a blue green color). It has a high molecular weight (>1300) and one of the largest amongst the commonly used histologic dyes.

It stains acid mucin specifically but not the neutral mucin. The intensity of stain depends upon the ionization of tissue component in a particular pH. It gives best with the alcian blue dyes when in a particular pH; the tissue component is fully iodized into acid groups. This property may be advantageous to identify, to separate the different acid mucins by using alcian blue solutions of varying pH. As for example sulfate esters reacts at a lower pH, compared to carboxylated.

In general, a pH 2.5 solution of alcian blue is satisfactory. The optimum pH for different mucins is given below:

- Strongly sulfated mucin: at lower pH (pH ≤1).
- Weakly sulfated mucin: pH 2.5–1.0.
- Hyaluronic acid and N-acetyl sialomucin: pH 3.2–1.7.
- N-acetyl-O-acetyl sialomucin: pH 1.5.

Though neutral mucin is not normally stained with alcian blue dyes, it can be done by different ways (Figs 3A and B). These include:

- By employing acid esterification using a periodic acid hydrochromic acid sequence.
- Treating with a ether-sulfuric acid mixture to introduce sulfate groups (SO_4^{--}).

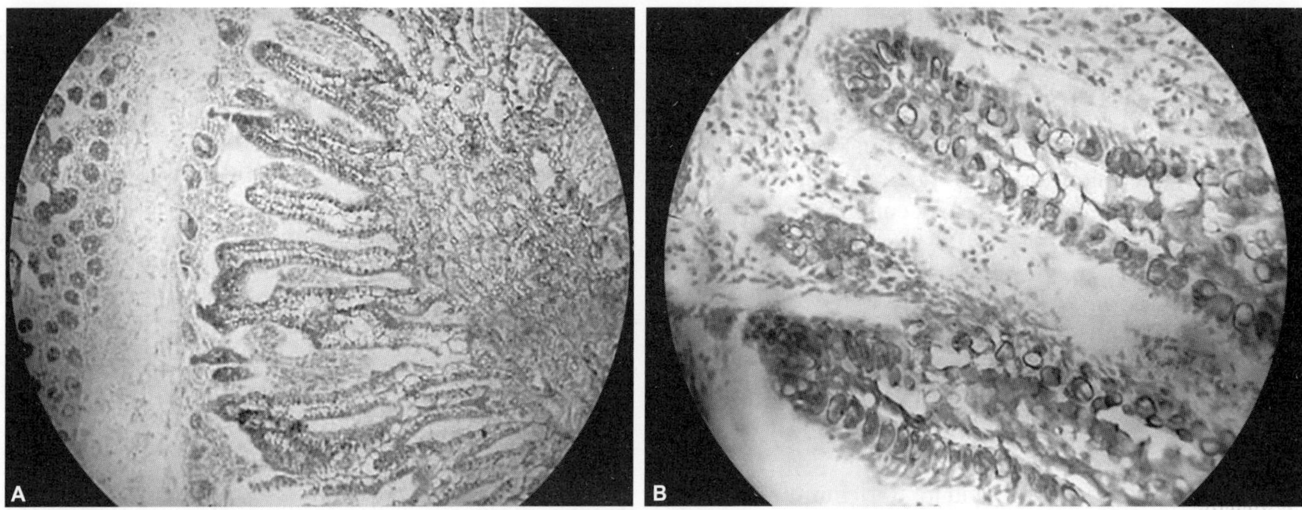

Figs 3A and B: Alcian blue, intestine, low and high power. Alcian blue stains acid mucins as blue *(For color version, see Plate 2)*

- Over oxidization of neutral mucin glycol groups to form aldehydes which subsequently produce carboxylic acid or acid groups needed for alcian dyes.

Preparation of Stain

- Alcian blue: 1 g
- 10% sulfuric acid yielding a pH of 0.2: 100 mL.
  Or
  0.2 M hydrochloric acid (yielding a pH of 0.5): 100 mL.
  Or
  0.1 M HCl (yielding pH of 1): 100 mL.
  Or
  3% acetic acid (yielding pH of 0.25): 100 mL.
  Or
  0.5% acetic acid (yielding pH of 3.2): 100 mL.

Mix it to prepare the alcian blue solution. This solution should be filtered before use. Old solutions lose staining power.

Staining Method

1. Deparaffinise the sections and bring to water.
2. Stain in alcian blue solution for 10–20 minutes.
3. Rinse in distilled water (or omit and blot dry if the pH of staining is critical).
4. Counterstain with 0.5% aqueous neutral red for 2–3 minutes.
5. Rinse in water.
6. Dehydrate rapidly in 95% and absolute alcohol.
7. Clear in xylol and mount in DPX or HSR resin.

Results

- Acid mucins (and most sulfated mucopolysaccharide): Blue.
- Nuclei: Red.
- Other tissue constituents: Red.

Notes:

- For general demonstration of acid mucins, alcian blue dissolved in 3% acetic acid (pH 2.5) is the solution of choice.
- Counterstain with a weak solution of neutral red (0.1–0.5%). Otherwise it will mask the alcian blue staining.
- Staining time will vary as per strength of solution used. As for example, if a 1% solution is used for 5 minutes, 0.1% of that solution needs more time say 30 minutes.

Combined Alcian Blue – PAS Technique

This technique separates acid mucins and neutral mucins. In this technique, firstly all acid mucins are stained with alcian blue but these stained acid mucins which are also PAS-positive would not react in the subsequent PAS stain. Only the neutral mucins will be stained with subsequent PAS stain.

Staining Method

1. Step 1–3 above, followed by steps 4–10 of PAS staining.

Results

- Acid mucin: Blue
- Neutral mucins: Magenta.

Points to Remember

- Avoid Ehrlich's hematoxylin as a counterstain as it stains certain types of mucin and hampers final staining method.
- Stain lightly with counterstain otherwise it will be difficult to distinguish the staining color of hematoxylin and alcian blue (both gives blue color).

SOUTHGATE'S MUCICARMINE METHOD (MAYER, 1896; MODIFIED BY SOUTHGATE, 1927)

Southgate's modification of Mayer's original method (which did not contain aluminium hydroxide) gives more consistent results. This stain demonstrates both gastric and epithelial mucin well.

Composition of Staining Solution

- Carmine: 1 g
- Aluminium hydroxide: 1 g
- 50% alcohol: 100 mL
- These constituents are mixed by shaking and then add:
- Aluminium chloride (anhydrous): 0.5 g.

Preparation

Boil the above mixture in water - bath for 2.5–3 minutes. Cool, filter and store at 4°C.

Staining Method

1. Deparaffinize histologic sections and bring to water.
2. Stain the nuclei with conventional hematoxylin (but not with Ehrlich).
3. Differentiate in acid alcohol and blue in tap water.
4. Stain with above staining solution for 20–30 minutes.
5. Rinse in distilled water.
6. Dehydrate in 95% and absolute alcohol.
7. Clear in xylene and mount in Canada balsam or DPX.

Results

- Mucin: Red
- Nuclei: Blue.

Points to Remember

- It is also useful to stain encapsulated fungi, e.g. Cryptococcus neoformans.

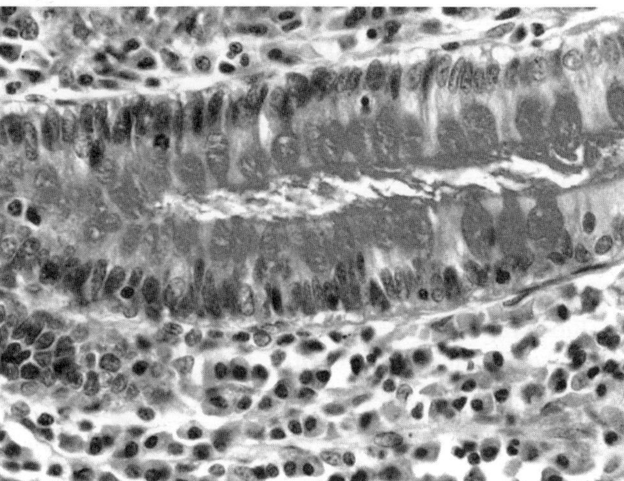

Fig. 4: Mucicarmine stains strongly sulfated or acid mucin as red *(For color version, see Plate 3)*

- In the modification of Southgate's staining method, aluminium hydroxide is added to improve the clarity of staining.
- Avoid Ehrlich's hematoxylin, as certain mucins will be stained and staining with mucicarmine will be hampered.
- The mucicarmine staining solution can be stored at 4°C for 5–6 months.
- The combination of alcian blue–PAS technique is superior to mucicarmine technique to demonstrate tissue mucins more consistently and informatively (Fig. 4).

Best Carmine Method (Best 1906)

Composition of Staining Solution

- Carmine stock solution:
  - Carmine: 2 g
  - Potassium carbonate: 1 g
  - Potassium chloride: 5 g
  - Distilled water: 60 mL
  - These reagents in a 250 mL flask should be gently boiled for 3–5 minutes until the color deepens. The deeper color will give deeper stain of glycogen. Cool the mixture and add 20 mL of concentrated ammonia. Filter it and store in a refrigerator at 4°C (0–5°C) or in a dark container at 4°C. Discard after 6–8 weeks.
- Carmine working solution:
  - Carmine stock solution: 12 mL
  - Fresh concentrated ammonia: 18 mL
  - Methyl alcohol: 18 mL

- Best's differentiating fluid:
  - Absolute alcohol: 20 mL
  - Methyl alcohol: 10 mL
  - Distilled water: 25 mL.

Staining Method

1. Dewax the histologic sections and bring to water.
2. Place in alum hematoxylin (Harris or Ehrlich) for 10–15 minutes to stain nuclei.
3. Rinse rapidly in 1% acid alcohol for differentiation to make the background clear.
4. Wash in running tap water to remove alcohol and blueing.
5. Stain with carmine working solution for 10–15 minutes.
6. Wash slide with Best's differentiating fluid for celloidine section. Use methyl alcohol for paraffin sections.
7. Flood with fresh alcohol or acetone.
8. Clear in xylol and mount in DPX or Canada balsam.

Results

- Glycogen: Deep red
- Nuclei: Blue
- Some mucin, fibrin: Weak red.

CHAPTER 7

Lipids

INTRODUCTION

The term "lipid" is used to describe all naturally occurring fats and fat-like substances. They are soluble in organic or fat solvents like chloroform, ether, acetone, benzene, petroleum and so on.

Definition: Lipids are "naturally occurring fat-like substances that are soluble in organic solvents but not in water". (Baker, 1946).

As per **Lovern's definition** (1955), lipids are 'actual or potential derivatives of free fatty acids and their metabolites'.

But this definition cannot be accepted too rigidly as there are some exceptions. As for example, lecithin is slightly soluble in water but insoluble in acetone. Lysolecithin is another lipid which is freely soluble in warm water and insoluble in ether. Cerebrosides and sphingomyelin when purified are not soluble in many fat solvents.

CLASSIFICATION OF LIPIDS

Group-I—Simple Lipids

Simple lipids are neutral esters of fatty acids (palmitic, linoleic or stearic) with alcohols. They are divided into:

- **Neutral lipids:** These are composed of fats and oils; and the alcohol is glycerol.
- **Waxes:** The alcohol is higher than glycerol like cholesterol esters.

Group II—Compound Lipids

Compound lipids contain other product besides fatty acid and alcohol.

- **Phospholipids:** They contain phosphoric acid molecule. Examples are lecithin, sphingomyelin, cephalin, plasmals (acetol phosphatides).
- **Cerebrosides:** These are lipid containing sphingosine, one fatty acids and a molecule of sugar (glucose or galactose). Examples are kerasine (cerasine), phrenosine, oxynervone and nervone.

Group III—Derived Lipids

These are lipids which derived from the Group I and II lipids, by hydrolysis. They are classified into:

- **Fatty acids:** They are derived from natural products. These can be saturated fatty acids like palmitic acid or stearic acid and unsaturated fatty acids like oleic acids.
- **Alcohols:** They are having high molecular weight and are derived from hydrolysis of waxes. Examples are sterols like cholesterol and straight chain cholesterols.

From histochemical stand points, lipids can be divided into hydrophobic and hydrophilic lipids.

Hydrophobic lipids: They have preponderance of non-polar groups, i.e. lacking polar groups and therefore, they are insoluble in water but soluble in organic solvents. It means surface tension of these lipids at lipid-water interface makes them globular or spherical in shape in water/aqueous solution. Hence, these lipids are impermeable to aqueous solutions. Examples are esters and unconjugated lipids.

Hydrophilic lipids: These lipids contain polar groups (phosphoryl) and basic groups; which make them water miscible. Examples are phospholipids and glycolipids (cerebrosides, gangliosides, sulfatides).

CLASSIFICATION OF LIPIDS BASED ON POLAR AND NONPOLAR GROUPS

- **Polar lipids or hydrophilic lipids (soluble in water/ aqueous solution):**
  - **Phospholipids:** It contains phosphoric acid, long chain fatty acids, polyhydric alcohol and nitrogen bases (variable).
    - Glycerol-based: Phosphatidylcholine (lecithin), phosphatidylserine, plasmalogens, cephaline (phosphatidylethanolamine)
    - Sphingosine-based: Sphingomyelins
  - **Glycolipids:** Cerebrosides, gangliosides, sulfatides.
- **Nonpolar lipids or hydrophobic lipids (soluble inorganic solvents)**
  - **Esters:** Cholesterol esters, waxes, mono-, di-, triglycerides.
  - **Unconjugated lipids:** Cholesterol and fatty acids.

Again the lipids can be divided into acidic, neutral and basic lipids based on presence of acid groups or basic groups in their molecules. These are usually polar lipids.

- **Acidic lipid:** Phosphatidyl serine, sulfatides, gangliosides
- **Neutral lipids:** Cerebrosides
- **Basic lipids:** Phosphatidylcholine (lecithins), phosphatidylethanolamine (cephalins), plasmalogens, sphingomyelins.

Fats and lipids are one of the normal constituent of cells. These can be found in the cells as free fat or combined with other compounds like carbohydrate (glycolipid), protein (lipoprotein), phosphates (phospholipids) and so on. Accumulation of fat in some tissues is the basis of certain pathologic conditions/diseases. As for example, fat embolism arises due to bone injuries and fractures and fat accumulates in lung, long bone's marrow and in circulation (vessels).

Fat is soluble in organic solvents like alcohol. So, histologic sections from routine paraffin embedding (which uses alcohol for processing) cannot demonstrate fats or lipids. As in the tissue processing, alcohols are used which will dissolve the fats/lipids. For demonstration of lipids, frozen section is ideal as it does not require tissue processing alcohol.

FIXATION OF LIPIDS

As already told frozen sections (cryostat) are the best way to demonstrate fats/lipids. But these also need some degree of tissue fixation, so that the section and lipids can withstand the harsh solvents or section cutting. Most useful fixatives for lipids are osmium tetroxide (OsO_4) and chromic acids. If formalin is to be used for lipid histochemistry, then 2% calcium acetate is added to 10% formalin, known as formal-calcium fixative.

Formalin may be oxidized to formic acid if it is stored for a long time, and this acid milieu is detrimental to lipids and causes hydrolysis of lipids if this fixative is used. Addition of calcium acetate act as a buffer (as good as phosphate buffer) and prevents formation of formic acid. Not only that, this added calcium makes a protective lattice complex of phospholipids with mucins and proteins and prevents dissolving of phospholipids. It has been confirmed that calcium ions reduce the solubility of myelin lipids (found in brain, myelinated nerve fibers). But addition of calcium acetate has one disadvantage—the calcium ions saponify (conversion of an oil or fat into a soap) free fatty acids to insoluble soap in acetone.

IDENTIFICATION OF LIPIDS

Histologic identification of lipids is usually based on the following:

- Solubility of lipid
- Reduction of osmium tetroxide
- Demonstration of fat soluble dyes
- Examination by polarized light
- Other staining and histological methods

1. Solubility of lipid: Keilig (1944) proposed that lipids may be differentiated by their solubility in various 'fat solvents'. He used Soxhlet extraction apparatus and blocks made from fresh human brain (<3 mm thikness). Lipids were extracted for 24 hours, with at least 3 changes of solvent. The continuous extraction with equal parts of methyl alcohol and chloroform may be used to identify that the extracted material substance is a lipid. After extraction of lipid, blocks are hydrated through descending grades of alcohol, then to water. Frozen sections are cut and stained by Sudan block B. The results of extraction of different lipids are shown in Table 1.

Flowchart 1 showing identification of unknown lipid based on solubility of lipids.

2. Reduction of Osmium tetroxide: Reduction of osmium tetroxide (OsO_4) to osmium dioxide (OsO_2) makes the colorless OsO_4 to OsO_2. It has little value as it does not react with all lipids. But may be used to identify unsaturated fatty acid (Oleic acid), but also secondary staining of fat due to presence of saturated fatty acids like palmitic acid and stearic acid.

3. Demonstration with fat soluble dyes: Fat soluble dyes are routinely used in histological laboratories to stain neutral fat. The first dye used for this purpose was Sudan III in 1896. Later on Lillie and Ashburn used oil red O in isopropyl alcohol, which gave more intense staining of lipids and minimal removal of lipid particles. Recently, Chiffelle and Putt advocated use of Sudan IV or Fettrot in propylene

Flowchart 1: Showing identification of unknown lipid based on solubility of lipids

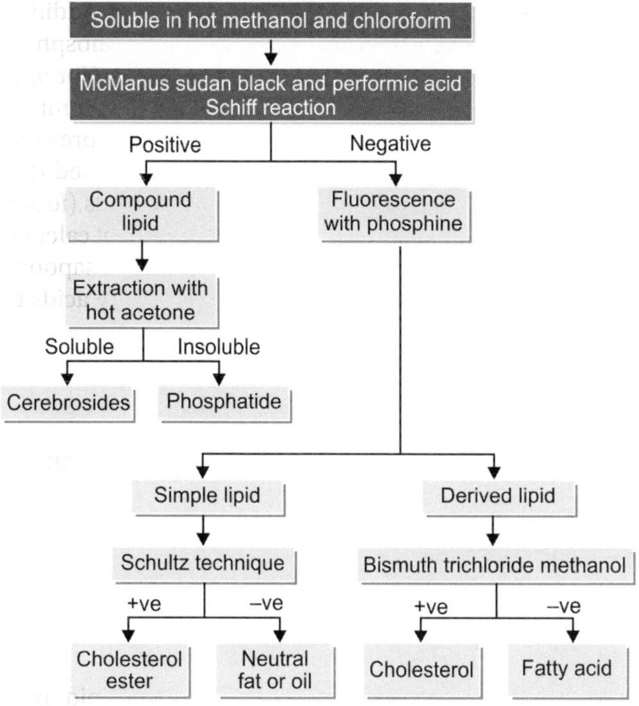

glycol, which gave best result so far and it does not remove even minute amount of lipids. Nowadays, this stain is widely used for routine histologic as well as research works.

4. Examination by polarized light: Most of the lipids are highly refractile and may be monorefringent or birefringent. By examining sections under polarized microscope, type of lipid can be determined, i.e. whether they are monorefringent (isotropic) or birefringent (anisotropic). But the information may often be ambiguous and it has little diagnostic value.

Monorefringent (isotropic)—seen in neutral fats, cholesterol and fatty acids in any state.

Birefringent (anisotropic)—found in any lipid in crystalline state.

5. Other staining or histochemical methods: The Nile blue sulfate method is used for differentiating neutral fat and fatty acids. Baker's acid hematin method is used to demonstrate phospholipids and cerebrosides.

CONTROL SECTIONS

Control sections should be stained during lipid staining. This is particularly important if that particular staining method is not used regularly. Negative control is used to exclude the possibility interference of other nonlipid compounds. Positive control helps to standardize particular staining method.

Negative controls: Negative control sections are made after total extraction of lipids from the sections or making delipidized sections.

Total extraction of lipids can be done, after putting the control sections in the following solution:
- Chloroform: 66 mL.
- Methanol: 33 mL.
- Distilled water: 4 mL.
- Concentrated HCl: 1 mL.

Ratio of chloroform: Methanol is 2:1(v: v) addition of water (4%) facilitate extraction of phospholipids and addition of concentrated HCl (1%) release bound lipids. The solution can be used for 1 hour at room temperature.

Acetone is also widely used for extraction of hydrophobic lipids (nonpolar lipids). If the dry sections are kept in anhydrous acetone (devoid of water) at 4°C for 20-25 minutes, it will selectively remove cholesterol and fats. This anhydrous acetone (dried over anhydrous calcium chloride or $CaCl_2$) cannot extract acetone insoluble phospholipids. But the commercial acetone which contains water also, extracts a major portion of phospholipids.

Positive controls: Most of the types of lipids are commercially available in its pure form. So, whenever a positive control of a particular type of lipid is needed, then that particular lipid applied to the filter paper and can be regarded as a tissue section in a staining technique.

Otherwise, sections are made from tissues from known lipid storage disorder (either at biopsy or during autopsy). In another method of making of positive control slides, lipid is suspended in gelatine and is allowed to set, fixed. After that a block is prepared to cut cryostat section.

For future use, multiple sections can be prepared from composite blocks and kept at -20°C.

Control sections:
- Fatty liver → triglycerides, free fatty acids
- Brain → myelin (phospholipids)
- Adrenal glands → free cholesterol, esterified cholesterol.

Sudan IV Stain

Sudan IV dye is soluble in fat but insoluble in water, like oil red O or Sudan black B. As the dye Sudan IV is dissolved in fat, it gives coloration and makes them fat-colorants. This stain is applied in the aqueous-alcoholic or alcoholic-acetone phase, because in this phase the stain is soluble. When the dye penetrates the tissue, it clearly has affinity for lipids but not for water. Some authors prefer other organic solvents like propylene, ethylene or isopropyl alcohol over

Table 1: Identification of different lipids by different staining techniques

Method of staining	*Simple lipid*		*Compound lipid*							*Derived lipid*		
	Waxes	*Neutral lipids*	*Phospholipids*				*Cerebrosides*			*Fatty acids*		*Higher alcohol*
	Cholesterol esters	*Neutral fat and oils*	*Lecithin*	*Cephalin*	*Sphingomyelin*	*Acetyl phosphatides*	*Nervone*	*Phrenosine*	*Kerasine*	*Unsaturated fatty acid*	*Saturated fatty acid*	*Cholesterol*
1. Fat soluble stain (Sudan IV, oil red O)	+ †	+++	+	+	+	–	+	+	+	+	+	+ †
2. Sudan black B (McManus)	–	–	+*	+*	+*	–	+*	+*	+*	–	–	-
3. Blue with Nile blue sulfate	–	–	+	+/-	+/-	+/-	–	–	–	+	+	-
4. Performic acid-Schiff	–	–	+	+	+	+	+	+	+	–	–	-
5. Fischler's method	–	–	–	–	–	–	–	–	–	+*	+*	-
6. Schultz technique	+	–	–	–	–	–	–	–	–	–	–	+
7. Periodic acid-Schiff (PAS)	–	–	+	+	+	–	+/-	+	+	–	–	-
8. Acid-hematin pyridine	–	–	+	+	+	–	+ (pale)	+ (pale)	+ (pale)	–	–	-

Abbreviations: +, positive; –, negative; *, a negative result is not diagnostic; †, gives positive results only when lipid is melted, negative in room temperature.

ethanol or acetone. To demonstrate fat by Sudan IV stain fresh cryostat section is preferred, but 10% buffered formalin (addition of 2% calcium acetate) can also be used.

Composition of Staining Solution

- **Sudan IV stain:**
  - Sudan IV: 1 g
  - Acetone: 50 mL
  - 70% ethanol: 50 mL

  Dissolve the Sudan IV dye in acetone and alcohol mixture. A supersaturated solution of the dye may be used for more intense staining (which may require more amount of Sudan IV dye). But supersaturated solution of Sudan IV dye may cause precipitate over the tissue sections and also it is less dependable.
- Harris hematoxylin staining solution
- Glycerine jelly.

Staining Method

1. Cut frozen sections.
2. Wash in water and rinse in 70% alcohol (ethanol).
3. Stain in Sudan IV stain for 10–20 minutes.
4. Differentiate in 70% alcohol to remove excess stain.
5. Rinse in water.
6. Counterstain the nuclei in Harris hematoxylin for 2–3 minutes.
7. Differentiate quickly in 1% acid alcohol.
8. Blueing in tap water.
9. Mount in glycerine jelly.

Result

- Fat and lipids: Orange to red
- Nuclei: Blue.

Sudan Black B Stain

Sudan black B is known as the most sensitive lipid stain. It was introduced by Lison and Dagnelie in 1935. Unlike the other Sudan dyes, it can stain both phospholipid and neutral fat (compound lipids). It also can stain myelin and mitochondria.

The ability of formalin and calcium to make these lipids insoluble in acetone and other reagents used in paraffin processing, make them unsuitable for Sudan III or osmium tetraoxide staining. But Sudan black B stain can be used. Ideal sections for Sudan IV staining are unfixed cryostat sections, short fixed frozen sections and cryostat sections post-fixed in formol-calcium. Use of solvents like ethanol or acetone is not recommended for this dye, as these solvents remove a significant portion of the lipid. So small fat droplets are dissolved out and are not detected by stain. Propylene, propylene glycol, isopropyl alcohol or ethylene glycol are better as a solvent. But 70% ethanol is still used for general purpose.

Staining Method

1. Rinse cryostat sections in 70% ethanol.
2. Stain the slides in saturated Sudan black B in 70% ethanol for 30–120 minutes. Sections of routine formol saline-fixed tissue should be stained for 30–180 minutes at 60°C.
3. Rinse in 70% ethanol to remove excess surface dye.
4. Wash in tap water and differentiate in 70% alcohol (or in 85% propylene glycol solution for 2–3 minutes).
5. Wash in distilled water.
6. Counterstain in Mayer's carmalum for 2–3 minutes. (Mayer's carmalum: Dissolve 2 g of carmine in 100 mL of 5% ammonium alum by boiling for 1 hour. Add few crystals of thymol to prevent fungal growth, filter before use).
7. Wash well in water.
8. Mount in glycerine jelly.

Results

- Compound lipids (phospholipids, cerebrosides): Blue-black
- Nuclei: Red.

Oil Red O Stain

For this staining technique, cryostat sections, short-fixed frozen sections, unfixed or post-fixed in formol-calcium is chosen.

Staining Solution

A saturated solution of oil red O (0.25–0.5%) in isopropyl alcohol is kept in stock. Working solution is made by adding 6 mL of stock solution with 4 mL of distilled water. Allow the mixture to stand for 5–10 minutes and then filter it.

Staining Method

1. Cut frozen sections (relatively thick section of 8–10 μm).
2. Wash well in distilled water.
3. Rinse in 70% ethanol.
4. Stain in oil red O staining solution for 10–35 minutes.

5. Differentiate in 70% alcohol to remove excess stain.
6. Counterstain nuclei lightly in Harris hematoxylin for 1–2 minutes.
7. Blue in tap water (alternatively, ammonia water may be used).
8. Mount in glycerine jelly.

Results

- Lipids: Orange to red.
- Nuclei: Blue.

Nile Blue Sulfate Method

Preparation of Staining Solution

Add 10 mL of 1% H_2SO_4 to 200 mL of 1% Nile blue sulfate in water. Boil this mixture in a flask for 2 hours. Maintain the pH of the final solution at pH_2.

Staining Method

1. Cut frozen sections and dry it.
2. Stain in Nile blue sulfate staining solution for 30–40 minutes at 60°C.
3. Differentiate in 1% acetic acid for 1–2 minutes.
4. Wash well.
5. Counterstain nuclei with 1% chloroform-washed methyl green for 3–5 minutes.
6. Wash in tap water.
7. Mount in glycerine jelly.

Result

- Phospholipids: Blue
- Free fatty acids: Pink to blue.
- Unsaturated hydrophobic lipids: Pink.

Performic Acid-Schiff Method (for Phospholipids and Cerebrosides)

Tissue fixation: Formol saline or Zenker-formol should be used.

Reagent

- Performic acid: Mix 40 mL of 98% formic acid with 4 mL of 30% hydrogen peroxide (100 vol.). Allow to stand it for 1½ to 2 hours. Do not store and prepare fresh reagent for use.
- Peracetic acid: Commercially peracetic acid (40%) is available in the market like formalin (40%).
- Schiff reagent (see PAS staining in Carbohydrates Chapter at page 36).

Staining Method

1. Place frozen sections or paraffin sections in water (remove mercury precipitate if any).
2. Blot the slide.
3. Oxidise with performic acid or peracetic acid for 3–5 minutes.
4. Immerse in Schiff reagent for 20–30 minutes.
5. Wash in warm running water for 5–10 minutes.
6. Mount in glycerine jelly.

Result

Phospholipids and cerebrosides (lipids with unsaturated bonds): Red.

Baker's Acid Hematin Method

Baker's acid hematin method (used in conjunction with pyridine extraction test) is a superior technique to demonstrate phospholipids and cerebrosides. But the staining procedure is long and time consuming, Hence, not used for lipid stain commonly.

Reagents

- **Fixative:** Formol calcium.
- **Dichromate calcium solution:**
  - Potassium dichromate: 5 g
  - Calcium chloride: 1 g
  - Distilled water: 100 mL.
- **Acid hematin**: Dissolved 0.05 g of hematoxylin in 40 mL of distilled water. Then add 1 mL of 1% sodium iodide. Heat the mixture in a flask until it boils. Cool it and now add 1 mL of glacial acetic acid. Solution is now ready for use but it cannot be stored for future use.
- **Borax ferricyanide differentiator:**
  - Borax (sodium tetraborate, 10 H_2O): 0.25 g
  - Potassium ferricyanide: 0.25 g
  - Distilled water: 100 mL
  - Mix these things and keep the solution in the dark.

Staining Method

1. Small pieces of tissues are fixed in formol calcium for 6–8 hours.
2. Transfer the fixed tissues into dichromate calcium solution for 18 hours at room temperature.
3. Again transfer them to dichromate calcium solution for 24 hours at 60°C.
4. Wash well in distilled water.
5. Cut frozen sections (thickness 8–10 μm).
6. Mordant sections in dichromate calcium solution for 1 hour at 60°C.

Table 2: Lipid and carbohydrate accumulation in different storage disorders

Name of the disease	*Enzyme deficiency*	*Major accumulating metabolite*	*Organs involved*
A. Glycogen storage disease			
1. Type I (Von Gierke's disease)	Glucose-6-phosphatase	Glycogen	Kidney, liver
2. Type II (Pompe's disease)	Acid α-glucosidase (acid maltase)	Glycogen	Heart, skeletal muscle
3. Type III (Forbe's/Cori's disease)	Amyloglucosidase (debrancher)	Limit dextrin	Heart, skeletal muscle
4. Type IV (Anderson's disease)	Amylo-trans-glucosidase (brancher)	Amylopectine	Liver
5. Type V (Mc Ardle's disease)	Muscle phosphorylase	Glycogen	Skeletal muscle
6. Type VI (Hers' disease)	Liver phosphorylase	Glycogen	Liver
7. Type VII	Phosphofructokinase	Glycogen	Muscle
8. Type VIII	Phosphorylase kinase	Glycogen	Liver
B. Sulfatidoses			
1. Gaucher's disease	Glucocerebrosidase	Glucocerebrosides	Liver, spleen, bone marrow
2. Niemann-Pick disease	Sphingomyelinase	Sphingomyelin	Liver, spleen, bone marrow, lungs, lymph nodes
3. Krabbe's disease	Galactocerebrosidase	Galactocerebrosides	Kidney, nervous system
4. Fabry's disease	α-galactosidase	Ceramide	Kidney, spleen, heart, skin
C. Mucopolysaccharidosis			
1. Type I (Hurler)	α-L-iduronidase	Dermatan sulfate, heparan sulfate	Liver, spleen, bone marrow, cornea, heart
2. Type II (Hunter)	L-iduronate sulfatase	Dermatan sulfate, heparan sulfate	Liver, spleen, heart
D. Gangliolipidosis (Gangliosidosis):			
1. GM1—Gangliosidosis (infantile and juvenile form)	GM1—ganglioside galactose	GM1—ganglioside	Liver, kidney
2. GM2—Gangliosidosis (Tay-Sachs, Sandhoff disease)	Hexosaminidase	GM2—ganglioside	Liver, kidney, spleen, heart, brain

7. Wash in distilled water.
8. Stain in acid haematin for 5 hours at 37°C.
9. Rinse in distilled water.
10. Differentiate in borax ferricyanide for 18 hours at 37°C.
11. Wash in water.
12. Mount in glycerine jelly.

Results

- Phospholipids and nucleoprotein: Dark blue to black.
- Cerebrosides: Pale blue to blue-black.
- Mucin, fibrinogen: Dark blue.

Lipid and carbohydrate accumulation in different storage disorders are summarized in Table 2.

CHAPTER 8

Proteins and Nucleic Acid Staining

INTRODUCTION

Proteins are a group of complex organic compounds containing carbon, hydrogen, oxygen, nitrogen and sulfur. Proteins are major constituent of different cells in the tissues. They are principal constituents of protoplasm of the cell and have high molecular weight. Proteins consist of alpha amino acids joined by peptide linkages. Twenty different amino acids are commonly found in proteins. Each protein has a unique genetically defined amino acid sequence which determines its basic shape and function. They serve as structural elements, enzymes, hormones, immunoglobin, etc. Proteins are involved in oxygen transport (like myoglobin), muscle contraction (myofilaments like actin and tropomyosin), electron transport and other activities.

Proteins may be alone in the tissues or they may be conjugated to other components to form conjugated proteins. When they combine with lipid they form lipoproteins. Likewise they form mucoproteins (mucopolysaccharide + protein) and nucleoproteins (nucleic acid + proteins). When it comes to identify the lipoproteins or mucoproteins in tissues, usually stains are used to demonstrate lipid or mucopolysaccharide respectively. In this chapter we will discuss staining procedures of simple proteins and nucleic acids of nucleoprotein (DNA and RNA).

Simple proteins are composed of albumin, globulin, fibrous structural proteins (like collagen, elastin, reticulin, etc.), complements, enzymes and others. Demonstration of simple proteins and nucleoproteins can be divided into the following groups:

- Histophysical methods
- Amino acid histochemical methods
- Enzyme histochemical methods
- Immunohistochemical methods
- Fluorescent methods.

HISTOPHYSICAL METHODS

Fibrous proteins like collagen, reticulin, fibrin, elastin, and amyloid can be demonstrated by simple techniques/stains by using their physical configuration rather than chemical composition of these proteins. Different small or large molecule dyes are used like trichrome stains for collagen, silver stain for reticulin, van Gieson stain for elastic fibers, phosphotungstic acid hematoxylin (PTAH) for fibrin and Congo red stain for amyloid proteins.

AMINO ACID HISTOCHEMICAL METHODS

In these techniques usually some of constituent amino acids are demonstrated and not the whole protein component. The techniques/stains to demonstrate these amino acids are based on linkages within the amino acids and identification of particular exposed groups:

- Phenyl groups, e.g. in tyrosine
- Indole groups, e.g. in tryptophan and tryptamine
- Protein bound amino groups, e.g. in lysine
- Guanidyl groups, e.g. in arginine
- Disulfide and sulfhydryl linkages, e.g. in cysteine and cysteine.

Ninhydrin-Schiff Method for Amino Groups

Fixative: Neutral buffered formalin, freeze dried tissue, formaldehyde vapor.

Histologic sections: Paraffin, cryostat or freeze dried.

Composition of Staining Solution

- Solution A: 0.5% ninhydrin in absolute alcohol
- Solution B: Schiff's reagent.

Staining Method

1. Place the histologic sections in 70% ethyl alcohol.
2. Treat the slides with solution A (Ninhydrin solution) overnight at 37°C.
3. Wash in running tap water.
4. Treat with solution B (Schiff's reagent) for 45–60 minutes.
5. Wash in running tap water.
6. Counterstain the nuclei with Harris or other alum hematoxylin.
7. Wash in running tap water.
8. Dehydrate through graded alcohol in ascending order.
9. Clear in xylene and mount in Canada balsam/DPX.

Results

Amino groups: Pinkish-purple.

Performic Acid-Alcian Blue Method for Disulfides

Fixative: Neutral buffered formalin, freeze dried tissue, formaldehyde vapor.

Histologic sections: Paraffin, cryostat or freeze dried.

Composition of Staining Solution

- Performic acid solution
  - 98% formic acid: 40 mL
  - Hydrogen peroxide: 4 mL
  - Concentrated sulfuric acid: 0.5 mL
- Alcian blue solution
  - Alcian blue: 1g
  - 98% sulfuric acid: 2.7 mL
  - Distilled water: 47.3 mL

Staining Method

1. Place the histologic sections into water and blot to dry (remove excess water).
2. Treat with performic acid solution for 4–5 minutes.
3. Wash well in tap water for 8–10 minutes.
4. Dry the slides at 60°C.
5. Rinse in tap water.
6. Stain in alcian blue solution for 45–60 minutes at 37°C (room temperature).
7. Wash in running tap water.
8. Counter stain if necessary (used neutral red not hematoxylin as it gives blue color).
9. Wash in tap water.
10. Dehydrate through graded alcohol in ascending order.
11. Clear in xylene and mount in Canada balsam or DPX.

Results

Disulfides: Blue.

Points to Remember

- Hair bearing skin has abundant keratin which has many disulfide containing amino acids. So they may be used as positive control.
- The intensity of stain or blue color will depend on the amount of disulfide present.
- Performic acid solution is to be used fresh but before use it, stand for 1–2 hours.
- Histologic sections should be washed carefully. It may be washed away after performic acid treatment following vigorous washing.

Diazotization-Coupling Method for Tyrosine

Fixative: Neutral buffered formalin, formaldehyde vapor, freeze dried tissue.

Histologic sections: Paraffin, fixed cryostat, celloidin and freeze dried.

Composition of Staining Solution

- Incubating solution A
  - Sodium nitrite: 3.5 g
  - Concentrated acetic acid: 4.4 mL
  - Distilled water: 47 mL
- Incubating solution B
  - Ammonium sulfamate: 0.5 g
  - Potassium hydroxide: 0.5 g
  - 8 amino-1-naphthol-5-sulfonic acid: 0.5 g
  - 70% alcohol: 50 mL.

Staining Method

1. Place the histologic sections into water.
2. Place sections in incubating solution A for 24 hours in the dark at 4°C.

3. Rinse in water at 4°C.
4. Place the sections in solution B for 1 hour in the dark at 4°C.
5. Wash in light acid (0.1 m HCl, three to four changes) each change 4–5 minutes.
6. Rinse in running tap water for 8–10 minutes.
7. Counterstain if necessary (Harris or other alum hematoxylin).
8. Dehydrate through graded alcohol in ascending order.
9. Clear in xylene and mount in DPX or Canada balsam.

Results

Tyrosine containing proteins: Purple and red.

ENZYME HISTOCHEMICAL METHODS

Enzymes have specific actions on its substrates. So proteins which act as enzymes can be demonstrated based on their actions on its specific substrates. This will be discussed in the enzyme histochemistry and the histochemical stains.

IMMUNOHISTOCHEMICAL METHODS

Recent advent of antibodies against a wide array of antigens including protein like immunoglobulins, enzymes and hormones has revolutionized the detection of these antigens in tissues/different parts of body. The concept of immunohistochemistry (IHC) comes from detection of antigen-antibody complex following treatment with a substrate or chromogen (like avidin-biotin). The details will be discussed in the subsequent chapter.

FLUORESCENT METHODS

Nucleic acids can be demonstrated by fluorescent method. The most common stain used to demonstrate nucleic acid by fluorescent method is acridine-orange. It stains DNA yellow green and RNA red. But acridine-orange is not suitable for paraffin embedded tissue. Also the stains are temporary. So, it is not popular stain as in routine histologic work paraffin embedded tissue are used. But this stain can be used in alcohol-fixed tissue and in exfoliative cytology.

Acriflavine is another fluorochrome which can be used to demonstrate nucleic acids. Following acid hydrolysis, acriflavine can be used as a 0.01% alcohol solution. It can be used as an alternative to basic fuchsin in Schiff's reagent. Here also it needs acid hydrolysis before the staining steps. Both these procedure will stain the DNA into fluorescent yellow. Of these two procedures the second one has better specificity and is preferred.

NUCLEIC ACIDS

Nucleic acids are high molecular weight polymeric substances composed of nucleotides that constitute the acidic groups of the nucleoproteins and contain phosphoric acid, sugars plus purine and pyrimidine bases.

Nucleoproteins are composed of nucleic acids and proteins. The two nucleic acids are DNA and RNA. DNA is located in the nucleus of the cell whereas RNA is located in the ribosome of the cytoplasm.

DEOXYRIBONUCLEIC ACID

In the year 1869, Friedrich Miescher isolated a substance from the nuclei known as nuclein. This nuclein was later named as deoxyribonucleic acid (DNA). In 1914, Robert Feulgen showed color test for DNA in a test tube. But he described the method of staining DNA in chromosome in a much later year of 1924. There are four nitrogen bases in DNA—adenine and guanine are two purines and thymine and cytosine are two pyrimidines. DNA molecules are composed of alternate five carbon sugar (deoxyribose), phosphate group and a nitrogen base which is attached to sugar group. The chain of DNA may be subdivided into smaller units known as nucleotide. Each nucleotide consists of phosphate-sugar and a base. Multiple units or series of such units are called polynucleotide.

RIBONUCLEIC ACID

In ribonucleic acid (RNA), the sugar moiety is ribose and nitrogen bases are adenine, guanine, cytosine and uracil. They are also attached to a phosphate group as in DNA to form polynucleotide chain. As already said this RNA is mainly seen in the ribosomes of endoplasmic reticulum. Besides, it can be seen in the nucleolus and the cells which are actively synthesizing protein.

General Notes on Nucleic Acid Staining

- **Acid hydrolysis:** When nucleic acids are hydrolyzed, it will form three substances: (a) phosphate; (b) sugar; (c) nitrogenous base. The staining procedure of nucleic acids depends on the reaction of dyes with phosphate group or production of aldehydes from the sugar deoxyribose. But nitrogen bases are not stained by histochemical method.
- **Fixative:** Good fixatives are alcoholic and acidic fixatives, e.g. Carnoy's fluid which contain both alcohol and glacial acetic acid. Formalin is not ideal as nucleic acid fixative. If formalin is to be used, then tissue should

be fixed in neutral buffer formalin at 4°C which prevents DNA degradation in nucleus by DNA nucleases. It can give acceptable staining of the nucleic acid.

- **Basophilia:** DNA as well as RNA is stained by cationic dyes. As for example methylene blue at pH 3.0–4.0 can selectively stain nucleic acids. Simple cationic dye (methylene blue, neutral red) and complex ionic dye (alum hematoxylin) link with nucleic acids differently. These formation of link between two types of cationic dyes can be differentiated. If simple cationic dye staining, prior treatment with acid will reduce the staining intensity. But staining with alum hematoxylin will be hardly affected by prior treatment with acid.
- **Decalcification:** If decalcification is needed (bony tissue, calcified tissue) then treats with organic acids (formic acid) for short period of time. Application of strong inorganic acids (HCl, HNO_3) is not recommended. EDTA is probably the best decalcifying agent. One disadvantage of using acid for prolonged period is that it will denature DNA making the nuclei pyrinophilic (red in color). So when stained with methyl green pyronin this will give nuclei red rather than giving green colored DNA material in normal condition.

Techniques Specific for DNA

- **The Fuelgen reaction:** It has been used extensively for the demonstration of DNA particularly for cytomorphometric applications. The procedure depends on the reaction of aldehyde or ketone groups with Schiff's reagent (fuschin-sulfuric acid). In these staining techniques, DNA is treated with hydrochloric acid which breaks the purine-deoxyribose bonds and aldehyde group is formed. This aldehyde group reacts with Schiff's reagent to give red-purple color. But if the sections are treated with hydrochloric acid for a prolonged time it will give negative Fuelgen reaction as there is breakdown of DNA (depolymerization). RNA does not give positive Fuelgen reaction as it is completely hydrolyzed by the hydrochloric acid. Fluoroscent dyes like acridine-orange or auramine O, may also be used in place of Schiff's reagent.
- **Acid hydrolysis:** As regards to acid hydrolysis, time is very crucial. An increasing stronger reaction is obtained as the hydrolysis time is increased until the optimum time is reached. Beyond this time the reaction will weaken and may even become negative. As a fixative, Bouin's fluid is unsuitable as it causes overhydrolysis of nucleic acid during fixation. Bauer in 1932, proposed following optimum time for acid hydrolysis (1M HCl at 60°C) for different fixatives.

Fixative Time in Minutes

Carnoy fluid	8
Chrome-acetic	14
Flemming	16
Formalin	8
Formaldehyde vapor	30–60
Helly	8
Regaud	14
Susa	18
Zenker	5
Zenker-formol	5
Bouin's fluid	Unsuitable

Fixatives: Preferably a nuclear fixative should be used like Carnoy's fluid. But other fixatives may also be used as stated above but the optimum hydrolysis time should be used. If only nuclei are to be examined formol-saline gives good result. Methanol or Clarke's fixative is preferred when smears from tissues are to be examined.

Feulgen Nucleal Reaction for DNA

Composition of Staining Solution

- Hydrochloric acid (1M)
  - Concentrated HCl: 8.5 mL
  - Distilled water: 91.5 mL
- Schiff's reagent (*see* page in carbohydrate, Chapter 6)
- Potassium meta-bisulfite solution
  - 10% potassium metabisulfite: 5 mL
  - 1M hydrochloric acid: 5 mL
  - Distilled water: 90 mL

Staining Method

1. Place the section in water.
2. Rinse them in 1M HCl at room temperature.
3. Then transfer the sections in 1M HCl at 60°C for optimum time (*see* previous Table).
4. Rinse in 1M HCl for 1–2 minutes at room temperature.
5. Treat the sections with Schiff's reagent for 45–60 minutes.
6. Rinse them in potassium metabisulfite solution for 1–2 minutes.
7. Repeat wash in potassium metabisulfite solution twice for 1–2 minutes.
8. Rinse well in distilled water.
9. Counterstain in 1% light green if required for 1–2 minutes.
10. Wash in water.
11. Dehydrate in graded alcohol in ascending order.
12. Clear in xylene and mount in DPX or Canada balsam.

Results

- DNA: Red-purple
- Cytoplasm: Green.

Naphthoic Acid Hydrazide Reaction (Feulgen NAH)

Feulgen reaction though used routinely to demonstrate DNA, it is not highly specific. Because the aldehyde-leuco fuchsin compound which is formed due to Feulgen reaction may diffuse and attach with other protein components. Use of both Feulgen and Feulgen NaH overcomes this problem as the latter reacts to aldehyde group released by acid hydrolysis in a different way. So, if the material gives positive result with both Feulgen and Feulgen NaH, it should be none other than DNA.

Composition of Staining Solution

- Hydrochloric acid (1M)
  - Concentrated HCl: 8.5 mL
  - Distilled water: 91.5 mL
- NaH solution
  - 2-hydroxy-3-naphthoic acid hydrazide: 100 mg
  - Ethyl alcohol: 95 mL
  - Acetic acid: 5 mL
- Fast blue B salt solution
  - Fast blue B salt: 100 mg
  - Veronal acetate buffer, pH 7.4: 100 mL.

Staining Method

1. Bring sections in water and rinse briefly in 1M HCl.
2. Place sections in 1M HCl at 60°C (pre-heated).
3. Rinse sections in 1M HCl at room temperature for 1 minute.
4. Rinse sections in distilled water for 1 minute.
5. Rinse sections in 50% alcohol for 1 minute.
6. Transfer to a Coplin jar containing NaH solution for 3–6 hours at room temperature.
7. Rinse in 3 changes of 50% alcohol, keeping sections for 10 mintues each time.
8. Rinse sections in distilled water for 1 minute.
9. Transfer to fast blue B salt solution (freshly prepared) for 2–3 minutes.
10. Wash in water.
11. Counterstain if required.
12. Dehydrate, clear and mount in DPX.

Results

- DNA: Bluish purple
- Cytoplasmic and other proteins: Pinkish red.

RNA STAINING

RNA can be demonstrated by following methods:

- Methyl-green-pyronin method
- Acridine-orange method
- Gallocyanin-chrome alum technique.

Of these methods, methyl-green-pyronin is the technique of choice. Methyl-green-pyronin will stain both DNA and RNA. It was first reported by Pappenheim (1899) and modified by Unna in 1902. Pure methyl green is prepared by removing methyl violet from impure methyl green dye by washing in chloroform.

The methyl green binds with the DNA whereas pyronin component binds with the RNA. There is a spatial arrangement between phosphate groups on DNA and the NH2 groups of the methyl green dye. So, this dye is specifically attached to DNA. But pyronin has no such spatial alignment and does not have specificity. So any negatively charged constituent of the tissue will be stained as red. As for example, acid mucins/sialomucin or cartilage will be stained red.

Pyronin Y more selectively stains RNA than pyronin B. Also pyronin Y has better differentiation and is less diffusible. pH of the staining solution and concentration of the two dyes are very important. Some authors suggested that better results are obtained by washing in ice-cold water first, then to differentiate it in tertiary butanol.

The selective staining of nuclei by methyl green is related to the texture of DNA and dye size. The differential staining is based on the competition of the dyes for anionic sites of differing accessibilities. Pyronin also stains osteoid, granules of leukocytes and acid mucins.

Preparation of pure methyl green: A 2% aqueous solution of methyl green is washed with chloroform in a separating funnel to remove the impurity, methyl violet (a breakdown product of methyl green). This removal of methyl violet is continued until the washings are colorless. This pure methyl green can be stored for 6–9 months.

Methyl Green Pyronin Method

Fixative: Carnoy's fluid (formalin is second choice).

Composition of Staining Fluid

Two types of staining fluids can be used. Either of these staining solutions can be used and staining technique is also the same.

- Trevan and Sharrock's methyl green pyronin
  - 2% aqueous methyl green (washed): 10 mL
  - 5% aqueous pyronin: 17.5 mL
  - Distilled water: 250 mL.

Mix well and dilute with equal quantity of acetate buffer pH 4.8 before use.

- Jordan and Baker's methyl green-pyronin
  - 0.5% aqueous methyl green (washed): 13 mL
  - 5% aqueous pyronin Y: 37 mL
  - Acetate buffer (pH4.8): 50 mL

  The above solutions can be stored for 2–3 months. As already said, any of these two staining solutions can be used.

Staining Method

1. Bring section to water.
2. Pour staining solution over the slide and keep it for 15–60 minutes.
3. Rinse quickly in distilled water and blot it.
4. Flood slide with acetone for 1–2 seconds then again flood with acetone.
5. Flood slide with acetone xylol (equal parts).
6. Flood with xylol until it becomes clear.
7. Mount in DPX or neutral mountant.

Results

- DNA: Green/green-blue
- RNA: Red.

Gallocyanin-Chrome Alum Technique

This staining method stains both DNA and RNA. For specific demonstration of either DNA or RNA one has to take the help of RNAse or DNAse for removal of RNA or DNA.

Composition of Staining Solution

- 5% aqueous solution of chrome alum: 100 mL
- Gallocyanin: 0.15 g.

This is known as Elmarson's gallocyanin chrome alum.

Preparation of stain: Shake the above two well and slowly increase the temperature up to boiling point. Boil it for 4–5 minutes, cool it and filter it. Add distilled water through filter paper to make the filtrate volume 100 mL. This staining solution has pH of 1.64 and it can be stored for 4–5 weeks.

Staining Method

1. Bring sections to water.
2. Stain it with staining solution in a Coplin jar for 48–50 hrs at room temperature.
3. Wash in water for 2–3 seconds.
4. Dehydrate through graded alcohol in ascending order.
5. Clear it and mount in DPX.

Results

- Nucleic acid: Deep blue
- Cartilage: Red.

Enzyme Digestion Method for Nucleic Acids

Specific enzyme will digest DNA or RNA in tissue sections. While pure deoxyribonuclease (DNAse) will digest DNA pure ribonuclease (RNAse) will digest RNA. If the enzymes are pure, it won't digest the other nucleic acid.

Enzyme Extraction of DNA

Fixative: Use fixative other than potassium dichromate (it will inhibit digestion of deoxyribonuclease or DNAse).

Composition of Extraction Solution

- Deoxyribonuclease: 5 mg
- 0.2M TRIS buffer, pH 7.6: 5 mL
- Distilled water: 25 mL.

Mix well to make the extraction solution (30 mL).

Extraction Method

1. Place both test and control sections into water.
2. Place test section in extraction solution and control section in TRIS buffer for 4 hours at 37°C.
3. Wash in running tap watere for 4–5 minutes.
4. Stain both test and control sections by the Feulgen method to stain DNA.

Results

- Test section: DNA negative
- Control section: DNA red/red purple.

Enzyme Extraction of RNA

Fixative: Use fixative other than potassium dichromate and mercuric chloride.

Composition of Extraction Solution

- Ribonuclease: 8 mg
- Distilled water: 10 mL.

Mix well to make extraction solution (10 mL).

Extraction Method

1. Place both the test and control sections into water.
2. Place test section in extraction solution and control section in distilled water for 1 hour at 37°C.

3. Wash in distilled water.
4. Stain both test and control sections by methyl green pyronin method to stain RNA.

Results

- Test section: RNA negative, DNA: green/green blue
- Control section: RNA red, DNA: green/green blue.

Acridine Orange Stain for DNA and RNA

Acridine orange is a basic dye which can be used to demonstrate DNA and RNA. With this technique DNA appears green and RNA exhibits red fluorescence. This type of staining pattern is known as fluorescence metachromasia. The orthochromic form of the dye fluoresces green and the metachromatic form has a red fluorescence. As there is an overlap between red and green fluorescence, treatment of sections with RNAse improves the coefficient of variation between the fluorescence readings of acridine orange-stained nuclei.

CHAPTER 9 Connective Tissue Staining

INTRODUCTION

The connective tissue is named so because this tissue binds or connects other tissues of body. But that does not mean that this type of tissue has only supportive function. It has many subtypes like general or ordinary connective tissue, hemopoietic tissue (which includes blood) and specialized connective tissue like bones, cartilage, joints, etc. The connective tissue is derived from embryonic mesoderm.

The connective tissue has two components—cellular component and intercellular substance. Now, we will discuss about components of general or ordinary connective tissue.

CELLULAR COMPONENT

The main type of cells are:
- Fibroblasts
- Macrophages or histiocytes
- Plasma cells
- Mast cells
- Reticular cells
- Pigment cells
- Fat cells.

FIBROBLASTS

These cells are numerous in number. They derive from undifferentiated mesenchymal cells. When they become old, they become inactive and are converted into fibrocytes.

Functions

- Major role of fibroblasts is to produce collagen fibers by synthesizing tropocollagen proteins and taking these tropocollagens outside extracellular space.
- Fibroblasts have a significant role in wound healing. During the healing process there is proliferation of fibroblasts which is converted into fibrocytes. They also form granulation tissue when enmeshed in vascular stroma.

MACROPHAGES OR HISTIOCYTES

Tissue macrophages are called histiocytes. In active state; macrophages are free and take ovoid shape. They also have amoeboid movements when they are active. These cells can be stained when they are alive by dyes like India ink, tryptan blue, lithium carmine, etc. If these dyes are introduced locally or in systemic circulation, these dyes are phagocytosed by macrophages. Now, these stains or dyes are visualized as cytoplasmic granules. Macrophages are derived from the monocytes of the blood, from fibroblasts or from undifferentiated mesenchyme.

Functions

- The macrophages phagocytose foreign bodies, particulate organic material, invading microorganism and digest them. Hence, they destroy these elements from their harmful effects.
- Sometimes, nonspecific antigens are ingested by macrophages. These antigens are either destroyed or they are modified and transformed to the immunocompetent T or B lymphocyte.

Distribution in the Body

- Blood: Monocyte
- Connective tissue: Histiocyte
- Liver: Kupffer cell

- Bone: Osteoclast
- CNS: Microglia
- Lung: Alveolar macrophages or 'Dust cell'
- Placenta: Hofbauer cells
- Kidney: Mesangial cell
- Spleen: Littoral cell
- Synovium: Type A lining cell
- Lymphoid tissue and lymph node: Reticular cell.

PLASMA CELLS

Plasma cells are seen in abundance in mucosa and submucosa of the gastrointestinal tract and in the greater omentum. They appear in post-natal life and are not seen at birth.

Functions

- They secrete different antibodies to counteract antigens and thus help in defence mechanism.
- As these cells are almost absent at birth, antibody formation in the newborn is minimum.

MAST CELL

Mast cells are found along the blood vessels, in the fibrous capsule of the liver, in the synovial membrane and in the other parts of the body. These cells have many closely packed large membrane-bound granules in their cytoplasm. These granules can be metachromatically stained by methylene blue or toluidine blue.

Functions

- They liberate heparin which acts as anticoagulant.
- Mast cells produce histamine and smaller amount of serotonin (5-hydroxytryptamine). These chemicals have role in anaphylactic or allergic reactions and in inflammation.

PIGMENT CELLS

Pigment cells are also known as melanocytes. It is found in the epidermis of skin, in the iris and choroidal tissue of eye. Melanocytes within the epidermis are responsible for the production of melanin, a brown pigment that protects against potentially injurious ultraviolet (UV) radiation in sunlight.

RETICULAR CELLS

Reticular cells are present in the reticular connective tissue. These cells produce reticular fibers to which the cells are attached.

Functions

- Phagocytic: the cells ingest and remove the bacteria.
- They also act as stem cells and produce cellular constituents of blood.

FAT CELLS

Fat cells are found in the adipose tissue. When the adipose tissue is processed and stained with hematoxylin and eosin (H and E stain), the fat is dissolved in solvent/alcohol. So, the fat cell resemble 'signet ring'. By special method, the fat may be fixed with osmium tetroxide and it can be stained by oil red O, Sudan black, Sudan III and IV, etc.

INTERCELLULAR SUBSTANCE

The intercellular substance or matrix is a nonliving material and is synthesized by the connective tissue cells, particularly by the fibroblasts. As per AW Ham, "The body is an effice of intercellular substance in which cells live as residents".

The nature of intercellular substance varies as per tissue's function. It may be soft (as in umbilical cord) or it may be very hard (as in cortical bone). Like the texture, microscopical appearance also varies. Intercellular substance may be grouped as:

- Amorphous or gel type or ground substance
- Formed or fibrous type.

AMORPHOUS ELEMENT

Amorphous elements or ground substances are composed of mucopolysaccharides (polymers of carbohydrates conjugated with proteins). The amorphous element or ground substance is a viscous, semifluid material 'which lie between the cells and fibers'. The mucopolysaccharides are mostly synthesized by fibroblasts. When a person becomes old, the ground substance diminishes and fibrous element increases.

Compositions

- Water, mostly bound to mucopolysaccharides.
- Protein—glycoproteins, albumin, globulin, soluble proteins.
- Electrolytes.
- Mucopolysaccharides: Sulfated and nonsulfated type, hyaluronic acid, chondroitin sulfate. Hyaluronic acid possesses long and feathery carbohydrate molecules and holds much water. Hyaluronic acid keeps the ground substance in solid form and makes the tissue soft and pliable. On the other hand, chondroitin sulfate keeps the ground substance in gel form and is found in cartilage.

Functions

- It makes framework of the tissue and provides morphology.
- It acts as a mechanical barrier and checks spread of infection by offending organisms or bacteria.
- It helps in storage of water and in the diffusion of the metabolites between the capillaries and the cells.

Staining of Ground Substance

As the ground substance contains abundant water, it can be stained by freeze-dried PAS reagent, alcian blue or by toluidine blue (metachromatic stain).

FIBROUS ELEMENT

In the intercellular component, the proteins are frequently organized to form fibers. There are three types of fibers:
- White or collagen fibers
- Reticulin fibers
- Yellow or elastic fibers.

Collagen Fibers

It is the most common animal protein among animals and provides the extracellular framework for all multicellular organisms. At present, there are 27 types of collagen. Each collagen fiber is composed of three chains forming a trimer in the shape of triple fibrillar and nonfibrillar collagens. Type I, II, III, V and XI are fibrillar collagens. Here, the triple-helical domain is uninterrupted for > 1000 residues and these proteins are found in the extracellular fibrillar structures. On the other hand, type IV collagens have interrupted triple-helical domain but are long. They form sheets rather than fribls; hence they are nonfibrillar collagen. Collagen swells in acetic acid. It is digested by pepsin. On boiling collagen produce gelatine. Collagen fibers are stained pink in H and E stain, due to eosin, red in van Gieson's stain due to acid fuchsin and blue in Mallory's stain due to aniline blue (Table 1).

Table 1: Common types of collagen, their distribution in body and genetic disorders

Collagen type	*Tissue distribution*	*Genetic disorder*
Type I collagen	Bulk of body's collagen, most of the organic matrix of bases, abundant in soft tissue and also in structural protein of lung	Osteogenesis imperfecta, Ehler-Danlos syndrome (arthrochalasias type I)
Type II collagen	Hyaline and elastic cartilage, vitreous, intervertebral disc	Spondyloepiphysea dysplasia syndrome, Achondrogenesis type II
Type III collagen	Found in tissue which also contain type I collagen (liver, lung, kidney, spleen, etc.), soft tissue, reticular fibers	Ehler-Danlos syndrome (vascular type)
Type IV collagen	Basement membrane	Alport syndrome
Type V collagen	Blood vessels, soft tissues	Ehler-Danlos syndrome (classic type)
Type VI collagen	Microfibrils	Bethlem myopathy
Type VII collagen	Anchoring fibrillar protein at dermo-epidermal junction	Dystrophic epidermolysis bullosa
Type IX collagen	Intervertebral discs, cartilage	Multiple epiphyseal dysplasias

Reticulin Fibers

It can be distinguished from collagen fibers. Reticulin fibers are gram-negative, colored black by silver stain and isotropic (not birefringent), whereas collagen fibers are slight gram-positive, stained brown to mauve by silver stain and is anisotropic (birefringent). Reticulin fibers form a delicate supporting framework for highly cellular organs like lymph nodes, liver and endocrine glands.

Reticular fibers are fine and delicate fibers which are found along with a stronger and coarser collagen fiber, i.e. type III collagen fiber.

Reticular fibers are commonly found in reticular connective tissue, particularly in association with basement membrane. Here, these delicate fibers form a network and are bound to a special carbohydrate moiety of amorphous ground substance. These fibers can branch and anastomose. Like collagen fibers, they also show axial periodicity. So; they also can be called pre-collagen.

Stains

- In paraffin sections, by argyrophil-type silver impregnation technique.
- In frozen sections, by PAS stain.

Elastic Fibers

Elastic fibers are found throughout the body but most common locations are in skin, respiratory systems (lung, pleura), urinary bladder, ligaments, circulatory system (blood vessels). Under light microscope, their appearance vary according to location. In the upper dermis , the elastic fibers are fine and single whereas in the large arteries, elastic membranes have small holes or fenestra (Latin word, means window). These fenestra permits diffusion of materials. Recently, high resolution microscopic examination reveals elastic fibers have two components: elastin and elastic fiber-microfibrillar protein (EFMP). Elastin is an amorphous substance and biochemically resemble a protein. EFMP is microfibrillar in nature and shows a periodicity of 4–13 nm.

Elastic fibers are arranged in a plexus. They can branch and anastomose.They are resistant to chemical treatment. As these fibers are elastic, they can be stretched easily and again recoils its original position when pressure is released. It has protein subunits, known as tropo-elastin (rich in amino acid valine). They are synthesized by fibroblasts and probably also by smooth muscle of blood vessels. Elastic fibers are congophilic (stained by Congo red), acidophilic (eosinophilic or pink in H and E), and refractile. They are unaffected by boiling, acetic acid or pepsin unlike the collagen fibers. But elastic fibers are digested by trypsin.

As the age advances, the elasticity is reduced. There are changes in two components (elastin and EFMP). There are splitting and fragmentation, increase in glutamic acid, aspartic acid and calcium. So, ratio of EFMP and elastin is altered. Because of this alteration, skin of elderly persons becomes wrinkled. Elastic arteries lose their elastic properties.

FIBRIN AND FIBRINOID MATERIALS

Fibrin

It is formed by polymerization of fibrinogen. Fibrin is insoluble fibrillar protein whereas fibrinogen is soluble fibrillar protein. When there is a tissue damage or acute inflammation, plasma fibrinogen from blood vessels comes to extracellular space. Here, they polymerize to form fibrin. So, fibrin may be found outside the vessels in inflammatory exudates.

Fibrinoid Materials

It is usually seen in immune reactions involving blood vessels. The antigen-antibody complexes or immune complexes get deposited in the blood vessels and also leaked out to surrounding tissue. In H and E stain, it appears bright-pink and amorphous. It is seen in acute damage of blood vessels (necrotizing vasculitis) or in plugs of capillaries.

MASSON TRICHROME STAIN

'Trichrome stain' is a general term and three dyes were used in earlier technique—smaller molecule dyes, medium size dye and larger dye. The smaller dye will penetrate collagen, muscle, fibrin and erythrocyte and it will stain all these type of tissues. The medium size dye will penetrate collagen and muscle and will stain them. The larger dye will only stain collagen, they cannot penetrate muscle or erythrocytes.So, based on the permeability and pore size of fixed tissue—the stain was used to differentiate three tissue types, i.e. collagen, muscle and erythrocyte (Table 2).

Factors of Trichrome Stains

- **Heat:** It increases the tissue penetration of dyes and increases the rate of staining.
- **pH of staining solution:** Low pH is preferred (pH 1.5–3).
- **Fixative:** Routine formalin-fixed tissues are not ideal for trichrome stain. Preferred fixative are Bouin's fluid or Zenker's fluid, Formol-mercury or picro-mercuric alcohol can also be used as alternative. In case formalin-fixed tissues are to be used, treatment with picric acid or mercuric chloride solution (or both) should be done.
- **Nuclear stain:** Weigert iron hematoxylin or other iron hematoxylin are used as they are resistant to acidity of dye solution used in trichrome stain. Alum hematoxylin are unsuitable because they are easily decolorized in acid solutions.

Masson trichrome is the most popular technique among the trichrome stains.

Ideal fixatives are Bouin's fluid or Zenker's fluid overnight.

Table 2: Common stains used for different connective tissues and its color

Tissue type	*Masson trichrome*	*Reticulin silver*	*Methanamine silver*	*van Gieson*	*PTAH*	*H and E*	*PAS*
Collagen	Blue green	Pale grey	Unstained	Red	Orange red	Deep pink	Pale pink
Reticulin fibers	Blue green	Black	Unstained	Yellow	Orange brown	Unstained	Pink
Elastic fibers	Pale red	Unstained	Unstained	Yellow	Orange brown	Pink	Unstained
Fibrin	Red	Unstained/grey	Unstained	Variable yellow	Variable blue	Pink	Pink or unstained
Muscle	Red	Pale grey	Pale grey	Yellow	Blue	Deep pink	Pale pink
Cartilage	Variable	Variable	Variable	Variable	Variable	Purple	Pink
Basement membrane	Blue green	Pale grey	Black	Yellow	Orange	Pink	Magenta

Abbreviations: PTAH, phosphotungstic acid hematoxylin; H and E, hematoxylin and eosin; PAS, periodic acid-Schiff.

Staining Method

1. Bring sections to water.
2. Remove mercury pigment with iodine-sodium thiosulfate sequence if required.
3. Stain with Weigert's iron hematoxylin for 20–30 minutes (Refer to routine hematoxylin and eosin staining).
4. Differentiate in 1% acid-alcohol until only nuclei are stained.
5. Wash in running tap water for 10 minutes until sections are blue.
6. Stain in 1% Ponceau 2R in 1% acetic acid for 5 minutes.
7. Rinse quickly in distilled water.
8. Mordant for 10–15 minutes in phosphomolybdic acid-phosphotungstic acid solution if aniline dye is to be used. Mordant for 5–15 minutes in 5% aqueous phosphotungstic acid if light green is to be used. Discard acid solution after use.
9. Drain and counterstain in 2.5% aniline blue in 2% acetic acid for 5–10 minutes. Or 2% light green in 2% acetic acid for 5 minutes.
10. Differentiate in 1% acetic acid solution for 2–5 minutes to remove excess blue or green.
11. Dehydrate in 95% alcohol, followed by absolute alcohol.
12. Clear in xylene and mount in Canada balsam or DPX.

Results

- Nuclei: Blue black or black
- Muscle, cytoplasm, keratin: Red
- Collagen, cartilage, mucus: Blue (if aniline blue is used) or green (if light green is used).

Verhoeff's van Gieson Method

Composition of Staining Solution

- Verhoeff's staining solution
  - Stock 5% alcoholic hematoxylin: 20 mL
  - 10% ferric chloride: 8 mL
  - Verhoeff's iodine (iodine 2 g, potassium iodide 4 g, water 100 mL) : 8 mL
  - Reagents are added as given above, then mix well; solution should be freshly prepared before use.
- Van Gieson's staining solution
  - Saturated aqueous solution of picric acid: 100 mL
  - 1% acid fuchsin: 10 mL
  - Freshly prepared solution is better.

Staining Method

1. Bring histologic sections to water.
2. Stain in Verhoeff's staining solution for 15–30 minutes until sections are jet-black.
3. Differentiate in 2% ferric chloride until elastic fibers are clearly visible (Rinse in water and examine under low power microscope).
4. Wash in water.
5. Place in 95% alcohol to remove iodine staining.
6. Wash in water for 5–10 minutes.
7. Counterstain in van Gieson's staining solution for 3 minutes. Blot it.
8. Dehydrate in graded alcohol.
9. Clear in xylene and mount in DPX.

Results

- Elastic fibers and nuclei: Black to blue black
- RBC, cytoplasm, background and muscle: Yellow
- Collagen: Red.

Note: Do not wash the sections after van Geison's staining (step 7). Put them directly in graded alcohol for dehydration. Otherwise, it will impair staining quality (if washed in water).

Van Gieson Technique

Composition of Staining Solution

- **Celestine blue solution:**
  - Celestine blue B: 2.5 g
  - Ferric ammonium sulfate: 25 g
  - Glycerine: 70 mL
  - Distilled water: 500 mL

  The ferric ammonium sulfate is dissolved in cold distilled water with stirring. Then Celestine blue B is added to this cold solution. Now, the mixture is boiled for 2–3 minutes. Cool it and filters it. Then add glycerin to this filtrate. The stain is prepared and it can be stored for 4–5 months.
- **Van Gieson solution:**
  - Saturated aqueous picric acid solution: 5 mL
  - 1% aqueous acid fuchsin: 0.9 mL
  - Distilled water: 5 mL
  - Mix them well.

Staining Method

1. Bring the dewaxed sections in water.
2. Hydrate in graded alcohol.
3. Stain in Celestine blue solution for 5–10 minutes.
4. Rinse in distilled water.
5. Stain in Mayer's another alum hematoxylin for 5–10 minutes.
6. Wash in tap water-until sections are blue.

7. Differentiate in acid alcohol (0.5–1% HCl for 1–2 minutes)
8. Wash in tap water.
9. Stain in van Gieson solution for 3 minutes. Blot it.
10. Dehydrate in graded alcohol in ascending order.
11. Clear in xylene and mount in DPX.

Results

- Nuclei: Blue/black
- Collagen: Red
- Elastic fibers, reticular fibers, basement membrane, RBC: Yellow.

Gomori's Aldehyde Fuchsin Method for Elastic Fibers

Fixative: Formol saline is the best. Other fixatives are also suitable.

Composition of Staining Solution

- Basic fuchsin: 1 g
- 70% alcohol: 200 mL
- Concentrated HCl: 2 mL
- Paraldehyde: 2 mL.

The fuchsin is dissolved first in 70% alcohol. Then add conc. Hydrochloric acid and paraldehyde. Mix well and keep the solution at room temperature for 24–48 hours until it turns blue. The solution is now ready for use. The solution can be stored in refrigerator for 2–3 months.

Staining Method

1. Place the dewaxed sections in water.
2. Treat in Lugol's iodine for 20–30 minutes.
3. Place in 5% sodium thiosulfate for 3–4 minutes.
4. Wash in running tap water for 2–3 minutes.
5. Rinse in 90% alcohol.
6. Stain with staining solution for 5–10 minutes.
7. Rinse in 90% alcohol.
8. Counterstain with orange G, light green or Masson trichrome stain.
9. Dehydrate in graded alcohol.
10. Clear in xylene and mount in DPX.

Results

- Elastic fibers: Deep purple.

Note: This is a progressive stain and it can stain other tissue elements apart from elastic fibers. Though staining color is same, i.e. deep purple but staining time varies.

- 5–10 minutes staining time: Mast cell granules
- 10–30 minutes staining time: Mucin and gastric chief cells
- 15–30 minutes staining time: β cell of pancreas
- 30–120 minutes staining time: β cell of pituitary.

Gomori's Silver Impregnation Method for Reticulin

General notes on silver impregnation technique: Silver impregnation method is widely used to demonstrate reticulin fibers. The pattern of deposited reticulated fibers in a tumor is sometimes characteristic enough to diagnose a particular tumor. In addition; mild degree of fibrosis can also be demonstrated by reticulin stain.

Reticulin fibers have an affinity for silver and subsequently stained with ammoniacal solution. The silver impregnation method needs perfection and any fault in the technique will lead to unstaining of the reticulin fibers. So, some precaution must be taken.

- Care should be taken to remove dust. This is perhaps most important factor in the deterioration and precipitation of silver solutions.
- Use well washed glassware (wash with 10% nitric acid) and rinse them in distilled water.
- Avoid using metallic forceps; plastic forceps are preferred.
- Glass rods should be washed when they are used in between solutions.

Fixatives: Formalin is the preferred fixative for silver impregnation technique. But other fixatives may also be used. If mercury fixatives are used then remove the mercury deposit by bringing the sections in water. But the histologic sections may be detached from slide as the silver solution is highly alkaline. To overcome this problem, use slide which is well coated with albumin as adhesive. Alternatively, treat the section with 1% celloidin (parlodin) in an ether-alcohol mixture. But it should be done after deparafinizing the section and treating them with absolute alcohol. Then soak the slides in 1% celloidin (parlodin) for 5 minutes. Wash off the excess celloidin. Immerse the celloidin film in 80% alcohol for 5 minutes, then to water to harden the celloidin film.

Preparation of Gomori's Silver Solution

In a test tube or flask, add 4 parts of 10% aqueous silver nitrate and 1 part of 10% potassium hydroxide. The potassium hydroxide will cause silver to deposit. Mark the volume of the fluid with a pencil/marker. Remove the supernatant fluid and wash the deposit several times with distilled water to make up to its original volume (previously marked by pencil/marker). Now, add strong ammonia drop by drop until the deposit is just dissolved. Again add 10% silver nitrate solution, to produce a light precipitate. Make the volume of this solution twice with addition of distilled water. Store in a dark bottle. Filter before use. Preferably, solution should be freshly prepared but it can be used for 24–35 hours.

Staining Method

1. Bring the deparaffinized sections to water.
2. Oxidize with 1% potassium permanganate for 1–2 minutes.
3. Rinse in tap water.
4. Decolorize with 3% potassium metabisulfite for 1 minute.
5. Rinse in tap water.
6. Sensitize in 2% iron alum for 1 minute.
7. Wash in tap water for 2–3 minutes, then rinse in distilled water 2–3 changes.
8. Impregnate in silver solution for 3 minutes.
9. Rinse quickly in distilled water.
10. Reduce in 10% formalin in tap water for 3 minutes.
11. Wash in running tap water for 3–4 minutes, then rinse in distilled water.
12. Tone in 1:500 gold chloride (yellow) for 5–15 minutes.
13. Rinse in distilled water.
14. Place in 3% potassium metabisulfite for 1 minute to reduce toning.
15. Rinse in distilled water.
16. Fix in 3% sodium thiosulfate for 1 minute.
17. Wash in water.
18. Dehydrate through graded alcohol.
19. Clear in xylene and mount in DPX.

Results

- Reticulin fibers: Black (Figs 1A and B)
- Collagen fibers: Purple
- Nuclei and cytoplasm: Grayish/shades of gray.

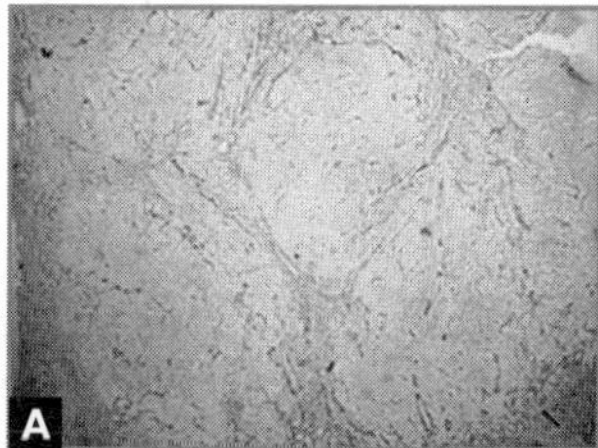

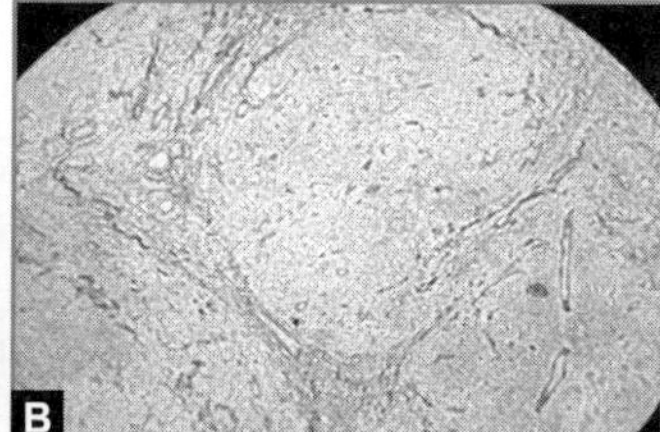

Figs 1A and B: (A) Microphotograph showing reticulin fibers in cirrhotic nodules of liver (Reticulin stain, low power view, 100×); (B) Microphotograph showing retculin fibers in a cirrhotic nodule (Reticulin stain, high power view, 400×) *(For color version, see Plate 3)*

Gordon and Sweet's Silver Impregnation Method

Composition of Staining Solution

- **Silver solution:** 5 mL of 10% aqueous silver nitrate solution add concentrated ammonia, drop by drop, until the precipitate, which is first formed, is just dissolved. Take care so that there is no excess of ammonia. Add 5 mL of 3% sodium hydroxide solution. Redissolve the precipitate by adding strong or concentrated ammonia, drop by drop, until the solution retains a trace opalescence. Make up the solution to 50 mL by adding distilled water.
- Acidified potassium permanganate
  - 0.5% potassium permanganate: 95 mL
  - 3% sulfuric acid: 5 mL.

Staining Method

1. Bring the dewaxed/deparaffinized sections to water.
2. Oxidize in acidified potassium permanganate for 1–5 minutes.
3. Wash in water.
4. Bleech in 1% oxalic acid for 3–5 minutes.
5. Rinse in distilled water.
6. Wash in tap water, and then in 2–3 changes of distilled water.
7. Mordant in 2.5% iron alum for 10 minutes to 2 hours (average 15 minutes).
8. Wash well in several changes of distilled water.
9. Place in silver solution in a Coplin jar for 1–2 minutes.
10. Rinse in several changes of distilled water.
11. Reduce in 10% aqueous formalin solution for 2 minutes.
12. Rinse in tap water, then in distilled water.
13. Treat with 5% sodium thiosulfate solution for 3–5 minutes.
14. Rinse in tap water.
15. Tone in 0.2% gold chloride for 5–15 minutes.
16. Rinse in distilled water.
17. Counterstain as desired (eosin or van Gieson).
18. Dehydrate through graded alcohol.
19. Clear in xylene and mount in DPX.

Results

- Reticulin fibers: Black
- Nuclei: Unstained or black
- Other elements: According to counterstain.

Notes:

- Silver solution should not be poured over the slide; it will cause precipitation on the slide. Use silver solution in a Coplin jar, precipitate will settle down in the bottom, not over the slide.

- For nuclear staining, iron alum solution should be used for more than 10 minutes, lesser time (<5 minutes) will give faint coloration of nuclei.

Phosphotungstic Acid Hematoxylin (PTAH)

Composition of Staining Solution

- Hematin: 1 g
- Phosphotungstic acid: 20 g
- Distilled water: 1000 mL.

Preparation: Dissolve the hematin in distilled water in a container using mild heat. In another container, dissolve phosphotungstic acid in distilled water using mild heat. Cool both the containers containing solutions. Now mix the two solutions when they are cool. Make volume up to 1000 mL by adding distilled water.

Ripening can be done by two ways

- Exposing to light and warmth for 6–8 weeks
- For immediate use, add 0.177 g of potassium permanganate (chemical ripening).

Staining Method

1. Bring dewaxed sections to water.
2. Treat with 0.5% iodine in 80% alcohol or Lugol's iodine for 3 minutes.
3. Drain and rinse in water.
4. Transfer to 3% sodium thiosulfate and left for 3 minutes.
5. Rinse in distilled water.
6. Place in 0.25% aqueous potassium permanganate for 4–5 minutes.
7. Wash in water for 2–3 minutes, then rinse in distilled water.
8. Place in 5% oxalic acid for 10–15 minutes.
9. Rinse in distilled water.
10. Wash in water for 4–5 minutes, then rinse in distilled water.
11. Stain in PTAH staining solution for 12–20 hours.
12. Dehydrate in 95% alcohol first, then in absolute alcohol.
13. Clear in xylene.
14. Mount in DPX or Canada balsam.

Results

- Fibrin: Blue
- Cross striation of skeletal muscle: Blue
- Neuroglia, myoglia, fibroglia, centrioles, nuclei: Blue
- Reticulin, collagen and ground substance: Yellow to brick red.

TAKE HOME MESSAGE

- In van Gieson stain, elastic fibers, reticular fibers red blood cells and muscle appear yellow whereas collagen becomes red. Trichrome method provides additional discrimination of tissue component. In the Masson trichrome method; muscles, fibrin and RBC are red whereas collagen and reticulin fibers are blue (aniline blue) or green (light green). In the Mallory trichrome technique, muscle and fibrin become red, whereas collagen and reticulin are stained blue.
- Reticulin fibers mainly consist of type III collagen in a glycoprotein complex. It can be stained by several techniques but Gordon-Sweet technique is most sensitive and most widely used stain for reticulin fibers. In this method, hydroxyl groups of adjacent hexose sugars are oxidized to aldehydes by potassium permanganate. These newly formed aldehydes then reduce silver diamine ion to metallic silver. This reaction can be further modified by use of silver chloride as a toner.
- Basement membrane can be stained by PAS technique. Basement membrane becomes PAS positive as the lamina rara zone is composed of complex carbohydrates, which are PAS positive. Thin basement membrane of normal glomeruli can be well visualized by the hexamine silver method (the Jone's technique). The collagenous component of basement membrane can be demonstrated by trichrome stains.
- Elastic tissues consist of elastin and glycoprotein. Both van der Waals forces and hydrogen bonding are responsible for staining of elastic tissue by different stains/dyes. In the Verhoeff technique, elastic fibers are stained black due to formation of metallic (iron)–dye (hematin)–lake. Weigert's resorcin fuchsin is also used as a elastic fiber stain (elastic fibers become blue to black). In aldehyde fuchsin, elastin fibers are stained purple and it becomes dark brown in Orcein stain.
- Fibrin stains positively with Mallory's PTAH and exhibits a positive reaction with DMAB due to high content of tryptophan. Fibrinoid material is variably metachromatic with toluidine blue. In PTAH, fibrin is uniformly blue stained, on the contrary the fibrinoid material stains orange-yellow to blue.

CHAPTER 10

Pigments and Minerals

INTRODUCTION

Pigments are colored substances, some of which are normal constituents of cells (like melanin), while others are abnormal or pathological and accumulate in cells only under special circumstances.

Pigments can be defined in biology as substances occurring in living matter which absorb visible light. All pigments absorb electromagnetic energy within a narrow spectrum (approximately 400–800 nm).

The pigments encountered in normal or pathological conditions may be classified as (Table 1):

- **Endogenous pigments:**
  - Hematogenous or blood-derived pigments: Hemoglobin, hemosiderin, bile pigments, porphyrins.
  - Nonhematogenous pigments: Melanin, lipofuscins, ceroid type lipofuscins, Dubin-Johnson pigments, pseudomelanosis (melanosis coli), Hamazaki-Wesenberg bodies.
  - Endogenous minerals: Iron, calcium, copper, uric acid and urates.
- **Exogenous pigments and minerals:** Carbon, silica, asbestos, lead, silver and tattoo pigments.
- **Artifact and artefactual pigments:** Formalin, mercury, chromic oxide, malarial and schistosome.

HEMOGLOBIN

Hemoglobin is a conjugated protein, which is composed of red pigmented **heme component** and a colorless protein **component globin**. Four molecules of heme are attached to every globin molecule. Hemoglobin transports oxygen and carbon dioxide within the bloodstream.

Pathologically, hemoglobin is seen in kidney diseases/glomerulonephritis, as renal casts/RBC casts. They appear as granules or yellow or yellow-brown within the casts.

Stains

- Peroxide technique like benzidine-nitroprusside method.
- Amido black technique.
- Tinctorial method.
- Kiton-red-almond green technique.

HEMOSIDERIN

It is a hemoglobin-derived golden-yellow to brown, granular or crystalline pigment. Hemosiderin is a breakdown product of hemoglobin which is composed of ferric iron and protein. When there is a local or systemic excess of iron, ferritin forms hemosiderin granules. Hemosiderin pigment represents aggregates of ferritin micelles.

Small amounts of hemosiderin can be seen normally in mononuclear phagocytes/histiocytes of bone marrow, liver and spleen. Local excess of iron leading to hemosiderin deposition is seen in hemorrhage in tissues, systemic overload of iron causing hemosiderin deposition is seen in a disease called hemosiderosis.

Stains

- Perls' Prussian blue reaction.
- Schmeltzer's method for ferrous and ferric iron.
- Hukill and Putt's method for ferrous and ferric iron.

Table 1: Name of different pigments in histologic sections and their staining properties

Name of pigment	*Sites*		*Perl's Prussian blue*	*Schmorl's reaction*	*Bleaching by ammoniacal silver*	*Bleaching by other methods*	*Other important staining methods or tests*
	Normal	*Pathological*					
1. Endogenous							
a. Hematogenous							
i. Hb	RBC	Renal cast or RBC cast	–	–	–	–	Patent blue method, Tinctorial method
ii. Hemosiderin	Phagocytes (small amount)	Hemorrhage in tissues	+	–	–	–	Hukill and Putt's method
iii. Bile pigment (Hematoidin)	Liver	Bile duct obstruction, HCC	–	–	–	–	Modified Fouchet's technique, Gmelin technique
b. Nonhematogenous							
i. Melanin	Skin, hair, eyes	Nevus, melanoma	–	+	+	+	–
ii. Lipofuscin	Adrenals	Heart, liver, testes, ganglion	–	+	+	+	Long Ziehl-Neelsen technique, Sudan black-B, PAS
iii. Argentaffin	Stomach, Intestine, Appendix	Neuroendocrine/ carcinoid tumor	–	+	+	–	–
iv. Chromaffin	Adrenal medulla	Pheochromocytoma	–	+	+	+	Toluidine blue, Giemsa
2. Exogenous							
i. Carbon	–	Lungs and associated LN	–	–	–	–	Insoluble in conc. H_2SO_4, not bleached by Mayer's chlorine
ii. Silica	–	Lungs and associated LN	–	–	–	–	Anisotropic (birefringent and resistant to micro-incineration)
iii. Asbestos	–	Lungs and associated LN	+	–	–	–	–
iv. Silver	–	Subcutis, nasopharynx	–	–	–	+	Okamoto and Utamura method, blackened by ammonium sulfide
v. Tattoo pigment	–	Skin, LN	–	–	–	–	–
3. Artifact							
i. Formalin		Tissue containing blood					
ii. Mercury	All tissues		–	–	–	–	–
iii. Malarial pigment (Hematozoin)		Bone marrow, liver, spleen, LN and brain	–	–	–	–	Treatment with saturated alcoholic picric acid will remove the pigment

Abbreviations: RBC, red blood cell; HCC, hepatocellular carcinoma; LN, Lymph node; PAS, periodic acid-Schiff.

BILE PIGMENTS

Bile pigments are a group and represent conjugated and unconjugated bilirubin, biliverdin and hematoidin. Bile pigments are formed normally by the breakdown of red blood cells at the end of their lives (after 120 days) in the liver. Pathologically, excess of bile pigments are seen in bile duct obstruction, rare congenital enzyme disorders, liver cell death and regeneration and hepatocellular carcinoma.

Stains

- Modified Fouchet technique.
- Gmelin technique.

PORPHYRIN PIGMENTS

Porphyrins are the precursors of the heme portion of hemoglobin. It is seen in disorders like porphyrias and protoporphyrias. In hematoxylin and essin (H & E) section, they appear as dense dark brown pigment. In frozen section they exhibit brilliant red fluorescence.

MELANIN PIGMENTS

Melanin is derived from Greek (*melas* mean black). It is an endogenous, nonhemoglobin derived brown-black pigment. It is normally present in skin, eye and hair. Pathologically, it can be seen in tumor forming excess melanin pigments like nevus and malignant melanoma.

Stains

- Masson-Fontana silver technique.
- Schmorl's reaction.

Bleaching of melanin pigments can be done by 20 volume hydrogen peroxide or by Mayer's technique, which is described below:

- At the bottom of Coplin jar, place a thin layer of potassium chlorate. Then fill the Coplin jar with 70% alcohol.
- Wash the slides in water, again place the slides in the jar.
- Now, add 1 mL of concentrated hydrochloric acid to the bottom of the jar.

This will produce nascent chloride by chemical reactions and this chlorine will bleach melanin within few hours. If there is excess melanin, add more hydrochloric acid.

LIPOFUSCINS

It is an insoluble pigment, also known as lipochrome or wear-and-tear pigment. It is derived from lipid peroxidation and is composed of polymers of lipids and phospholipids in complex with protein. The term comes from Latin word *fuscus* meaning brown. In H and E stained tissue section, it appear as yellow-brown, finely granular, cytoplasmic often perinuclear pigment. This pigment is seen in the elderly or aging patients in liver and heart and also known as 'brown atrophy pigment'. It may be seen in cancer cachexia and severe malnutrition.

Stains

- Schmorl reaction.
- Periodic acid-Schiff (PAS) technique.
- Sudan black B.
- Long Ziehl-Neelsen method (prolonged carbol-fuchsin method).

DUBIN-JOHNSON PIGMENTS

This pigment is seen the centrilobular hepatocytes in Dubin-Johnson syndrome, which is caused by a defect in hepatocellular excretion of bilirubin glucuronides across the canalicular membrane. It is characterized by conjugated hyperbilirubinemia. This pigment appears as a brownish-black, granular, intracellular pigment (located in the lysosomes).

PSEUDOMELANOSIS (MELANOSIS COLI)

The use of purgatives unscrupulously may result in melanosis coli or pseudomelanosis. In histologic sections, there are mucosal histiocytes which contain granular black or brown pigment. Initially, only histiocytes beneath the surface epithelium are affected. Later on entire mucosa and even submucosa and mesenteric lymph nodes are affected. In severe cases, the colonic mucosa including that of appendix, may be uniformly black. This pigment has some features of melanin as it takes up silver stains and can be bleached by hydrogen peroxide. But unlike melanocytic tumors, they are HMB45 and Melan A/Mart-1 negative.

Stain

Prussian blue.

HAMAZAKI-WESENBERG BODIES

These appear as small, yellow-brown, spindle-shaped structures which are found in the sinuses of lymph nodes as cytoplasmic inclusions or singly (lying free). These bodies were first described in lymph nodes of sarcoidosis patients. It may also be found in melanosis coli and other conditions. Histochemically, they resemble lipofuscin but ultra-structurally they are giant lysosomal residual bodies.

IRON

Metallic iron deposits or iron ore pigments may be seen in the lungs as occupational health hazards (e.g. miners). This pigment may be black, blue, red or yellow based on their composition. Most of the deposits of iron in tissue are ferric salt. Rarely, it may be found as ferrous salt.

Stains

- Perls' Prussian blue stain for ferric iron.
- Turnbull's blue reaction for ferrous iron.
- Hukill and Putt, Schmeltzer's method for both ferrous and ferric iron.

CALCIUM

Pathologic calcification is the abnormal deposition of calcium salts, together with smaller amounts of other mineral salts like iron, magnesium, etc. There are two forms—dystrophic calcification and metastatic calcification. Dystrophic calcification occurs in dying tissues or in areas of necrosis, atheroma of advance atherosclerosis, aging or damaged heart valves, tuberculous lymph nodes, etc. Here, serum level of calcium is normal. In contrast, metastatic calcification occurs in otherwise normal tissues and result from hypercalcemia secondary to calcium metabolism disturbances. Examples are hyperparathyroidism, multiple myeloma, leukemia, breast cancer, Paget's disease, Vitamin D toxicity, renal failure, etc. Calcium deposit in these conditions are as carbonates and phosphates.

Stains

- Von Kossa.
- Alizarin red S (thought to be specific).

COPPER

Copper accumulation may be seen in Wilson's disease, primary biliary cirrhosis and other hepatic disorders.

Stains

- Rubeanic acid method.
- Modified rhodamine technique.
- Mallory and Parker's hematoxylin method (fresh alkaline hematoxylin method).

LEAD

Lead poisoning may occur from contaminated food, water and air. It is also found from environmental lead like mining, batteries and spray painting.

Stains

Mallory and Parker's hematoxylin method.

URIC ACID AND URATES

The high level of uric acid in blood occurs in gout. Deposition of monosodium urates occurs in subcutaneous tissues as nodules (tophi), synovium, joints and kidney. Pseudogout or chondrocalcinosis mimics gout, but in these cases there is deposition of calcium pyrophosphates.

Stains

Lithium carbonate extraction—hexamine silver technique.

CARBON

Carbon occur as black particles and is found in lungs and associated lymph glands. It may be rarely found in liver and skin. Black pigmentation of the lung (anthracosis) is seen as a result of heavy deposition of carbon in coal workers and some city dwellers. It is also seen in tobacco smokers who inhale particulate carbon.

Carbon is distinguished from formalin pigment, malarial pigment and melanin by its insolubility in concentrated sulfuric acid (which dissolve other pigments) and the inability of bleaching by Mayer's chlorine method.

SILICA

Silica is found in lungs and associated lymph glands of stone grinders (silicosis), coal miners. Silica is seen as greyish crystal and may be demonstrated by its resistance to micro-incineration. Silica is anisotropic (doubly refractile).

ASBESTOS

It is a special form of silica and is found in the lung and associated glands of asbestos workers. 'Asbestos bodies' may be found as beaded particles, which are Prussian blue positive.

SILVER

It is rarely seen in the skin of silver nitrate workers, as occupational hazard known as argyrea. It may also be found in kidney or other parts of body due to medical treatment and other investigations. In H and E sections, silver appears as fine dark brown granules located in basement membrane and sweat glands. It may be blackened by ammonium sulfide.

Stains

Okamoto and Utamura method.

TATTOO PIGMENT

Tattoo pigments are usually confined to the skin which has been tattooed and any adjacent lymph nodes. Tattoo pigments may be of various types of colored pigments.

FORMALIN PIGMENTS

This pigment is seen as brown or brownish-black precipitates/deposits in the tissues. It may be seen if the tissues are fixed for a prolonged period in acidic formalin or tissues taken out sometime after death. These deposits are commonly seen in blood rich tissues such as spleen, large blood vessels or hemorrhagic lesions. It appear as microsatellite deposit, which is birefringent or anisotropic. Use of buffered neutral formalin will prevent this.

Removal of Formalin Pigment

- Treating unstained tissue sections with saturated alcoholic picric acid or picric alcohol.
- 1% alcohol solution of sodium or potassium hydroxide.

MERCURY PIGMENTS

This pigment may be seen in tissues, which are fixed in mercury based fixatives like Zenker's or Helly's fluid. Mercury pigment appear as brownish-black extracellular crystals. Most of the time, they are monorefringent, though they may be birefringent occasionally.

Removal of Mercury Pigment

- Treating the sections with iodine solution like Lugol's iodine, then bleaching with weak sodium-thiosulfate or hyposolution.
- Incorporating iodine in the dilute alcohols used during dehydration stage.

CHROMIC OXIDE

Very rarely seen and appears as fine yellow-brown particulate deposits in tissues.

Removal of Chromic Oxide

Treatment with 1% acid alcohol.

MALARIAL PIGMENT (HEMOZOIN PIGMENT)

This pigment may be seen in persons suffering from malaria. Common locations are brain capillaries (falciparum malaria), bone marrow, liver, spleen and lymph nodes. This pigment is morphologically similar to formalin pigment and is anisotropic or birefringent. But unlike formalin pigment, it is not seen in whole of the tissue section and is found within phagocytic cells.

Removal of Malarial Pigment

Treatment of sections with saturated alcoholic picric acid for 12–24 hours.

SCHISTOSOME PIGMENT

It is occasionally seen in tissue of persons suffering from schistosomiasis. This pigment has the property of both formalin and malarial pigment.

PERL'S PRUSSIAN BLUE REACTION (FOR FERRIC IRON)

Fixative

Alcohol fixative or buffered formol saline. Avoid acid fixatives. Chromates interfere with preservation of iron.

Sections

Paraffin, frozen or celloidin sections.

Principle of the Technique

Acid ferrocyanide solution reacts with tissue iron and unmask the ferric iron as ferric hydroxide [Fe $(OH)_3$] form with the help with hydrochloric acid. Diluted potassium ferrocyanide then reacts with ferric iron and produces an insoluble blue compound, composed of ferric ferrocyanide (Prussian blue).

Composition of Staining Solution

- 2% aqueous potassium ferrocyanide: 10 mL.
- 2% hydrochloric acid: 10 mL.

Prepare freshly just before use by mixing those two things (equal volume).

Positive Control Section

Preferably use a positive control section. Postmortem lung tissue would be ideal as it contains many iron containing macrophages (hemosiderin laden macrophages).

Staining Method

1. Bring test and control sections to distilled water.

2. Treat the sections with staining solution (acid ferrocyanide) for 10–30 minutes. If there is doubt, carry out the reaction at 60°C, which will hasten the reaction but it is not necessary always.
3. Wash thoroughly in several changes of distilled water.
4. Counterstain the nuclei lightly with 1% neutral red or safranin for 10–15 seconds.
5. Wash rapidly in distilled water.
6. Dehydrate in graded alcohol and clear in xylene.
7. Mount in Canada balsam, DPX or Euparal.

Results

- Ferric iron: Blue.
- Nuclei: Red.

Notes:
- Timing for counterstain should be short (10–15 seconds). Otherwise faint positive reaction will be masked by overstaining.
- Staining time will vary depending upon the amount of ferric iron present in tissue sections.
- Euparal is more lasting mountant than DPX or Canada balsam.
- Sometimes in positive reaction, the deposit of ferric ferrocyanide may be dissolved by the hydrochloric acid. To overcome this problem, use lighter 5% acetic acid instead of 2% hydrochloric acid in staining solution.

TIRMANN-SCHMELZER'S TURNBULL BLUE TECHNIQUE (FOR FERROUS AND FERRIC IRON)

Staining Method

1. Bring sections to distilled water (test and control sections).
2. Treat the sections with a diluted solution of yellow ammonium sulfide for 1-3 hours.
3. Rinse in distilled water.
4. Treat with a freshly prepared solution of equal parts of 20% potassium ferrocyanide and 1% hydrochloric acid. Filter it 10 minutes before use.
5. Wash thoroughly in several changes of distilled water.
6. Counterstain-nuclei lightly with 1% neutral red or safranin for 10–15 seconds.
7. Rinse in distilled water.
8. Dehydrate, clear and mount.

Results

- Ferrous salt and converted ferric to ferrous salt by ammonium sulfide: Deep blue.
- Nuclei: Red.

Note:
- In stage 2, ferric salts are converted to ferrous salts by ammonium sulfide and ferric salts are also stained. To differentiate between ferrous and ferric salts, two parallel sections are taken and stage 2 is performed on one of them (this will only demonstrate ferrous salt).
- Tirmann in 1898 first demonstrated ferrous iron by this method.

HUKILL AND PUTT'S METHOD (FOR FERROUS AND FERRIC IRON)

Composition of Staining Solution

- Bathophenanthroline (4, 7-diphenyl-1, 10-phenanthroline)—100 mg
- 3% aqueous acetic acid: 100 mL.
- Mix them and place them in an oven at 60°C for 24 hours. Cool it at room temperature and filter it. Add 0.5% thioglycolic acid just before use (0.5 mL in 100 mL solution).

Staining Method

1. Bring sections to distilled water.
2. Stain the slides with staining solution for 2–3 hours at room temperature.
3. Rinse in distilled water.
4. Counterstain in 0.5% methylene blue for 2–3 minutes.
5. Rinse in distilled water.
6. Drain the sections and dry them in incubator at 37°C.
7. Mount them (preferably synthetic resin).

Results

- Ferrous iron: Red.
- Nuclei: Blue.

****Notes:***
- In this staining method, there is no dehydration by graded alcohol before mounting as it will remove the red color formed by the ferrous iron.
- The staining solution is stable for 3–4 weeks. Thioglycolic acid is added just before use as it rapidly undergoes oxidation.

MODIFIED FOUCHET TECHNIQUE FOR BILE PIGMENTS

Composition of Staining Solution

Fouchet's solution: Dissolve 25 g of trichloroacetic acid in 100 mL of distilled water (25% acid solution). Dissolve 1 g of ferric chloride in 10 mL of distilled water (10% solution) in a separate container. Mix them and store in a dark bottle.

Staining Method

1. Bring sections to distilled water.
2. Treat them with Fouchet's solution.
3. Wash in running tap water for 8–10 minutes.
4. Rinse in distilled water.
5. Counterstain in van Gieson solution (Refer to page 59) for 2 minutes (this step is optional but accentuate the staining color).
6. Rinse in distilled water.
7. Dehydrate, clear and mount in resins.

Result

- Bile pigments: Emerald green to blue green.
- Collagen: Red.
- Muscle: Yellow.

****Note:*** It will stain only liver bile pigments. Other bile (like gallbladder bile or in RA sinus) will not be demonstrated.

GEMELIN TECHNIQUE FOR BILE PIGMENTS

Staining Method

1. Bring paraffin or frozen sections to water.
2. Mount in water by putting coverslip and avoiding air bubbles.
3. Place the water mounted section on microscope stage and focus it.
4. Now with the help of a pipette, place 2–3 drops of 50% nitric acid at one end of the cover slip. On the opposite end of the coverslip, apply a small piece of filter paper to draw the nitric acid over the section.
5. Remove excess solution and watch for unidentified pigments which are changing colors.

Results

- Bilirubin and hematoidin (bile pigment) if present will change color.
- First Yellow→Green→Blue→Purple→Purple-red→Red.

Notes:

- It will stain all the bile (liver, gallbladder, hematoidin) unlike the Fouchet technique, which stains bilirubin/ bile of liver origin only.
- The technique is not very reliable and false-negative cases are common. So, before issuing a negative result, perform the test at least three times.
- This stain is impermanent, so cannot be stored.
- Sulfuric acid can be used as an alternate to nitric acid.
- Lillie and Pizzolato in 1967, used bromine in carbon tetrachloride as an oxidant which gave good result.

MASSON-FONTANA METHOD FOR MELANIN

Fixatives

Formalin or formol-saline is probably best. Zenker-formol also gives good results. But mercuric chloride or chromate fixative should not be used.

Sections

Paraffin, frozen or celloidin.

Composition of Staining Solution

Preparation of silver solution (after Fontana): To 10 mL of 10% aqueous silver nitrate add strong ammonia drop by drop in glass flask until the precipitate which first formed disappears. The end point of titration is seen when a faint opalescence is found, then add equal amount, i.e. 10 mL of distilled water to this solution. Filter it and store in a dark bottle in a refrigerator. It can be used for 4–6 weeks.

Staining Method

1. Bring test and control sections to water.
   For control section, histologic section of epidermis of skin of black people, choroidal tissue of eye or known case of nevus or melanoma (melanotic) should be used.
2. Treat the sections with ammoniacal silver solution in a Coplin jar at room temperature overnight or at 56°C for 30–40 minutes. Remember, the Coplin jar should be covered with aluminum foil so that light should not pass through.
3. Wash the sections in distilled water (several changes).
4. Transfer to 3% sodium thiosulfate for 3 minutes.
5. Wash well in running tap water for 2–3 minutes.
6. Counterstain in 0.5% aqueous neutral red for 5 minutes or in 1% safranine for one minute.
7. Wash in tap water for 30–40 seconds.
8. Dehydrate, clear and mount in resin or Canada balsam of DPX.

Results

- Melanin pigments: Black.
- Argentaffin and chromaffin granules: Black.
- Nuclei: Red.
- Other cytoplasmic constituents: Shades of red and pink.

Notes:

- Titration of silver nitrate with ammonia is very crucial. The end point should be properly judged and best seen by using reflected light against a black background. If there is addition of excess ammonia, then add few more drops of 10% silver nitrate to restore the desired opalescence.
- Always use clear glassware, otherwise silver solution will react with the contaminant or other residues.
- Prolong reaction at 56°C may form fine deposit. So, try to maintain the reaction time as advocated.
- The above technique may be substituted by using hexamine silver solution instead of Fontana silver solution, known as Gomori-Burtner methenamine (hexamine) silver solution. Here, stock solution is prepared by adding 5 mL of 5% silver nitrate to 100 mL of 3% methenamine (hexamine) in distilled water. A precipitate forms which again redissolved immediately. Keep this stock solution in a cool dark place for many weeks (8–12 weeks). For working solution, add 4 mL of Holmes' boric acid-borate buffer, pH 7.8–15 mL of stock solution. [Holmes' buffer, pH 7.8-: M/5 boric acid 80 mL + M/20 borax 20 mL = 100 mL].

SCHMORL'S REACTION FOR MELANIN

Composition of Staining Solution

- Freshly prepared 1% aqueous potassium ferrocyanide: 4 mL.
- Freshly prepared 1% aqueous ferric chloride: 30 mL.
- Distilled water: 6 mL.
- Mix well, use this solution within 15–30 minutes.

Staining Method

1. Take solution to distilled water.
2. Treat them with staining solution of ferric-ferrocyanide (freshly prepared) for 10–20 minutes.
3. Wash in running tap water for 5–10 minutes.
4. Counterstain nuclei lightly with 1% neutral red or Safranine for 15–30 seconds.
5. Dehydrate, clear and mount in Canada balsam or DPX.

Results

- Melanin: Dark blue.
- Lipofuscin, Argentaffin cells, bile, thyroid colloid: Dark blue.
- Chromaffin cells (after dichromate fixation): Greenish blue.
- Nuclei: Red.

Notes:

- Sections may be differentiated with 1% potassium hydroxide in 50% alcohol after step 2. Reaction of differentiation will be stopped by rinsing in 70% alcohol and distilled water. Next steps (3, 4 and 5) will proceed as usual.
- This staining method is preferred by many over the conventional method of Masson-Fontana, as it is easier to perform and background staining is minimal.
- Staining reaction will vary depending upon the substance to be stained. As for example, melanin reacts quickly compared to lipofuscin. So, for demonstration of lipofuscin will take longer staining time than melanin.

LONG ZIEHL-NEELSEN METHOD FOR LIPOFUSCIN

Staining Method

1. Bring sections to water.
2. Keep the slides in a Coplin jar containing filtered carbol fuschin in a water bath, at 60°C for 3–4 hours.
3. Wash well in running tap water.
4. Counterstain nuclei with 0.5% aqueous methylene blue or Carazzi's hematoxylin for 1–2 minutes.
5. Dehydrate, clear and mount.

Results

- Lipofuscin: Megenta.
- Nuclei: Blue.
- Background: Pale blue to pale magenta.

VON KOSSA'S TECHNIQUE FOR CALCIUM

Staining Method

1. Bring sections to water.
2. Keep sections in citrate buffer, pH 4.5 for 20–30 minutes.
3. Wash the slides well in distilled water.
4. Put the slides in open bright sunlight or in ultraviolet light for 10–20 minutes. Alternatively, a 60 Watt electric bulb may be used for 40–60 minutes at a distance of 4–5 inches.
5. Wash in distilled water (several changes).
6. Treat with 5% sodium thiosulfate for 3–4 minutes.
7. Counterstain with 1% neutral red (2–3 minutes) or safranine (1 minute).
8. Dehydrate, clear and mount in Canada balsum or DPX.

Result

Calcium deposits: Black.

ALIZARIN RED S METHOD FOR CALCIUM

Staining Solution

About 2% aqueous alizarin red S titrated with 10% ammonium hydroxide to make pH 4.2.

Staining Method

1. Bring sections to distilled water.
2. Put the slides in a Coplin jar containg staining solution of Alizarin red S for 2–5 minutes. Check the slides in a microscope for required staining time.
3. Blot the slides and rinse them in acetone for 20–30 seconds.
4. Treat the slides with a mixture of equal volume of xylene and acetone for 15–30 seconds.
5. Rinse in xylene and mount it (resin, Canada balsum or DPX).

Result

Calcium deposit: Orange-red.

Notes:
- Calcium deposit if present will be birefringent in this technique.
- Staining time will vary depending on amount of calcium. More amount of calcium in sections will take more staining time.
- End point of staining is checked microscopically, which is denoted by orange red coloration of calcium deposits. Do not put the slide in staining solution, more than required time, otherwise the staining color will diffuse to rest part of the tissue section.

MODIFIED RHODAMINE TECHNIQUE FOR COPPER

Composition of Staining Solution

- **Rhodamine stock solution:**
  - 5-p-Dimethylaminobenzylidene rhodanine (DMABR): 0.1 g
  - Absolute ethanol: 50 mL

  Mix well and store this stock solution. For working solution, take 1 mL of stock solution and add 16 mL of distilled water.
- **Borax solution**:
  - Disodium tetraborate: 0.1 g
  - Distilled water: 20 mL.

Staining Method

1. Bring the sections to water.
2. Stain the slides with rhodamine working solution for 3 hrs at 56°C with the help of an incubator.
3. Rinse in distilled water (several changes).
4. Stain the nuclei in Carazzi's hematoxylin for 3–4 minutes.
5. Rinse in distilled water.
6. Treat them with borax solution immediately for 10–15 seconds.
7. Dehydrate, clear and mount.

Results

- Copper and copper associated protein: Red/orange-red.
- Nuclei: Blue.
- Bile: Green.

MALLORY AND PARKER'S METHOD FOR LEAD AND COPPER

Composition of Staining Solution

Dissolve 5 mg of hematoxylin with few drops of 95% of alcohol. To it, dissolve 5 mL of filtered 2% potassium hydrogen phosphate.

Staining Method

1. Bring histologic sections to water.
2. Stain in freshly prepared staining solution of hematoxylin (mentioned above) for 2–3 hours at 56°C.
3. Wash in running tap water for 10 minutes.
4. Dehydrate in 95% alcohol.
5. Clear in terpineol and mount in terpineol-balsam.

Results

- Lead: Dark gray-blue.
- Copper: Blue.
- Nuclei: Blue.
- Formalin fixed hemosiderin: Brown.
- Alcohol fixed hemosiderin: Black.

CHAPTER 11

Bone and Decalcification

INTRODUCTION

Bone is a specialized connective tissue. In adult human two types of bone are seen microscopically.

- **Cortical or compact bone:** It is hard, solid and very strong bone. It forms long bones like femur, humerous, tibia, etc. and external surface of flat bones like skull, ribs, etc.
- **Trabecular or cancellous or spongy bone:** It is found in the epiphysis, diaphysis and marrow cavities of long bones. Also found in vertebrae and central portion of flat bones.

Constituents of bone: Bone is composed of cells and intercellular substance or matrix.

- **Bone cells**: Two types
  - Fixed cells or osteocytes.
  - Temporary or embryonic cells—osteoblasts and osteoclasts (giant cells).
- **Intercellular substance:** Two types viz. organic and inorganic.
  - Organic substance: Organic matrix or osteoid tissue composed of collagen fibers and cement substance.
    - Collagen fibers: It accounts for most of the organic controls.
    - Cement substance: Comprises of mucoprotein, glycoprotein, proteoglyans, mucopolysaccharides like chondroitin sulfuric acid.
  - Inorganic substance: Bone salts predominantly calcium hydroxyapatite crystals. Others are magnesium, phosphate, carbonate, chloride, fluoride and citrate.

In the bone the extracellular components or matrix are mineralized. This mineralized matrix gives strength and marked rigidity, at the same time provides some degree of elasticity. Rigidity is maintained by inorganic or mineral salt, which accounts for 2/3rd of bone by weight. These mineral salts make the bone radiopaque. Elasticity is maintained by organic materials, which accounts for 1/3rd of bone.

Organic extracellular matrixes of collagen fibers are different from other collagens in the body. Though it is mainly composed of type: I collagen but is has a property to become mineralized. This mineral is laid down in bands or lamellar pattern which is almost parallel to one another. This bone is now known as *lamellar bone.*

In certain pathologic conditions and in immature bone, there is absence of lamellar mineral or calcium salt deposition. The nonlamellar collagen fibers are coarse and the bone is known as *woven bone.*

Three types of cells are found in immature bone: Osteoblast, osteocytes and osteoclasts. Osteoblasts and osteocytes are derived from mesenchymal-type cells called osteoprogenitor cells. Osteoblasts synthesize and secrete organic component of the extracellular matrix of new bone, which is known as osteoid or osteoid tissue. This osteoid rapidly undergoes mineralization to form mineralized bone or lamellar bone. Active obteoblasts which are responsible for organic matrix synthesis usually are located on the surface of osteoid tissue. But when it is transformed into bone, osteoblasts become trapped within bone and now is known as osteocytes. These osteocytes are responsible for maintenance of the bone matrix. Osteoclasts are multinucleated gain calls which are responsible for bone resorption and bone remodeling.

Bone becomes brittle due to mineralization and is very difficult to cut into ordinary histologic sections. For routine histologic sections, minerals are removed by the process of decalcification first. For this, bones are put in acid solutions or other declicifiers prior to sectioning and staining.

By the above method, the cellular details and organic component of matrix are preserved but the stains are taken up less readily. Recently, use of acrylic as embedding bone with prior decalcification becomes popular in the study of the mineralization process and its disorders. In this method, diamond edges knives are used for section cutting.

BONE TECHNIQUES

There are many techniques to demonstrate bone and its constituents. They include:

- For decalicified bone: Paraffin, frozen, transmission electron microscopy (TEM).
- For mineralized bone: Paraffin, frozen, plastic, scanning and transmission electron microscopy.

The above mentioned sections may be used for microscopic, radiographic and morphometric studies. It may also be used for fluorescence microscopy and polarized microscopy.

SPECIMENS AND BIOPIES

Size of the bone specimen may vary. It may be as short as few millimetres as in needle biopsy or it may be very long as in amputation of whole lower limb or pelvis.

- For the diagnosis of bone tunors, infections, etc: These are treated like soft tissues. But minerals are removed before making paraffin sections.
- For diagnosis of metabolic bone diseases: For the diagnosis of metabolic bone diseases, the iliac crest is the site of choice for biopsy. Tissue is removed with a Jamshidi needle or with a large trepheine; making a core of bone measuring near about 7 × 20 mm. Preferably, a plastic embedding medium like methyl methacrylate (MMA) is used for this purpose.
- Amputated specimens: It is done in cases of tumors, long standing osteomyelitis, gangrene, etc. Most or all the skin is stripped off, muscular tissue is removed and the bone is placed under the saw or joint disarticulated below the bone lesion. The representative bony tissue containing the lesion is now put in a fixative. If the amputated limb or specimen should be attended later on, then it is kept in a mortuary refrigerator at 4°C (preferably with a fixative).
- Resection and replacement surgery bone specimens: Benign or low grade malignant bone tumors are treated as large biopsy specimens. In replacement surgeries like knee replacement, hip replacement or femoral head replacement, usually the whole, specimen is received. A wedge shaped sample is cut from the whole specimen, either prior to or after some fixation. A bone saw or heavy duty knife is good for this purpose. Then the cut wedge-shaped bone specimen is put into fixative for 24–48 hours. After that specimen is decalcified, processed and sectioned.

FIXATIVES FOR BONE SPECIMENS

Like other specimens, bone specimens also follow general rules for fixation. Complete fixation prevents the damaging effects of acid decalcification. As a routine fixative, formalin is suitable and 10% neutral buffered formalin (NBF) is preferred. For trephine/bone marrow biopsies, best fixative is Zenker or Zenker's formalin. For methyl methacrylate (MMA) embedding, fixative of choice is 10% NBF.

Large bone specimens should be bisected or reduced in size by sawing into multiple slabs. Then, immerse these pieces into fixative immediately, or within 48 hours after initial fixation. Once cut into small pieces, these should be immersed into fresh fixative.

Fixative	*Not suitable for*	*Reasons*
Alcohol based	Acid decalcification	Slow or prevents decalcification
Mercury based or chloroform	Radiography	Make bone radiopaque

Cook and Ezra Chon (1962) had shown that tissue damage during acid decalcification was approximately four times greater compared to unfixed bone tissue.

SAWS IN BONE CUTTING

For bone histology, proper sawing by a good saw is essential. Thin slices of bone are made using fine-toothed bone saw or hacksaw. Other than surgical saws, there are other saws like handyman's bench saws and hobby shop which cut through stones, plastic and some thin metals. These saws are used to cut cortical bone slowly with a maximum depth of 7.5 cm. Unlike other saws, water-cooled saws are capable of full-length cuts through long bones (femur, humerous, tibia) and they prevent heat damage to bone due to high-speed sawing.

Larger saw blades have 1.25 cm width with 6 tpi (teeth per inch) while smaller saws have 0.5 cm width with 12–16 tpi (teeth per inch). Soft tissues and fibrous tissue should be removed from the specimen before sawing. The first cut should be made through the mid-plane. Then, parallel cut sections are made which are 3–5 mm thick. The cut bone slabs should be cleaned to remove bone dust or debris. Now, these bone slabs are fixed for an additional 24–48 hours (especially if they are partially fixed or pinkish-red).

DECALCIFICATION

The presence of calcium salts and other minerals in bone and other calcified tissues prevents the preparation of good histologic sections by routine methods. Incomplete removal of these minerals results in ragged and torn sections and in damage to the cutting edge of the microtome knife.

Decalcification is a routine procedure which makes bone and calcified tissue compatible with the embedding media for cutting a microslide and the subsequent staining. The most ubiquitious media is paraffin wax. Decalcification adjusts the hard substance of bones to the softness of paraffin. Some media, like resins do not require decalcification at all. Bones are the main object of decalcification but other surgical specimens like calcified tumors, atheromatous plaques, calcified heart valves also require decalcification.

The technique of decalcification, may be divided into the following stages:

- Section of tissue and section cutting (sawing)
- Fixation
- Decalcification
- Neutralization of acid decalcifier
- Thorough washing

There are two formulas in grossing of bone and calcified surgical specimens.

- Fixation → cutting/sawing → decalcification → processing → sections.
- Cutting/sawing → fixation → decalcification → processing → sections.

The second formula is most widely accepted. Unless some safety issues and precautions, as in AIDS or TB; bone cutting in the fresh state is desirable as it assures better bone-soft tissue relationships. It also provides even fixation and decreases turnaround time (TAT). Through there are some exceptions, as in metallic prosthesis that is cemented in the extremity/long bones. In this case, the bone should be cut properly without decalcification after preliminary fixation. Grossing a long bone specimen with osteosarcoma after chemotherapy is another exception.

Classification of Decalcifying Agents

- Acid solutions:
  - Strong or inorganic acids: Nitric acid (HNO_3), hydrochloric acid (HCl), formalin-nitric acid, Perenyi's fluid.
  - Weak or organic acids, aqueous formic acid, formic acid-formalin, buffered formic acid, others like acetic acid and picric acid as components in Bouin's, Carnoy's or Zenker's fixatives.
- **Chelating agents**: Ethylenediaminetetraacetic acid (EDTA), formalin-EDTA.
- Ion-exchange resins
- Electrophoretic method or electrolytic ionization
- Microwave technique.

Decalcification is a chemical process. The goal is to extract calcium and other minerals. Calcium in bones and in pathologic calcification is in carbonate and phosphate salts together with small amounts of other minerals salts which are almost insoluble. Strong acids like 5–10% nitric acid or hydrochloric acid and weak acids like 5–10% formic acid (HCOOH) form soluble calcium salts in an ion-exchange chemical process that moves the calcium in tissues to the decalcifying solutions. The same final effect makes 14% EDTA (C_{10}, H_{12}, N_2O_8.2Na)-that sequesters metallic irons, including calcium in aqueous solutions as a chelating factor.

All these methods are greatly accelerated by application of heat and also by agitation. Decalcification if carried out at 56–60°C, causes swelling of tissues which is undesirable though the procedure (decalcification) is rapid. Even, a temperature of 37°C also has some disadvantages like swelling of tissues and impairment of subsequent staining. So, use of heat is not recommended.

An *ideal decalcifier* should have some properties like:

- Complete removal of calcium salts and other minerals
- Reasonable speed for decalcification
- Absence of damage to tissues
- Nonimpairment of subsequent staining methods.

Choice of Decalcifying Agent

A combination of formalin with a decalcifier (formic acid or EDTA) is not recommended. In combined formalin-declacifier solutions, both penetrate fast (Table 1). Formalin's penetration is 12 times faster than binding, which in turn is about four times faster than cross-linking

Table 1: Bone decalcification solutions for surgical specimens

Type of bone specimens	*Strong acid (nitric or hydro-chloric acid)*	*Strong acid + EDTA*	*Weak acid (formic acid)*	*Weak acid + EDTA*
Compact or cortical bone	++	+	–	–
Spongy or cancellous bone	+	++	+	+
Bone needle biopsy or trephine biopsy	–	+	++	++

'++', very good or optimal; '+', good or satisfactory; '–', negative which is needed for fixation. That means acid starts its work before formalin fixation is complete. Decalcification with fixation is used by some workers although it should be used with some reservations. But works of fixative and acid are not simultaneous as the penetration coefficient of acids is always higher than that of fixatives.

EDTA's ubiquity makes it popular as decalcifier and some regard it as 'magic' decalcifier. The optimal pH for EDTA is 7–7.4. It works too slowly under pH 5, owing to its insolubility and after pH 8, the solution becomes tissue unfriendly due to alkaline sensitive protein bonds. It does not work in formic acid with pH 3 as a decalcifier. When EDTA is used, the solution can percipitate loads of undistributed calcium at the bone surface. So, it needs more intensive agitation and vigorous post-decalcification rinsing.

In general, the above mentioned three groups of decalcification solutions completely satisfy the surgical pathology practice. When strong acids are used as decalcifier, the calcium is removed fastly and there is less damage to tissue artigenicity excepting immunoglobulin. So, strong acids may be used for immunohistochemisty (IHC) in bone histology. But EDTA is a better choice. If routine histologic staining is bad, then IHC staining will be impaired.

The EDTA decalcification, however completely satisfies the requirements for an in-situ hybridization (ISG) technique. The same can be said about IHC and enzyme histochemistry. EDTA takes longer time, but is the best decalcifier for these studies. EDTA does not have problems like pale nuclei with H and E staining, as 'overdecalcification' is practically impossible.

Strong Acids (Nitric or Hydrochloric Acid)

Aqueous nitric acid

Nitric acid: 5–10 mL
Distilled water: 100 mL

Von Ebner's fluid

(hydrochloric acid)
Concentrated HCl: 15 mL
Sodium chloride (NaCl): 175 g
Distilled water: 1000 mL

Formalin (formol) nitric acid

- Formalin: 10 mL
- Distilled water: 80 mL
- Nitric acid: 10 mL

Percenyi's fluid

- 10% nitric acid: 40 mL
- Absolute alcohol: 30 mL
- 0.5% chromic acid: 30 mL

Aqueous nitric acid: It may be used as 5–10% solutions. They decalcify rapidly and not recommended longer than 24–48 hours as it causes poor staining quality. Only fresh nitric acid should be used as old yellow nitric acid will make the tissues also yellow. Addition of 1% urea as preservative will stabilize the solution. Decalcification time is less, as for example cross-section of human rib of 5 mm thickness will need 12–24 hours for decalcification.

Formalin (formol) nitric acid: As formalin is added in this formula, formaldehyde partially inhibits the tendency of maceration caused by nitric acid. Cross-section of human rib (5 mm thickness) will need 1–2 days for decalcification.

Perenyi's fluid: It is an excellent decalcifying solution for deposits of calcium but slow for decalcifying dense bone. It does not make the tissue hard and cytological preservations are good. In some laboratories, it is the decalcifying fluid of choice. A cross section of 5 mm thick rib will require 2–4 days but femur of same thickness will require 10–14 days.

Von Ebner's fluid (HCl): This decalcifying agent is moderately popular in action. But results are not satisfactory. Cross-section of 5 mm thick rib will require 36–37 hours for decalcification.

WEAK ACIDS (FORMIC, PICRIC, ACETIC ACID)

Formic acid is mainly used as decalcifier in this group. Others like picric acid and acetic acids are components of Bouin's, Carnoy's or Zenker's fixative and is used rarely when there is extreme urgency.

The use of 5–10% aqueous formic acid is good as decalcifying agent. Addition of formalin or a buffer is also in practice. Formalin is added for simultaneous effect of fixation and decalcification. Buffers are added to counteract the injurious effects of formic acid. 5–10% formic acid has a reasonable speed and minimum damage to tissue occurs. The increase of the formic acid concentration up to 22% will speed up the decalcification but at the cost of tissue damage or cellular detail.

Decalcification with 5% formic acid solution will be completed in 1–10 days depending upon the thickness of the tissue and degree of calcification. A cross-section of 5 mm thick human rib will require 36–48 hours. Formic acid (5%) is not suitable for decalcification of dense cortical bone. For dense cortical bone 15% formic acid (aqueous) or 4% hydrochloric acid and 4% formic acid mixture may be tried. Formic acid (5%) may be used as an alternative decalcifier for IHC but it has some tissue damaging effects.

Aqueous formic acid:

- 90% formic acid: 5–10 mL
- Distilled water: 100 mL

Formic acid-formalin (Gooding and Stewart's fluid)

- 90% formic acid: 5–10 mL

- Formalin: 5 mL
- Distilled water: 100 mL

Buffered formic acid (Evans and Krajjan fluid)

- 90% formic acid: 35 mL
- 20% aqueous trisodium citrate: 65 mL
- This solution has a pH of 2.3 approximately.

CHELATING AGENTS (EDTA)

Ethylenediaminetetraacetic acid (EDTA) is most commonly employed chelating agent. Though it is a nominal acid, but unlike strong or weak acids, it does form soluble calcium salts in an ion-exchange methods. It binds calcium and magnesium ions of which calcium is more important. EDTA binds to the ionized calcium on the outer side of the apatite crystal. As this layer becomes depleted due to sequestration of metallic ions, it is reformed by the calcium ions of inner tissue. So, the crystal becomes smaller and smaller as the decalcification progressively proceeds.

EDTA will not bind to calcium ion at a pH <3 and the binding becomes optimal at pH 8 but this higher alkaline pH damages the alkali-sensitive protein linkages present in the tissues. The optimal pH for working EDTA solution is in the range of pH 7–7.4.

EDTA may be used as tetrasodium salt (14%) or as disodium salt (10%) of which the first one is more commonly used. By convention, the tetrasodium salt is alkaline. So, the optimal pH of 7–7.4 is made by using concentrated acid. EDTA takes more than 6–8 weeks to decalcify dense cortical bone whereas less than a week is needed for small bones/spicules.

Hillemann and Lee (10–11% EDTA, disodium salt)

- EDTA, disodium salt: 5.5 g
- Formalin: 10 mL
- Distilled water: 90 mL.

Neutral EDTA (14% EDTA, disodium salt)

- EDTA, disodium salt: 125 g
- Distilled water: 875 mL

Neutral solution is made (pH 7) by adding approximately 12.5 g of NaOH (sodium hydroxide) to the above solution. This addition of NaOH also makes the cloudy solution clear.

ION EXCHANGE RESINS

Iron-exchange resins in decalcifying fluids may be used to remove the calcium ions from decalcifying fluid. For this, the resin used is an ammonium form of sulfonated polystyrene resin. This resin is layered on the bottom of the container which contains decalcifying fluid. The depth of the resin should be such that it is ≥10% of the total volume of the decalcifying fluid. A depth of 1/2 inch or 1.25 cm is good. Volume of the decalcifying fluid in this method should be 20–30 times of the volume of surgical specimen.

After its use for decalcification, the resin may be regenerated by washing 2–3 times with diluted hydrochloric acid (N/10 HCl) followed by 3–4 washes in distilled water. By this regenerating technique, resins can be reused for a long time. The use of resin along with decalcifying agent make the decalcifying process more rapid as the rate of solubility of the calcium from the tissue increases. X-ray should be used to determine the end point of decalcification because chemical tests are unsuitable for this purpose.

These resins cannot be used with every decalcifying agents like mineral or strong acids. But formic acid containing fluids give good results.

ELECTROPHORETIC METHOD OF DECALCIFICATION

This method was based on attraction of calcium ions to negative electrode. The electrolyte used in this method is equal parts of 8% hydrochloric acid and 10% formic acid. Brass plate is used as negative electrode and platinum wire as positive electrode. This platinum wire which acts as positive electrode is wrapped around the bone/surgical specimen with the coils not more than 4 mm apart. A 6 volt DC is applied. Decalcification should be checked by X-ray every 2–3 hours duration. A human rib of 5 mm thickness will need 6–8 hours for decalcification.

Speed of decalcification may be increased by moving the positive and negative electrodes closer or by increasing the temperature of the electrolyte to 40–45°C. But this method has been abandoned by most histological laboratories nowadays.

Microwave (Micro-oven) Technique

The microwave oven is ubiquitous multipurpose instrument used in histology laboratory. It accelerates the decalcification process. The decalcification becomes rapid but problem may arise to monitor time and temperature. The problem may be solved by using different programs. Employment of this technique requires triage of calcified materials and specific grossing technique for uniformity of section. Tissue with high content of calcified material can benefit from micro oven assisted decalcification. For this two things are needed.

- Specialized bone grossing table
- Portable microwave decalcification instrument.

Treatment of Hard Tissues

- **Perenyi's fluid:** It can soften like chitinous material. Immersion of hard tissue like calcified arteries, calcified glands/lymph nodes, thyroid etc. for 12–24 hours will make it soften and sectioning becomes easier.
- **Lendrum's technique**: After washing out the fixative, tissue is immersed in a 4% aqueous solution of phenol for 1–3 days. This technique will make hard tissue softer.

Treatment Following Decalcification

- **Neutralization of acid decalcifier:** Overnight washing in tap water or other more alkaline solutions. Culling advocated the use of washing in two changes of 70% alcohol over 12–18 hours before processing into dehydration step. Blotting or quickly rinsing in tap water, remove excess acid solution from their surfaces.
- **For frozen sectioning**: Tissues decalcified for frozen sectioning, should be stored in formal-saline or thoroughly washed in water before making frozen sections.
- **Tissues decalcified in neutral EDTA solution:** The decalcified tissue should be placed in formal saline overnight. It cannot be placed in 70% alcohol directly as the remaining EDTA in tissues form precipitates. Also a crystalline crust may be formed on the surface of the embedding block.

Test for Completion of Decalcification

There are three methods to determine the end point of decalcification:

- **Chemical methods:** Calcium oxalate test
- **Radiography:** Most efficient test for detecting presence of calcium
- **Physical methods:** Needling or probing, cutting or trimming, palpation, bending, squeezing, bubble test (carbon dioxide bubbles).

Of the three methods mentioned above, first two methods are reliable.

Calcium Oxalate Test (Chemical Test)

Solution

- Concentrated ammonia
- Saturated aqueous ammonium oxalate.

Test Method

1. Add a small piece of litmus paper to approximately 5 mL of decalcifying fluid (which was used for decalcification).
2. Add strong or concentrated ammonia drop by drop until the solution becomes neutral to the litmus paper, shake well after addition of each drop of ammonia.
3. Next add 5 mL of saturated aqueous ammonia oxalate and shake well.
4. Wait for 30 minutes to look for any turbidity.

Results

If precipitate of calcium hydroxide is formed after addition of ammonia, then more amount of undecalcified calcium is present in the tissue. If precipitation of calcium oxalate is formed after addition of saturated aqueous ammonium oxalate (step 3), then less amount of calcium is present. Longer it takes to form precipitate; lesser the amount of calcium is present. If the decalcifying fluid remains clear for ≥30 minutes, it is presumed that the decalcification process is complete.

Disadvantage

The above test is not suitable for acid decalcifiers with higher concentration like >10% nitric acid or formic acid. Diluting the acid to make less concentrated, will reduce the sensitivity of the test.

Radiography

As already mentioned, this is the most effective method to determine the end point of decalcification. The most satisfactory method is undoubtedly taking X-ray of the tissue. But remember tissues which have been fixed in a mercury fixative (like mercuric chloride) cannot be tested by this method.

Carbon Dioxide Method

Carbon dioxide is produced when tissue is treated with acid decalcifier. Carbon dioxide bubbles remain on the surface of tissue and it denotes presence of underlying calcium carbonate. Upon shaking it will disperse and again reappear on the surface, so long the tissue calcium is present. This is unreliable method to detect end point decalcification.

SURFACE DECALCIFICATION

Surface decalcification is needed in case of paraffin blocks of tissues containing unsuspected mineral deposits or incompletely decalcified paraffin blocks which prevent the production of satisfactory histologic section.

After trimming, the paraffin block is placed in an acid solution such as 1% HCl or HNO_3 for 15–60 minutes, so that the acid bathes the cut surface. Then a few histologic sections may be taken.

FACTORS OF DECALCIFICATION PROCESS

Concentration and Volume of Decalcifying Agent

Generally, more concentrated solutions decalcify tissue more rapidly but they have more harmful effects. The addition of additives like buffers will protect the tissue from harmful effects but slow the decalcifying process. So, optimal concentration is required.

Usually a large volume of decalcifying fluid/agent is added in a ratio of 20:1 (fluid: tissue = 20:1). Also, renewal of the fluid during the decalcifying process is required. For strong acids, 2–3 changes in 24 hours, daily changes for weak acids and weekly changes for EDTA is recommended.

Agitation

It is presumed that mechanical agitation will hasten the exchange of fluids within as well as around tissues. Some authors recommend manual agitation once or twice a day.

Temperature

Increase in temperature will hasten the decalcification process. But there is a fear of destroying bony tissue, which becomes macerated at 60°C, when acid is used as decalcifying agent. On the other hand, lowering the temperature will decrease the rate of reaction. The optimum temperature should be determined by the concerned laboratory.

Other Factors

Age of the patient, size of specimen, type of bone, etc. are also act as factors. As for example, elderly persons, especially women have lower bone density with lesser amount of minerals/calcium, so it requires lesser time for decalcification. Mature cortical bone requires more time than immature developing cortical bone or cancellous/trabecular bone. Tissue with larger size will require more time for decalcification.

PLASTIC OR SYNTHETIC RESIN EMBEDDING

An embedding medium which commensurate the hardness of the bone is required for undisrupted sections of bone (undecalcified). Synthetic resins (like GMA, MMA) work well for both light microscopy and electron microscopy. Epoxy EM resins are suitable only for ultra-thin sectioning of tiny/small bone tissue pieces.

Acrylic resins like methacrylate are used as supporting medium for undecalcified bone. Some favor an n-butyl/ethyl methacrylate mixture, i.e. methyl methacrylate (MMA) for this. MMA mixed with dibutyl phthalate or polyethylene glycol is softer and more elastic than MMA.

METHYL METHACRYLATE EMBEDDING PROCEDURE

Regents

- Monomer: Methyl methacrylate
- Polymer: Poly (methyl methacrylate) of low molecular weight, natural beads
- Catalyst: Benzoyl peroxide (supplied as damp because this is potentially explosive)
- For washing: 5% NaOH (sodium hydroxide)
- For drying: CaCl2, 8–16 mesh (calcium chloride).

Preparation of Resins

- **Stock catalyzed monomer:** In a separating funnel, place measured volume of monomer (methyl methacrylate). Then add an equal volume of 5% NaOH. Shake well this mixture and allow them to separate. The methacrylate will form in the upper layer. Discard the lower layer. Repeat the procedure twice more (So, a total of three washings in 5% NaOH). Now, wash the newly formed resins in distilled water thrice. Add 1g of benzoyl to every 100 g of monomer (methyl methacrylate). Filter it through calcium chloride. Store this stock monomer in an airtight bottle at 0–4°C.
- **Monomer-polymer embedding medium**:
  Poly (methyl methacrylate): 20 g
  Stock catalyzed monomer: 50 mL
  Mix the above two regents in a container on rotating mixer at room temperature for 24 hours. Store in an airtight container for shorter duration at 0–4°C. Remember before making mixture both the stored reagents must come to room temperature. This step will form partially polymerized methacrylate.

Processing of Surgical Specimens/Bone

- Dehydrate the undecalcified bone/surgical specimen in ascending graded alcohol (70%, 90% and three changes of absolute alcohol), duration 24 hours in each alcohol.

Table 2: Advantages and disadvantages of different decalcifying agents

Sl. no.	*Decalcifying agent*	*Advantages*	*Disadvantages*
1.	Nitric acid (5 to 10%) (aqueous)	• Rapid decalcification • Gives better nuclear staining	• Damage to tissue occurs if left for prolonged time • Decalcification time should be monitored
2.	Formalin-nitric acid, 5–10%	• Rapid decalcification • For urgent biopsies • It is not very destructive like aqueous nitric acid • Prevents maceration effect of nitric acid	• Requires neutralization by 5% sodium sulfate • Nuclear staining is not very good
3.	Formic acid 5–10% aqueous	• Fixation and decalcification occur simultaneously • Recommended for small pieces of bony tissue and teeth • Good nuclear staining • Minimal tissue damage	• Decalcification process is slow and requires more time • Some tissue damage may occur if sued in high concentration (close to 25%)
4.	Chelating agent (EDTA), pH 7–7.4	• No tissue damage • End point is determined easily	• Slight tissue hardening • Very slow process (6–8 weeks)
5.	Iron exchange resins	• Rapid process • Small quantity is adequate • Can be regenerated after use. So can be reused	• Strong acids cannot be used along with it. Only formic acid can be used • End point can not be assessed by chemical tests. X-ray may be required to do so
6.	Electrophoretic method	Rapid decalcification	• Not routinely used as it is cumbersome process and costly • Heat produced during the process, caused tissue damage

- Infiltrate with a mixture of equal parts of absolute alcohol and unwashed methyl methacrylate for 24 hours.
- Then three changes with unwashed methyl methacrylate, each of 24 hours duration.
- Now, infiltrate with partially polymerized methacrylate at 4°C for 24 hours.
- Embed the tissue in fresh partially polymerized methacrylate in a thin-walled flat-based container. Remember, the container should have appropriate depth, so that it allows shrinkage of tissue with embedding medium during cure step which cause evaporation.
- Cure at 37°C for 1–3 days, preferably in a water bath (this step cause evaporation and shrinkage).
- Store the embedding blocks in a dry place.

Points to Remember

- The above method is suitable for cancellous bone of 5 to 10 mm thickness. Longer processing time is needed for compact bone.
- The container should be thin-walled, so that heat produced is dispersed quickly.
- Embedding moulds should have a depth of 50 mm. Then, the methacrylate blocks can be directly clamped into the microtome or vice, for milling or sawing.
- The blocks are trimmed by sawing after hardening, so that sides are parallel and suitable for direct clamping.

Advantages and disadvantages of different decalcifying agents are summarized in Table 2.

CHAPTER 12

Nervous System

INTRODUCTION

The nervous system is divided into three main groups:

- Central nervous system (CNS) → brain, spinal cord.
- Peripheral nervous system (PNS) → peripheral nerves.
- Autonomic nervous system → consisting of autonomic nerves and ganglia.

The brain and spinal cord of CNS contain neurons, glial cells, meninges and blood vessels, neurons communicate with other via intercellular interfaces called synapses.

NEURONS

It is an excitable cell which accounts for processing and transmitting neurons. They have several components:

- Cell body or soma or perikaryon: It is located mainly in the gray matter of brain and spinal cord. They contain various organelles like neurofibrils, microtubules, Nissl bodies in the cytoplasm and are bounded by cell membrane.
- The nucleus: It is in the central position of cell body and it stores the cell's genetic code in DNA.
- The axon: It is an elongated fibrous process. In lower spinal cord, they are very long and innervate muscles of lower extremity. They transmit electrical impulses away from cell body to synapse.
- Dendrites (dendrons): These are cytoplasmic extensions of the cell bodies. They receive electrical impulse from other neurons at synapse.

GLIAL CELL

The name neuroglia (meaning nerve glue) is given as they act as supporting cells in CNS. The principal types are:

- Astrocytes (protoplasmic and fibrous type): Protoplasmic astrocytes are mostly found in gray matter and fibrous astrocytes are abundant in white matter. They are involved in repair after brain damage. It also acts as blood–brain barrier to protect the brain from harmful bloodborne substances.
- Oligodendroglia: These cells are small and they have no vascular feet or fibers unlike astrocytes. They are abundant in white matter and found along the myelinated fibers. But in the gray matter, they are concentrated around the blood vessels and nerve fibers.
- Microglia: These are small oval shaped cell which contain a deeply staining nucleus. A thick process arises from each end of cell and branches to give many small processes ending in terminal spines.

MENINGES

Menings cover the brain and spinal cord. They are composed of outer dura mater, the arachnoid mater and inner pia mater. The pia mater and arachnoid are jointly called as pia-arachnoid membrane as their attachment to each other is very close.

Central nervous system is divided into gray mater and white mater. The gray mater contains majority of cell bodies but little myelin. On the contrary, the white mater is composed of many myelinated axons but few neurons. Neuropil is the term used to describe the network of neuronal processes in which neuronal cell bodies reside.

MYELIN

It is a complex mixture of lipoprotein and when the lipid is depleted, the residual protein is known as neurokeratin (filaments like). The lipid component consists of cholesterol, lecithin, galactocerebrosides and phospholipids. The protein component of myelin is a basic protein. Myelin sheath consists of alternate arrangement of concentric layer of lipid and proteins.

NISSL SUBSTANCE (TIGROID OR CHROMIDIAL SUBSTANCES)

These are deeply stained angular bodies, stained with basic aniline dyes. They are evenly distributed throughout the cytoplasm except for the area immediately surrounding the origin of the axon because of the crowding of neurofiorils at the axon hillock. These substances are more numerous in motor nerve cells then in sensory cells. Damage to nerve fibers usually results in loss of Nissl substances.

Fixative

Formol saline is the best routine fixative.

Processing

Sections may be obtained from paraffin or celloidin embedded tissue or frozen tissue. Paraffin embedding requires extra care.

Paraffin Embedding

Tissues should be impregnated with paraffin wax for 12–16 hours. At least four changes of paraffin wax should be given during this time. Vacuum bath embedding is unsuitable as this method will make the sections brittle. Also the sections float off the slide during silver impregnation method or during staining.

Section Cutting

Sections are cut at a thickness of 7–8 µm. Routinely and for demonstration of myelin, the thickness should be 12 µm. For demonstration of dendrites and axons (complete neurons), the thickness should be 15–20 µm.

CRESYL FAST VIOLET STAIN (NISSL SUBSTANCE)

Fixative

Alcohol, formalin or Carnoy.

Sections

- 7–10 µm thick paraffin section to demonstrate only Nissl substance.
- 25 µm thick paraffin section to assess cortical neuronal density.

Reagents

- Cresyl fast violet solution
  - Cresyl fast violet: 0.5 g
  - Distilled water: 100 mL
  - Mix regents and filter.
- Differentiation solution
  - Glacial acetic acid: 250 µL
  - Alcohol: 100 mL
  - Mix well.

Staining Method

1. Deparaffinize histologic sections and bring them to water.
2. Cover the slide with filtered cresyl fast violet solution for 15–20 minutes.
3. Dip into differentiation solution (0.25% acetic alcohol) for 4–8 second to remove the stain.
4. Briefly pass through absolute alcohol and then into xylene.
5. Repeat step 3 and 4 as necessary (but time in step 3 will be less than step 4).
6. Rinse in xylene.
7. Mount in DPX or Canada balsam.

Results

- Nissl substance: Purple, dark blue.
- Neurons: Pale purple, blue
- Cell Nuclei: Purple blue.

LUXOL FAST BLUE – CRESYL VIOLET FOR MYELIN

Fixative

Formalin.

Section

10–15 µm paraffin.

Reagents

- **Luxol fast blue solution**
  - Luxol fast blue: 1 g
  - 95% alcohol: 1,000 mL
  - 10% acetic acid: 5 mL
  - Mix reagents and filter.
- **Cresyl violet solution**
  - Cresyle violet: 0.1 g
  - Distilled water: 100 mL

- **Lithium carbonate solution:** 0.1% lithium carbonate solution.
- **Cresyl violet differentiator**
  - 95% alcohol: 90 mL
  - Chloroform: 10 mL
  - Glacial acetic acid: 3 drops
  - Mix well.

Staining Method

1. Bring section to 95% alcohol.
2. Stain in Luxol fast blue solution overnight at 37°C.
3. Wash in 95% alcohol, then in distilled water.
4. Dip the slides into Coplin jar containing lithium carbonate solutions for 10–20 seconds.
5. Differentiate in 70% alcohol until the white and gray mater are well distinguished (30–60 seconds).
6. Rinse in distilled water. Check microscopically and repeat the steps 4, 5 and 6 if required (but now time will be reduced).
7. Wash in distilled water.
8. Stain in cresyl violet for 8–10 minutes at room temperature.
9. Wash in distilled water.
10. Wash in 70% alcohol.
11. Dip into cresy violet differentiator for 1–2 seconds.
12. Rinse in 95% alcohol to wash the differentiator.
13. Rinse in absolute alcohol.
14. Clear in xylene. Check microscopically the differentiation of nuclei and Nissl substance. Repeat step 11, 12 and 13 if required.
15. Mount in DPX .

Results

- Myelin: Blue
- Nuclei: Purple
- Cells: Violet-pink.

PAGE'S SOLOCHROME CYANINE TECHNIQUE (FOR MYELIN)

Fixative

Formalin.

Sections

Paraffin section (6–10 μm). Cryostat section (10 μm).

Preparation of Staining Solution

- Solochrome cyanine RS: 0.2 g
- 10% iron alum: 4 mL
- Distilled water: 96 mL
- Concentrated hydrochloric acid: 0.5 mL.

Staining Method

1. Bring sections to water.
2. Stain the slides in staining solution for 10–20 minutes at room temperature.
3. Wash in running water.
4. Differentiate in 5% iron alum and check microscopically, nuclei should be unstained. Wash in distilled water many times.
5. Wash in running tap water.
6. Counterstain in neutral red, van Gieson or neutral fast red if desired.
7. Dehydrate in graded alcohol.
8. Clear in xylene and mount in DPX.

Results

Myelin sheaths: Blue.

GLEES AND MARSLAND'S MODIFICATION OF BIELSCHOWSKY'S METHOD

Fixative

10% formol: Saline.

Sections

Paraffin 10–15 μm.

Reagent Preparation (Ammoniacal Silver Solution)

- 20% silver nitrate: 30 mL
- Absolute alcohol: 30 mL.

Add strong, ammonia drop by drop until the precipitate first formed is just dissolved. Then, add additional five drops of strong ammonia.

Staining Method

1. Deparaffinize (removal of paraffin wax) with xylene 30–60 seconds.
2. Rinse in absolute alcohol.
3. Flood the slide with 1% celloidin for 20 seconds.
4. Wipe of excess celloidin from back side of the slide. Flood with 70% alcohol to harden the celloidin for 1–5 minutes.
5. Wash well in distilled water.

6. Treat with 20% silver nitrate for 25–60 minutes at 37°C.
7. Rinse in distilled water.
8. Wash in 10% formalin twice each for 10–15 seconds. Sections should be pale yellow to brown now. Do not wash.
9. Flood the sections with ammoniacal silver solution and keep for 30 seconds.
10. Drain off the silver solution and flood slide with 10% formalin for 1–2 minutes.
11. Rinse in distilled water.
12. Fix in 5% sodium thiosulfate for 2–5 minutes.
13. Wash in tap water.
14. Blot and flood with absolute alcohol to remove celloidin film.
15. Clear in xylene and mount in DPX or Canada balsam.

Results

- Nerve cells (and neurofibrils), Axons and dendrites: Dark brown to black
- Background: Light brown.

EAGER'S METHOD FOR DEGENERATING AXONS

Fixative

Formol saline.

Sections

Frozen, 30 μm thick.

Reagents

- Ammoniacal silver solution
  - 1.5% silver nitrate: 40 mL.
  - Ammonia: 4 mL
  - 2.5% sodium hydroxide: 3.6 mL
  - 95% ethyl alcohol: 24 mL.
- Reducer
  - 1% citric acid: 27 mL
  - 10% formalin: 37 mL
  - Absolute alcohol: 90 mL
  - Distilled water: 810 mL.

Staining Method

1. Keep the frozen sections into 2% formalin.
2. Rinse them in distilled water.
3. Place them into 2.5% uranyl nitrate for 4–5 minutes.
4. Rinse in distilled water.
5. Place in ammonical silver solution for 5–15 minutes until it becomes brown.
6. Transfer directly (without washing) to reducer and leave until no further color changes occurs, for 2–5 minutes.
7. Rinse in distilled water.
8. Fix the slides in 0.5% sodium thiosulfate.
9. Wash and dehydrate in alcohol.
10. Clear in xylene and mount.

Results

- Degenerating nerve fibers: Brown to black
- Normal nerve fibers: Pale yellow.

MODIFIED BIELSCHOWSKY METHOD (FOR NEUROFIBRILLARY TANGLES AND PLAQUES)

Fixative

Formalin.

Sections

Paraffin, 6–8 μm.

Reagents

- **20% silver nitrate solution**
  - Silver nitrate: 20 g.
  - Distilled water: 100 mL.
- **Developer**
  - Formalin: 20 mL
  - Distilled water: 100 mL
  - Citric acid: 0.5 g
  - Concentrated nitric acid: 1 drop.
- **0.2% ammonia washing solution**
  - Ammonia: 0.2 mL
  - Distilled water: 100 mL.
- **'Hypo' solution:** 1% sodium thiosulfate.

Staining Method

1. Bring sections to water.
2. Place slides in 20% silver nitrate for 20 minutes at 4°C in a refrigerator.
3. Place the slide in distilled water and at the same time prepare following steps.
4. To the 20% silver nitrate, add ammonia drop by drop. Stir it vigorously until precipitate becomes clear. Add two additional drops of ammonia.
5. Return the slides from step 3 to this solution for 10–15 minutes at 4°C in a refrigerator.
6. Take 50 mL of ammoniacal silver solution (prepared in step 4). To it add three drops of developer solution. Keep

this solutions in a Coplin jar and wash the slide with 0.2% ammonia washing solution. Now place the slide in Coplin jar containing ammoniacal silver-developer solution for 2–5 minutes.

7. Rinse in distilled water.
8. Fix the section in 'hypo' solution for 5 minutes.
9. Wash in distilled water.
10. Dehydrate in alcohol and clear in xylene.
11. Mount in DPX.

Results

Neurofibrillary plaques: Black
Tangles: Black
Background: Brown.

CHAPTER 13

Some Special Stains

AMYLOID

Amyloid is a pathologic proteinaceous substance which is deposited in the extracellular space in various tissues and organs of the body in a wide variety of clinical settings. Amyloid is made up of nonbranching fibrils of indefinite length and a diameter of approximately 7.5–10 nm by electron microscope. X-ray crystallography and infrared spectroscopy demonstrate a characteristic crossed β-pleated sheet conformation responsible for birefringence.

STAINING FOR AMYLOID

- **Iodine staining:** It is used for unfixed specimen or histologic section. Amyloid gives mahogany brown color and if sulfuric acid is added, then amyloid turns violet.
- **Hematoxylin and Eosin stain:** Amyloid appears as eosinophilic extracellular substance.
- **Congo red:** Pink or red color under light microscope. This stain is most widely used and also it is very specific stain. Apple green birefringence under polarizing microscope.
- **Metachromatic stain:** Methyl violet or crystal violet gives rose pink appearance.
- **Fluorescent stains (Thioflavin T and S):** Give secondary immunofluorescence when seen with ultraviolet (UV) light. Amyloid appears yellow in color.
- **Periodic acid-Schiff (PAS) stain:** Amyloid is PAS positive (light magenta or pink color). But this is nonspecific stain.

Diagnosis

Diagnosis is done by microscopic examination from biopsy of rectum, kidney, gingiva and abdominal fat aspiration. The rectum is the best site for taking the biopsy material. The staining of abdominal fat aspirate is quite specific but not popular because of its low sensitivity. Grossly, the affected organ become enlarged and firm with a waxy appearance.

Choice of Procedure and Fixative

Amyloid is best demonstrated when examined the cryostat or free-floating frozen sections. These sections give intense staining which is frequently superior to that of paraffin-processed tissue sections. Most fixatives are useful like alcohol, mercuric chloride, etc. If formal saline fixative is used, then fixation should not be prolonged. The staining intensity becomes progressively less after few months. This is probably because in due course of time there is formation of methylene bridges, which block reactive groups.

WHAT IS BIREFRINGENCE?

Substances or crystals which are capable of producing plane-polarized light are called birefringent. This process is known as birefringence or dichroism. A birefringent substance or crystal split the light into two light paths which is determined by a different refractive index or RI and these two light paths vibrate in one direction only, i.e. polarized. But they vibrate at right angles to each other. The ray which has higher RI, has greater retardation. As the two rays have different RI, the two rays leave the birefringent substance at a different velocity. The ray which has higher RI and greater retardation is called **slow ray**. The ray which has lower RI and lower retardation is called **fast ray**. A birefringent substance (dichoic) when rotated in polarized light; changes of color and intensity are seen after rotating 90°. Further rotation in same direction (clockwise or anticlockwise) restores the original color. So, this birefringence is due to absorption of two rays (fast and slow rays) in some birefringent substances, depending upon the direction of the polarization.

Positive birefringence occurs if the plane of vibration of the slow ray (higher RI) is parallel to length of the fiber or crystal and negative if the plane of vibration of the slow ray is perpendicular to the length of the fiber.

Why does Amyloid Show Birefringence with Certain Dyes like Congo Red?

When amyloid is stained with Congo red, there is formation of pseudocrystalline structure due to orientation of linear dye molecule and β-pleated sheet configuration of amyloid fibril. This produces different light-absorbing characteristics along certain planes of the fibril. In Congo red staining, amyloid shows green birefringence. Toluidine blue shows red-to-blue dichroism and trypan blue shows colorless-to-blue dichroism.

Why does Amyloid Show Metachromasia with Certain Dyes like Methyl Violet?

Methyl violet and some other dyes produce metachromasia. Earlier it was thought that the mucopolysaccharide content of amyloid is responsible for this reaction which is now regarded as not correct explanation. Moreover, the red/purple coloration produced in this reaction is also nonselective as this coloration is also seen in mucin of rectal biopsies. Besides, methyl violet is a mixture of tetra, penta and hexa-parasaniline and the coloration of amyloid might be due to selective absorption of one of these colored fractions. Hence, polychromasia should be more appropriate terminology. In short, chemical rationale of this staining reaction is controversial and still remains unexplained.

ALKALINE CONGO RED TECHNIQUE

Fixative

Alcohol or Carnoy (Formalin or Zenker as alternative).

Reagents

- **Alkaline salt solution**: Take 50 mL of 80% alcohol which is saturated with sodium chloride. To it, add 0.5 mL of 1% aqueous sodium hydroxide. Filter and use immediately (10–15 minutes).
- **Stock stain solution**: 80% alcohol which is saturated with sodium chloride and Congo red.
- **Working solution**: Add 0.5 mL of 1% aqueous sodium hydroxide to 50 mL of stock stain. Filter and use immediately (10–15 minutes).

Staining Method

1. Bring sections to water.
2. Stain in hematoxylin for 5–7 minutes.
3. Rinse in distilled water.
4. Treat the slides in alkaline salt solution for 20 minutes.
5. Stain the slides in working solution of alkaline Congo red solution (working solution) for 20–30 minutes.
6. Dehydrate rapidly in absolute alcohol, thrice such changes.
7. Clear in xylene.
8. Mount in DPX.

Results

- Amyloid: Deep pink to red (Fig. 1)
- Elastic tissue: Pale pink
- Nuclei: Blue.

Points to Remember

- This alkaline Congo red technique does not need differentiation step unlike other methods. This is

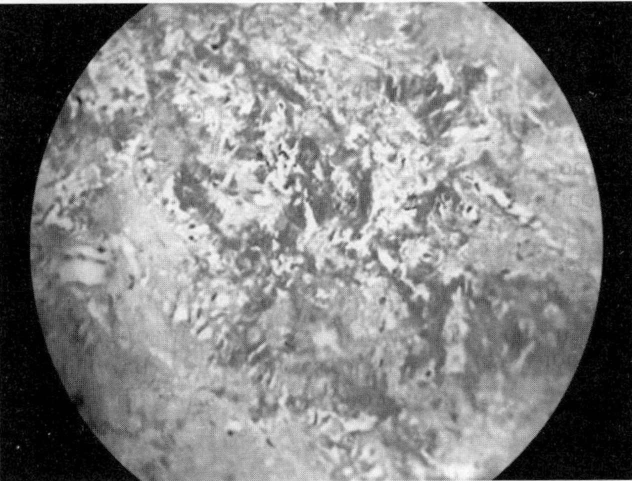

Fig. 1: Congo red stain, high power. Amyloids are stained by Congo red stain as deep pink to red *(For color version, see Plate 3)*

because of addition of high concentration of sodium chloride which reduces background electrochemical staining and enhances hydrogen bonding of Congo red to amyloid. This makes the staining method progressive as well as highly selective technique.
- Aqueous alkaline Congo red solution causes detachment of sections from slide. But alcoholic alkaline Congo red solution does not have this problem.
- The addition of sodium chloride gives more intense staining pattern.

THIOFLAVIN T METHOD

Fixative

Any fixative (alcohol, mercuric chloride, formal saline).

Reagent (Staining Solution)

1% aqueous thioflavin T.

Staining Method

1. Bring sections to water (remove mercuric or formalin pigment, if present).
2. Treat with alum hematoxylin solution for 2–5 minutes.
3. Wash in water.
4. Stain with 1% aqueous thioflavin T for 3–5 minutes.
5. Rinse in water.
6. Differentiate in 1% acetic acid for 20–25 minutes and remove excess fluorochrome from background.
7. Wash well in water.
8. Dehydrate in alcohol and clear in xylene.
9. Mount in nonfluorescent mountant (DPX or Canada balsam).

Results

- **Using blue light fluorescence** (quartz-iodine or mercury vapor lamp with BG12 exciter filter and K530 barrier filter): amyloid, elastic tissue, etc. gives yellow fluorescence.
- **Using UV light source** (mercury vapor lamp with UG1 exciter filter, K430 barrier filter and BG38 red suspension filter): amyloid, elastic tissue, etc. gives silver-blue fluorescence.

LENDRUM'S TECHNIQUE (METACHROMATIC STAIN)

- Bring sections to water.
- Stain in 1% aqueous methyl violet for 3–5 minutes.
- Differentiate in 70% formalin (or 1% acetic acid), check microscopically.
- Wash in running tap water for 1–2 minute.
- Flood with saturated aqueous solution of sodium chloride for 5 minutes.
- Rinse in water and mount (corn syrup or aqueous mountant).

Results

- Amyloid: Pink to red.
- Other elements: Violet.

Points to Remember

- Compared to 1% acetic acid, 70% formalin differentiator gives more stable results and stained slides can be stored for years.
- Methyl violet stained slides should be mounted using an aqueous mountant since dehydration destroys the staining reaction.

GRAM-TWORT STAIN

Sections

Formalin fixed paraffin sections.

Reagents

- Crystal violet solution (commercially available)
  - Crystal violet, 10% alcoholic: 1 mL
  - Distilled water: 9 mL
  - 1% ammonium oxalate: 40 mL

  Mix and store. Filter before use.
- Modified Gram's iodine (commercially available)
  - Iodine: 0.5 g
  - Potassium iodide: 1 g
  - Distilled water: 100 mL

  Dissolve potassium iodide in a small amount of the distilled water. Add iodine and dissolve it. To this, add remaining amount of distilled water.
- Twort's stain
  - 1% neutral red in ethanol: 9 mL
  - 0.2% fast green in ethanol: 1 mL
  - Distilled water: 30 mL

  Mix immediately before use.

Staining Method

1. Dewax the section and rehydrate in graded alcohol to water.
2. Stain in crystal violet solution for 3–5 minutes.

3. Rinse in running tap water gently.
4. Treat the sections with Gram's iodine for 3 minutes.
5. Rinse in the tap water. Blot it, then complete drying in a warm place.
6. Differentiate in acetic alcohol (2% acetic acid in absolute alcohol, preheated to 56°C). The color of section should be straw color or brownish.
7. Rinse in distilled water.
8. Stain in Twort's stain for 5–7 minutes.
9. Wash in distilled water.
10. Rinse in acetic alcohol until red color disappears (few seconds).
11. Rinse in fresh absolute alcohol.
12. Clear in xylene and mount in DPX or Canada balsam.

Results

- Gram positive organisms: Blue-black
- Gram negative organisms: Pink-red
- Elastic fibers: Black
- Red blood cells, cytoplasmic structures: Green
- Nuclei: Red.

ZIEHL-NEELSEN METHOD

Fixative

Formalin or others (not Carnoy's)

Sections

Paraffin sections.

Reagent (Carbol Fuchsin)

- Basic fuchsin: 1 g
- Absolute alcohol: 10 mL
- 5% aqueous phenol: 100 mL

First, dissolve the basic fuchsin in absolute alcohol. Then, add 5% phenol (aqueous).

Staining Method

1. Bring section to water.
2. Stain in hot carbol fuchsin. It may be done in two ways. Either flood the slides with stain and heat them until steam appears and leave it for 10 minutes. Or, the slides may be kept in a Coplin jar and put it in oven for 30 minutes at 56°C.
3. Wash in water and remove excess stain.
4. Differentiate in 3% hydrochloric acid in 70% alcohol for 5–10 minutes (Tissue becomes pale pink).
5. Wash in water.
6. Counterstain in 0.1% methylene blue for 10–15 seconds.
7. Wash in distilled water.
8. Dehydrate and clear in xylene.
9. Mount in DPX or Canada balsam.

Results

- Acid fast bacilli (Mycobacteria), Russell bodies, some fungus, Splendore-Hoeppli immunoglobulins around actinomyces: Red
- Nuclei: Blue
- Background: Pale blue.

Points to Remember

- Decalcification with strong acid will destroy acid-fastness property of bacteria. Use formic acid if decalcification is needed.
- Victoria blue or night blue can be used instead of carbol fuchsin. Safranine, tartrazine and picric acid (for color blind people) may be used as counterstain (in replacement of methylene blue).
- The blue counterstain is patchy if there are extensive areas of caseous necrosis.
- Do not counterstain for prolonged period, scant organisms will be difficult to find.

MODIFIED WADE-FITE METHOD FOR *M. LEPRAE* AND *NOCARDIA*

Fixative

10% neutral buffered formalin (NBF).

Section

Paraffin sections (4–5 μm).

Reagents

- **Carbol fuchsin**: as prepared in the previous method.
- 5% sulfuric acid in 25% alcohol
  - 25% ethanol: 95 mL
  - Concentrated sulfuric acid: 5 mL.
- **Methylene blue (commercially available) stock solution**
  - Methylene blue: 1.4 g
  - 95% alcohol: 100 mL.
- **Working methylene blue solution**
  - Stock solution of methylene blue: 5 mL
  - Tap water: 45 mL.
- **Xylene-peanut oil**: 1 part oil: 2 parts xylene.

Staining Method

1. Deparaffinise in xylene-peanut oil (two changes, 6 minutes each).
2. Drain the slide vertically and wash them with warm tap water for 3 minutes.
3. Stain the slides with carbol fuchsin for 25–30 minutes.
4. Wash in warm tap water for 3–5 minutes.
5. Keep the slides vertically to remove excess water on paper towel.
6. Decolorize with 5% sulfuric acid in 25% alcohol (two changes, 90 seconds each). At this stage sections become pale pink.
7. Wash in warm, running tap water for 5–7 minutes.
8. Counterstain with working methylene blue solution, 1–2 quick dip.
9. Wash in warm running tap water for 3–5 minutes.
10. Blot the slides and dry them in an oven for 5 minutes at 50–55°C.
11. After drying, 1–2 quick dips in xylene.
12. Mount it.

Results

- Nocardia, Mycobacterium leprae: Bright red (Figs 2A to D)
- Nuclei and other tissue elements: Pale blue.

GIMENEZ METHOD FOR *HELICOBACTER PYLORI*

Fixative

Formalin.

Sections

Paraffin sections.

Reagents

- Buffer solution (phosphate buffer, 0.1 M, pH 7.5)
  - 0.1 M sodium dihydrogen phosphate: 3.5 mL
  - 0.1 M disodium hydrogen orthophosphate: 15.5 mL

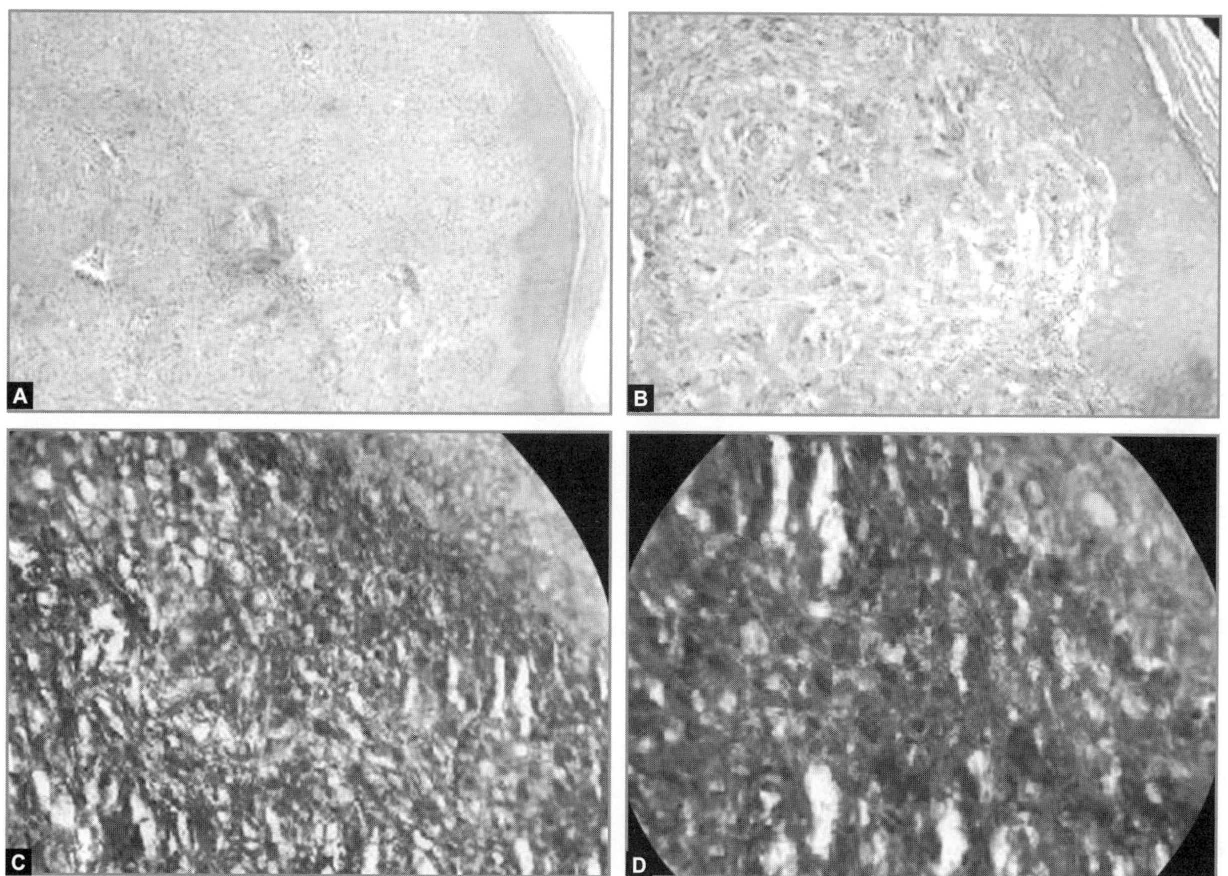

Figs 2A to D: (A) Low power view of skin lesion in lepromatous leprosy (H & E, ×100); (B) High power view showing sheets of foamy macrophages in dermis (H & E, ×400); (C) Modified Wade-Fite stain showing numerous red-colored lepra bacilli in dermis (×400); (D) Modified Wade-Fite stain showing red-colored lepra bacilli arranged in clusters and singly within foamy macrophages in dermis (×1000) *(For color version, see Plate 4)*

- Stock solution of Carbol fuchsin
  - Basic fuchsin: 1 g
  - Absolute alcohol: 10 mL
  - 5% aqueous phenol: 10 mL

  Mix and filter before use.
- Working solution of carbol fuchsin
  - Phosphate buffer: 10 mL
  - Stock solution of carbol fuchsin: 4 mL

  Mix and filter before use.
- Malachite green
  - Malachite green: 0.8 g
  - Distilled water: 100 mL.

Staining Method

1. Deparaffinize the section and rehydrate through graded alcohol to distilled water.
2. Stain in working carbol fuchsin solution for 2–3 minutes.
3. Wash well in tap water.
4. Stain in malachite green for 15–20 seconds.
5. Wash well in distilled water. Repeat the steps 4 and 5, until the section appears blue-green.
6. Blot the section, then dry it completely in air.
7. Clear it and mount it.

Results

- Helicobacter pylori: Red-magenta
- Background: Blue-green.

Points to Remember

- Be cautious during staining with malachite green, as overstaining or irregular staining is a common problem.
- This method is also useful to demonstrate Legionella bacillus in smears prepared from postmortem lung.

GIEMSA STAIN FOR PARASITES

Fixative

Preferably Zenker's or B5 (though other fixatives may be used).

Section

Thin paraffin embedded sections (3 μm).

Reagents

- Stock solution of Giemsa (commercially available)
  - Giemsa stain powder: 2 g
  - Methanol: 125 mL
  - Glycerol: 125 mL.

  Dissolve the Giemsa powder in glycerol with regular shaking at 60°C. Add methanol and shake well. Allow the mixture to stand for 7–10 days. Filter before use.
- Working solution of Giemsa
  - Giemsa stock solution: 1 mL
  - Distilled water with acetate buffer, pH 6.8: 24 mL.

Staining Method

1. Deparaffinize the section and rehydrate through graded alcohol, then to distilled water.
2. Rinse in acetate buffered distilled water, pH 6.8.
3. Stain in working solution of Giemsa, overnight.
4. Rinse in distilled water.
5. Wash in running tap water.
6. Blot it and quickly dehydrate in graded alcohol.
7. Clear in xylene and mount.

Results

- Protozoa and few other organisms: Dark blue
- Nuclei: Blue
- Background: Pink/pale blue.

PHLOXINE-TARTRAZINE TECHNIQUE

Fixative

Formalin.

Sections

Paraffin sections.

Reagents

- Phloxine solution
  - Phloxine: 0.25 g
  - Calcium chloride: 0.25 g
  - Distilled water: 50 mL

  Mix well.
- **Tartrazine:** A saturated solution of tartrazine in cellosolve or 2-ethoxyethanol.

Staining Method

1. Deparaffinize the sections and rehydrate through graded alcohol to distilled water.
2. Stain the nuclei in alum/Harris hematoxylin for 8–10 minutes.
3. Wash in running tap water for 5–8 minutes.
4. Stain in phloxine solution for 20–30 minutes.
5. Rinse in tap water.
6. Blot dry.

7. Stain in tartrazine until the viral inclusions give intense red coloration (checked by microscope). Usually, it takes 5–10 minutes.
8. Rinse in 95% alcohol.
9. Dehydrate in absolute alcohol.
10. Clear in xylene and mount.

Results

- Viral inclusions: Bright red
- Nuclei: Blue-gray
- Red blood cell: Variably orange-red
- Background: Yellow.

Points to Remember

- Initially all tissue components are stained red by phloxine solution. The tartrazine counterstain then acts as a differentiator by displacement and only the viral inclusions remain red.
- Russell bodies in plasma cells, Paneth cells in gastrointestinal tract and keratin retain this dye (phloxine) and remain red even after counterstaining with tartrazine. So, these substances may create diagnostic confusion.

CHAPTER 14

Enzyme Histochemistry and Histochemical Stains

ENZYMES

Enzymes are biocatalysts synthesized by living cells and they increase the rate of reactions without themselves being changed in the overall process.

HISTOCHEMISTRY

Histochemistry is defined by Pearse as " the identification, localization and quantification in cells and tissues and by chemical or physical tests, of specific substances, reactive groups and enzyme catalyzed substances". So any chemical procedure or technique that localizes a substance in cells or tissues for subsequent microscopy is a histochemical technique.

ENZYME HISTOCHEMISTRY

Enzyme histochemistry is the science that deals with immunologic and molecular biologic techniques in combination with histologic techniques.

The demonstration of enzymes in tissues is completely different from that of other inactive tissue components. Unlike other components, enzymes must be active to be demonstrated. Thus, demonstration of enzymes within cells, mainly depends on the action of enzymes on a specific substrate at the site of activity and formation of an insoluble substance. This insoluble substance, subsequently becomes colored or opaque.

For obvious reasons, tissues must be as fresh as possible and autopsy tissue/necropsy is usually unsuitable for demonstration of enzymes. If tissue cannot be processed for enzyme demonstration, then tissue should be kept in refrigerator. For most enzymes either fresh tissue (like cell cultures on cover slip) or frozen/crystal and freeze dried tissue sections are needed. But, some enzymes like alkaline phosphatase or acid phosphatase resist fixation, and hence their demonstration.

Fixatives

Refrigerator cooled acetone, buffered formol-saline or 95% alcohol are used. For most cases, cold acetone serves the purpose of enzyme demonstration.

PRINCIPLES OF ENZYME HISTOCHEMISTRY

Histochemistry procedures are based on biochemical reactions. Tissue or cells containing enzymes, when placed in a solution, they chemically react with the solution to produce a colored insoluble end product. The location and amount of the end-product can then be evaluated in the context of the cell or tissue.

CLASSICAL HISTOCHEMICAL REACTIONS

It is generally based on one of the four principles.

- Simple ionic interactions.
- Reactions of aldehyde with Schiff's reagent or silver compounds.
- Coupling of aromatic diazonium salts with aromatic residue.

- Conversion of substrate and enzyme to form a colored precipitate.

ENZYME TYPES

- **Oxidoreductase**: It is a large group and consists of following subgroups:
  - Oxidases: They catalyze oxidation of a substrate in the presence of oxygen.
  - Dehydrogenases: They catalyze oxidation of a substrate by removal of hydrogen.
  - Peroxidases: They catalyze oxidation of a substrate by removing hydrogen which combines with hydrogen peroxide.
  - Diaphoresis: They catalyze oxidation of NADH and NADPH by removal of hydrogen.
- **Hydrolases**: They catalyze the introduction of water of its elements into specific substrate bonds.
- **Transferases**: They catalyze the transfer of the radical of two compounds but without the uptake or loss of water.
- **Lyases**: They catalyze the removal of groups from substrates resulting in formation of double bonds of carbon. Decarboxylase is a subclass of this group.

TYPES OF HISTOCHEMICAL REACTION

There are four main types:

1. Simultaneous capture.
2. Post-incubation coupling (post-coupling).
3. Self-colored substrate.
4. Intramolecular rearrangement.

Simultaneous Capture

It is the most important technique for the demonstration of enzymes.

Principle

- Gomori's metal precipitate technique.
- Azo dye method.

Technique

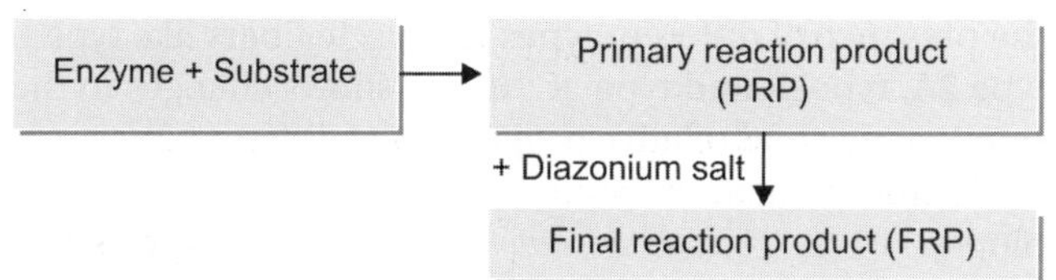

Primary reaction product (PRP): It is the product of the reaction of an enzyme on a substrate.

Final reaction product (FRP): It is the product of an insoluble uncolored PRP which has been rendered colored or opaque.

Example: The diazo technique for alkaline phosphatase.

Disadvantages of this Reaction

Diffusion of PRP (primary reaction product). This diffusion depends on following factors:

- The rate of coupling of the PRP and diazo salt.
- The rate of hydrolysis of the substrate.
- The diffusion coefficient of the PRP for the buffer.
- The pH of buffer medium and diazonium salt.

Post-incubation Coupling

Technique

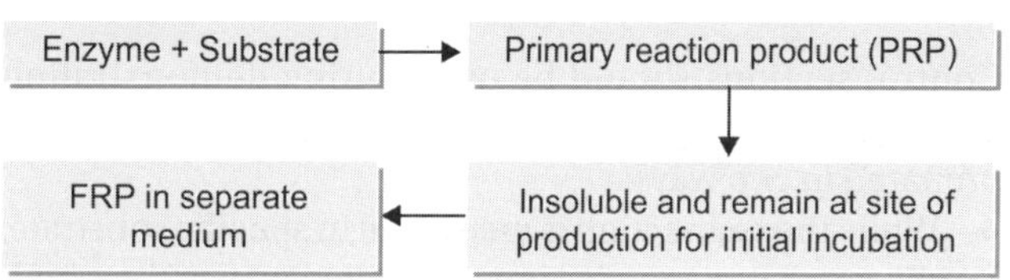

Example: The technique of Rutenberg and Seligman for acid phosphatase.

Advantages of this Reaction

- Cases where long first incubation is necessary because most diazonium salts slowly decompose when they remain in aqueous solution.
- Optimum pH for enzyme and for diazonium salt can be employed separately.

Disadvantages of this Reaction

- PRP is not completely insoluble.
- Some diffusion of PRP.

Self-colored Substrate

Technique

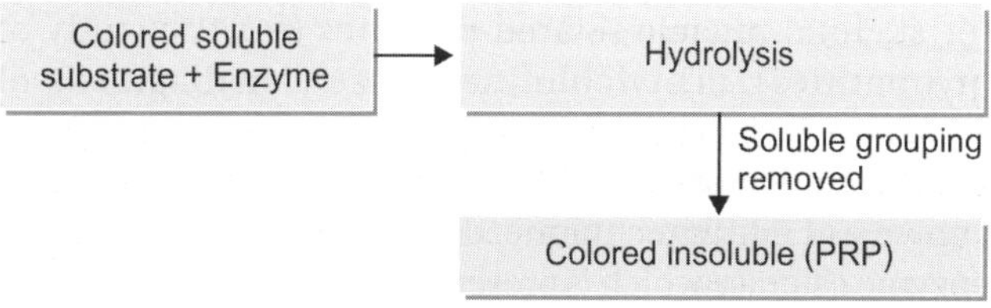

Example: The fluorescent technique of Burstone's for alkaline phosphatase.

Advantage

Diazonium salt coupling not required.

Intramolecular Rearrangement

Technique

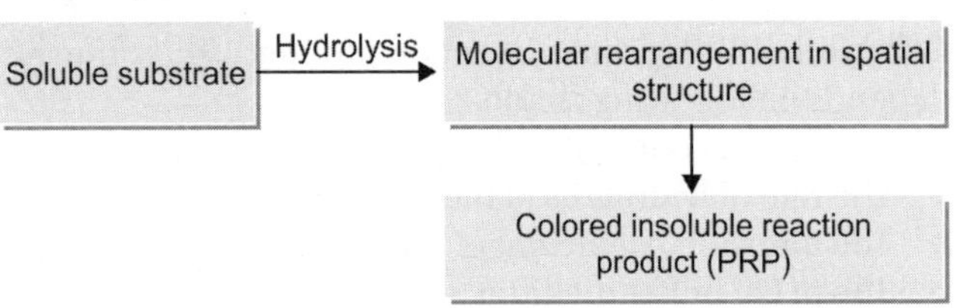

Example: The technique described by Nachlas for carboxylic acid esterase.

Control Sections

Control sections should be used during demonstration of enzyme activity in enzyme histochemistry. It can be prepared in two ways:

- While the test section is incubated in specific substrate, the control section is kept in distilled water. Then both the sections are taken through same remaining steps of technique.
- Additional control section may be obtained by keeping another test section in boiling water for 15 minutes (thus destroying the enzyme) or by incubating the section in M/100 sodium fluoride for 60 minutes at 37°C.

Diagnostic Applications

Enzyme hitochemical techniques are not widely applied to surgical and necropsy material for diagnostic purposes. This is because:

- Total or partial loss of enzyme activity, which occurs when a tissue is routinely fixed and processed into paraffin.
- The need for fresh tissue material.
- The relative nonspecificity of most of the reactions.
- The complexity of the technique.

Presently, the enzyme histochemical methods most commonly used for diagnostic purposes are those for skeletal muscle related enzymes (for the study of myopathies), acetylchlolinesterase (for diagnosis of Hirschsprung's disease) and chloracetate esterase (for demonstration of mast cells and myeloid cells). The latter, known as Leder's technique, depends on the fact that the enzyme esterase which is present in these cells, is one of the few enzymes which resist the effect of formalin fixation and paraffin embedding, is acid phosphatase.

Table 1: Applications of enzyme histochemistry

Enzymes	*Dye used to detect the enzyme*	*Positive results*
1. Acid phosphatase	Sodium β glycerophosphate (pH 5.0)	Black
2. Alkaline phosphatase	Sodium β glycerophosphate (pH 9.0)	Brown/ black
3. Tyrosinase (Melanoma)	L-tyrosine, DL-DOPA	Brown
4. Nonspecific esterase (for neural tumors)	α napthyl acetate	Reddish brown
5. Acetylcholinesterase (Hirschsprung's disease)	Acetylcholine iodide	Red brown
6. ATPase (Myopathy)	ATP	Dark

Another example of diagnostic application by this method is DOPA reaction in melanocytic cells to diagnose melanocytic tumors. This reaction depends on the enzyme tyrosinase and requires the use of fresh tissue. A modified version of this technique enables the demonstration of precipitation product in paraffin embedded material.

Following paraformaldehyde fixation, a plastic embedding technique has been described which combines preservation of various enzymes with good morphological detail. Even, at ultrastructural level (electron microscopy), enzyme histochemistry can also be carried out.

In short, current common uses of enzyme histochemistry in surgical histopathology are:

- Skeletal muscle biopsy.
- Rapid and easy detection of ganglia and nerves in cases of suspected Hirschsprung's disease.
- Demonstration of specific lactase or sucrase deficiency in jejunal biopsies in suspected celiac disease.
- Demonstration of white blood cells of myeloid lineage and mast cells (chloroacetate esterase technique).
- Miscellaneous (e.g. acid phosphatase in prostate carcinoma and alkaline phosphatase in vascular endothelial tumors) (Table 1).

SKELETAL MUSCLE BIOPSY

Cryostat sections of unfixed skeletal muscle demonstrate the presence of different types of muscle fibers like type I, type 2A, type2B and type 2C. It also shows changes in the number, size and relative proportion of different fibers.

Histochemical methods commonly used for muscle biopsy:

- Adenosine triphosphatase (ATPase)
- NADPH diaphorase

- Phosphorylase
- Cytochrome oxidase.

ADENOSINE TRIPHOSPHATASE (ATPase)

Sections: Unfixed cryostat.

Reagents

1. 0.1M glycine buffer:
   - Glycine: 375 mg
   - NaCl: 292.5 mg

   Make up to 50 mL with distilled water.
2. 0.1M glycine buffer with 0.75M $CaCl_2$:
   - 0.1 M glycine buffer (solution 1): 25 mL
   - 0.75 M $CaCl_2$ (calcium chloride): 5 mL (11.03 g $CaCl_2$. $2H_2O$ in 100 mL of distilled water)

   Mix well and add approximately 11 mL of 0.1 M NaOH to make a pH 9.4.
3. 0.1 M solution veronal-acetate buffer, pH 4.2 and pH 4.6.
4. Incubating solution:
   - ATP: 5 mg
   - Solution 2: 10 mL

   Adjust to pH 9.4 with 0.1 M NaOH or 0.1 M HCl as necessary.

Histochemical Method (at pH 9.4)

1. Incubate unfixed freshly cut cryostat sections in incubating solution 4 at 37°C.
2. Rinse well with distilled water.
3. Immerse the slides in 2% cobalt chloride for 5 minutes.
4. Rinse well with tap water, followed by three changes in distilled water.
5. Immerse in 1:10 diluted ammonium sulfide solution (in fume cupboard) for 30 seconds.
6. Rinse in running tap water.
7. Counterstain in Harris hematoxylin lightly.
8. Blueing in tap water.
9. Dehydrate in graded alcohol.
10. Clear in xylene and mount in DPX (alternatively, mounting may be done in glycerine jelly directly after step 8, bypassing dehydration and clearing).

Histochemical Method (at pH 4.2 and 4.6)

1. Incubate freshly cut sections in appropriate 0.1 M Veronal-acetate buffer (solution 3) at 4°C for 10 minutes.
2. Rinse in distilled water for shorter time.
3. Then proceed from step 1 in above mentioned method at pH 9.4.

Table 2: Skeletal muscle fiber at different pH in histochemical methods

Skeletal muscle fiber type	*ATPase pH 4.2*	*ATPase pH 4.6*	*ATPase pH 9.4*	*Dehydrogenase (SDH, LDH), NADH diaphorase*	*Phosphorylase*
Type 1	+++	+++	+	+++	±
Type 2A	–	–	+++	++	+++
Type 2B	–	+++	+++	+	+++
Type 2C	+	+++	+++	++	+++

Abbreviations: ATPase, adenosine triphosphatase; SDH, succinate dehydrogenase; LDH, lactate dehydrogenase; NADH, reduced form of NAD (Nicotinamide-adenine dinucleotide).

Results

- Strong staining pattern (dark or black): ++ or +++
- Light staining pattern (pinkish): +
- Negative (no staining).

Points to Remember

Muscle fibers are generally divided into groups based on their contractile properties, type 1 (slow -twitch) and type 2 (fast -twitch). Type 1 fibers have low levels of ATPase and high levels of mitochondrial oxidase enzymes, hence they are fatigue resistant.

Type 2 fibers have low levels of mitochondrial oxidative enzymes and high myophosphorylase activity so that they can utilize anaerobic glycolysis (Table 2).

CYTOCHROME OXIDASE

Section: Fresh cryostat sections.

Reagents (Incubating Solution)

- Catalase, 20 µg/mL: 1 mL
- Cytochrome C: 10 mg
- 0.1 M phosphate buffer, pH 7.4: 9 mL
- 3,3'-Diaminobenzidine tetrahydrochloride (DAB): 5 mg
- Adjust pH to 7.4 with the help of 0.1 M NaOH or 0.1 M HCl as necessary before use.

Histochemical Method

1. Incubate cryostat sections at room temperature for 2–3 hours.
2. Rinse in distilled water.
3. Fix in formal calcium for 15 minutes.
4. Counterstain briefly in hematoxylin for 15–20 seconds.
5. Wash and blue in tap water.

6. Dehydrate in graded alcohol.
7. Clear in xylene and mount in DPX.

Results

Brown reaction products → means tissue has cytochrome oxidase activity.

PHOSPHORYLASE

Section: Fresh unfixed cryostat section.

Reagent (Including Solution)

- 0.1M acetate buffer, pH 5.9: 50 mL
- 0.1M magnesium chloride: 5 mL
- Glucose-1-phosphate: 0.5 g
- Glycogen (rabbit/oyster liver): 10 mg
- ATP salt: 25 mg
- Sodium fluoride: 0.9 g
- Ethanol: 10 mL
- Polyvinyl pyrrolidine: 4.5 g

Mix the reagent in the above mentioned order and make the incubating solution. The solution should be kept in Columbia jar. After each incubation it is frozen. Discard when potency is diminished.

Histochemical Method

1. Incubate the sections in incubating solution for 90 minutes at 37°C.
2. Wash in 4% ethanol for 5 seconds and dry in air.
3. Fix in ethanol for 3–4 minutes, dry in the air.
4. Wash in Lugol's iodine (1:30 dilution) for 5 minutes.
5. Mount in 9:1 glycine jelly or Lugol's iodine.

Result

Phosphorylase activity: Blue/black.

DETECTION OF NERVES AND GANGLIA IN SUSPECTED HIRSCHSPRUNG'S DISEASE

In this disease, in children a variable segment of the rectum and colon is devoid of ganglionic cells which is called aganglionic segment. But in the normal rectum and colon, ganglion cells are present in the submucosa as well as in the myenteric plexus between the inner circular and outer longitudinal muscle of the bowel wall. These ganglia and their nerves are responsible for motility and peristalsis in healthy individuals.

The diagnosis of Hirschsprung's disease can be suspected clinically and radiologically. But the diagnosis may be confirmed by taking suction biopsy of the rectal mucosa and submucosa and subsequent demonstration of nerve fibers and ganglion cells with the help of histochemical method, acetylcholinesterase (absent in Hirschsprung's disease).

Acetylcholinesterase

Tissue Preparation

Snap-frozen tissue sections are cut in cryostat at thickness of 10 µm. They are air dried and fixed in formal calcium for 30 seconds (4% formaldehyde in 0.1 M calcium acetate).

Reagent (Incubating Solution)

- Acetylcholine iodine: 5 mg
- 0.1M acetate buffer, pH 6.0: 6.5 mL.
- 0.1M sodium citrate: 0.5 mL.
- 30 mM copper sulfate:1 mL
- Distilled water: 1 mL
- 4 mM iso-octamethyl pyrophosphoramide (iso-OMPA): 0.2 mL.

Add 1.0 mL 5 mM potassium ferricyanide just before use.

Histochemical Method

1. Rinse the sections in tap water for 10 seconds.
2. Incubate in the incubating solution for 1 hour at 37°C.
3. Wash in tap water briefly.
4. Treat with 0.05% p-phenylene diamine dihydrochloride in 0.05 M phosphate buffer, pH 6.8 for 45 minutes at room temperature.
5. Wash in tap water.
6. Treat the sections with 1% OsO_4 (osmium tetroxide fixative) for 10 minutes at room temperature.
7. Wash well in tap water for 5–10 minutes.
8. Counterstain lightly for 10 seconds in Carazzi hematoxylin or Mayer's alum hematoxylin.
9. Wash and dehydrate in graded alcohol.
10. Clear in xylene and mount in DPX.

Result

Nerve fibers and ganglion cells: Black/dark-brown containing acetylcholinesterase.

CONCLUSION

Enzyme histochemistry serves as a link between biochemistry and morphology. It is based on substrate metabolization by the tissue enzyme in its orthotopic localization (occurring at normal place). Visualization is accompanied with an insoluble dye product. But with the advent of immunohistochemistry and DNA oriented molecular pathology techniques, the potential of enzyme histochemistry currently tends to be under estimated. The most common histochemical stains are listed in Table 3 and discussed below; their results are also shown in Figures 1 to 3.

Table 3: Common histochemical stains

Stain	*Tissue element stained*	*Result (staining color)*
PAS	Neutral polysaccharide, glycogen, fungi and basement membrane	Magenta/Rose-red
Alcian blue, pH 2.5	All acid mucins/ mucopolysaccharides	Blue
Alcian blue, pH 1.0	Sulfated mucin only	Blue
Mucicarmine	Epithelial mucin, cryptococcal capsule	Red
Colloidal iron	Carboxylated and sulfated mucins, glycoproteins	Blue
PTAH	Muscle striations, fibrin	Deep purple
Trichome	Collagen, muscle, nuclei	Blue, red, black
Reticulin	Reticulin fibers	Black
JMS (Jone's methenamine silver)	Basement membrane	Black
Congo red	Amyloid	Deep pink/red
Thioflavin T	Amyloid	Yellow
Verhoeff-van Gieson	Elastic fibers	Black
Oil Red O	Fat	Red
Perls' Prussian blue	Iron	Blue
Rhodamine	Copper	Red to red-orange
Von Kossa	Calcium	Black
Alizarin red S	Calcium	Red
Luxol fast blue	Myelin	Red
Fontana -Masson	Argentaffin granules, myelin	Black
Hall's stain	Bile pigments	Black
Churukian-Schenk	Argyrophil granules	Black
Giemsa	Bacteria, mainly *H. pylori*	Blue
Steiner	Bacteria, mainly *H. pylori*	Black
Warthin-Starry	Spirochetes	Black
GMS (Grocott's methenamine silver)	Fungi	Taupe to black
Ziehl-Neelsen	Acid-fast bacilli (*M. tuberculosis*)	Red
Modified Wade-Fite	*Mycobacterium leprae*	Red
Gram stain	Differentiate gram (+) ve and Gram (–) ve bacteria	Gram (+): blue Gram (–): red
Bielschowsky	Nerve endings, tangles, plaques	Black

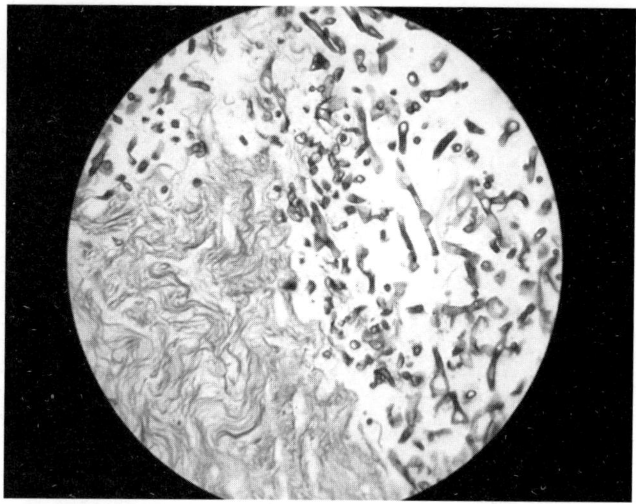

Fig. 1: Photomicrograph showing broad aseptate, ribbon-like hyphae of mucormycosis (Grocott silver methenamine stain, ×400) *(For color version, see Plate 4)*

AGYROPHIL STAINING

Agyrophil substances are present in the cell cytoplasm and they bind silver ions. They love silver ions (silver loving) but cannot reduce silver ions to its metallic form so as to visible. There are several methods for demonstration of agyrophil substances and all these methods chemically similar to the Warthin-Starry technique (used to demonstrate spirochetes). A solution of silver nitrate is used to impregnate the agyrophilic substances in the tissue. Then a reducing solution that contains hydroquinone is applied to reduce the bound silver ions to metallic silver. As a counterstain, nuclear fast red is often used. With this method, agyrophilic substances are stained black.

ARGENTAFFIN STAINING (MASSON-FONTANA METHOD)

Argentaffin substances bind silver ions like agyrophil substances, but they also reduce bound ionic silver to metallic silver without addition of a reducing substance (developer) unlike agyrophil substances. An ammoniacal silver solution is used to impregnate the argentaffin

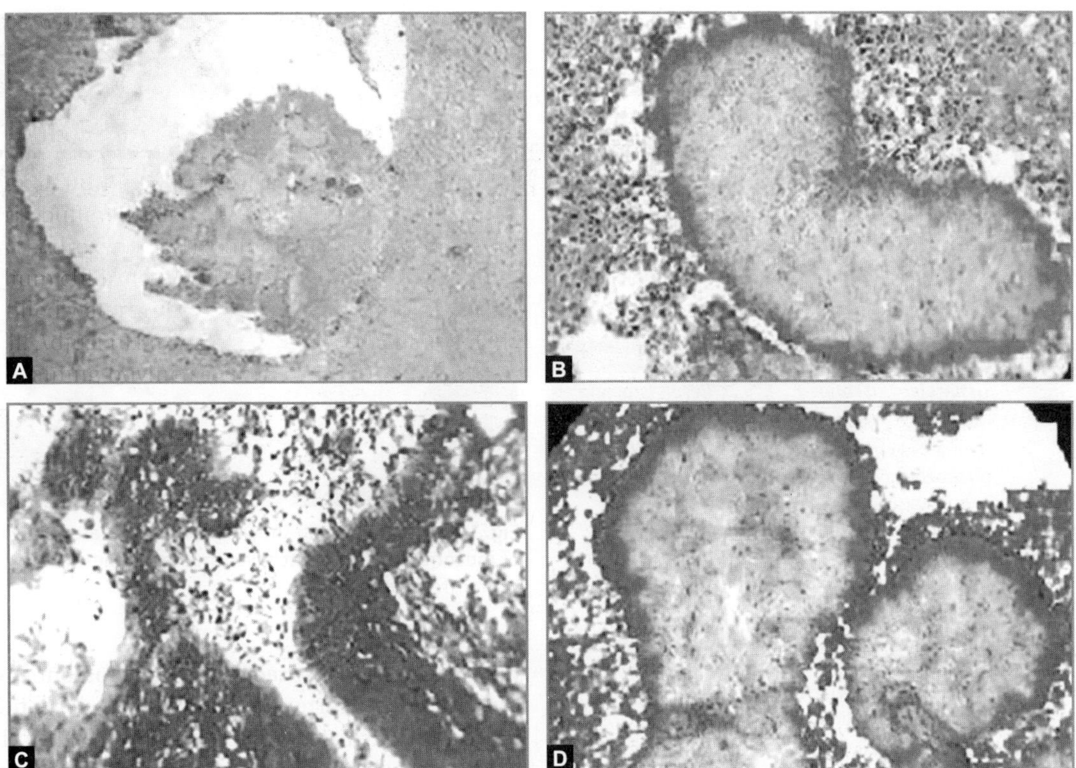

Figs 2A to D: (A) Microphotograph showing fungal mycetoma (eumycetoma) or "madura foot" (H & E, scanner view, 40×); (B) Microphotograph showing aggregates of fungal hyphae surrounded by neutrophils or microabscess and sulfur granules (PAS, low power view, ×100); (C) Microphotograph showing broader aseptate hyphae surrounded by neutrophils (PAS, high power view, 400×); (D) Microphotograph showing gram-negative organism/fungal element (Gram stain, high power view, 400×) *(For color version, see Plate 5)*

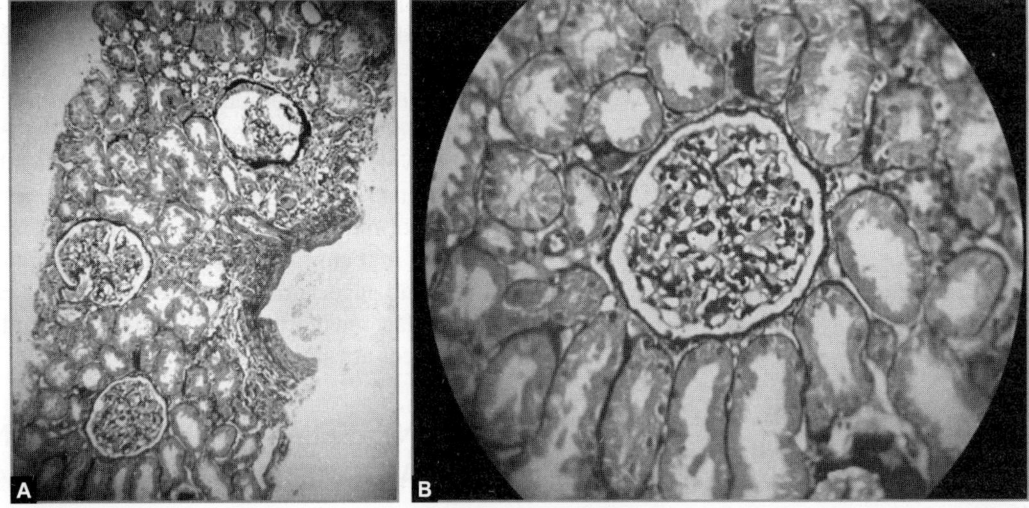

Figs 3A and B: Combined PAS and Jone's methenamine silver (JMS stain); kidney biopsy, low power and high power. PAS stains tubules as pink whereas JMS stains basement membrane surrounding Bowman's space and glomerular capillaries as black *(For color version, see Plate 5)*

substances in tissue sections. The argentaffin substances present in the tissue not only bind the silver ions in the solution but also reduce them to metallic silver. Gold chloride is usually used to tone this metallic silver from brown coloration to black. Nuclear fast red is the most popular counterstain. Melanin pigments like other argentaffin substances follow this property and can be stained with this method.

CHAPTER 15 Immunohistochemistry

DEFINITION

Immunohistochemistry is a method for demonstrating the distribution and location of tissue components or antigens by means of antigen-antibody reactions.

Immunohistochemistry, as the name implies is a marriage between two disciplines—immunology and histology. It is a powerful tool in the surgical pathologists' armamentarium (Table 1).

ANTIGEN

It is a molecule that induces the formation of monoclonal or polyclonal antibody directed against that particular antigen. Antigen bears one or multiple antibody binding sites.

EPITOPES

In the antibody binding sites of antigens, there are highly specific regions which are antigenic determinant groups or epitopes. They are composed of monosaccharide units or few amino acids. So, an epitope is an antigenic determinant of known antigenic structure.

ANTIBODY

They are basically immunoglobulins and belong to the class of serum proteins. There are five types: IgA, IgG, IgM, IgE and IgD. The monomer (a basic unit of antibody) has two light chains and two heavy chains. The monomer can be cleared by enzyme like pepsin or papain, resulting in the formation of Fab (fragment which binds antigen) and Fc (fragment which crystallize). Depending on the number of monomers or basic units it possesses, an antibody can be monomer, dimer, trimer, tetramer or pentamers.

SHORT HISTORY

The term 'antibody' was coined by Paul Ehrlich in 1891. Coons demonstrated immunofluorescence staining on frozen sections based on antigen-antibody interactions in 1940. Taylor and Burns developed immunohistochemistry (IHC) on routinely processed formalin fixed, paraffin-embedded (FFPE) tissue in 1974. Kohler and Milstein, in 1975 presented the hybridoma technique to produce monoclonal antibodies by fusing an antibody producing B cell with a myeloma cell which is selected for its capability to grow in tissue culture. Before the advent of hybridoma technique, polyclonal antibodies were used, which contain molecularly different antibodies that target multiple epitopes with varying specificity. This results in higher level of nonspecific background staining compared to use of monoclonal antibody (mAb). The use of mAb enables mere specification high quality staining.

DIFFERENT TECHNIQUES

Immunohistochemical techniques are a group of immunolabeling procedures which are capable of demonstrating various antigens or substances in cells and tissues. These techniques are based on the ability of specific antibodies to localize and bind to corresponding antigens or epitopes. This binding reaction is not visible unless the antibody is tagged with a label or conjugate that either

Table 1: Different immunohistochemical methods

1. Labeled antibody methods
   a. Direct methods
   b. Indirect methods
2. Unlabeled antibody methods
   a. (Strept) avidin-biotin method
   b. Hapten-labeled antibody
   c. Hybrid antibody
   d. Enzyme-antienzyme complex/peroxidase-anti-peroxidase (PAP) complex
   e. Immunoglobulin bridge
   f. Protein A label
   g. Labeled avidin D
3. Multiple staining techniques

absorbs or emits light and thus produces a contrast or a color. There are many labels which can be used (Table 1):

- Enzyme label
- Fluorescent label
- Colloidal metal label
- Radiolabel.

Enzyme Label

Enzymes are most commonly used label in immunohistochemistry (IHC). Incubation with a chromogen produces a colored end-product which is stable and visible under light microscope. Horseradish peroxidase is most widely used enzyme. The chromogen commonly used is 3, 3α-diaminobenzidine tetrahydrochloride (DAB). Alkaline phosphatase is another enzyme used as a label. Other chromogens are 3-amino-9-ethylcarbazole, α-naphthol pyronin, Hanker-Yates reagent, Kaplow and commercially available chromogens like Vector blue, Vector red, Vector VIP, etc. Horseradish is the choice of enzyme label for many reasons:

- The enzyme is easily obtainable.
- As the size is small, enzyme (label) tagged antibody easily binds to sites without blocking other adjacent sites.
- This enzyme is stable.
- Endogenous activity if any can be blocked easily.

Fluorescent Label

Fluorescent compounds when excited by ultraviolet light, emit light within the visible wavelengths. The color of the emitted light depends on the nature of the compound. As for example, fluorescein isothiocyanate emits green light whereas rhodamine emits red light or fluorescence. Texas red (emits red light) and R-Phycoerythrin (emits orange/red) are other fluorescein compounds. As a group, immunofluorescence methods require fresh tissue or fresh frozen tissue. The fluorescence is visualized on a dark background. Immunofluorescence cannot be performed on paraffin embedded or fixed tissue and also it lacks morphological details. It is therefore not very popular technique and has limited role in skin and kidney biopsies.

Colloidal Metal Label

Various metals such as iron, mercury, gold can be used as label in IHC methods. They produce sufficient electron opacity for visualization under light microscope as well as in electron microscopy. But the poor penetration of the metal conjugates to the specific site results in nonspecific deposition in the background. This is a serious drawback of this method. Among different metals, immunogold is probably the most popular method. It is used to localize particular substance like hormone ultrastructurally (electron microscope). The immunogold-silver staining method is very sensitive IHC procedure.

Radio Label

Sometimes radioisotopes are used as label and it requires autoradiographic facilities. But it is not very popular as internally labeled antibodies are not widely available.

In IHC, labels are either directly bound to the primary, secondary and tertiary antibodies or they are indirectly bound to antibodies with the help of other substances such as enzyme, biotin, haptens, protein-A, or polymers. Major categories of IHC methods are listed in the following table.

The first two methods detect only a single/particular antigen while the third method detects multiple (at least two) antigens in a single tissue or block.

LABELED DIRECT METHOD (TRADITIONAL METHOD)

In this method, primary antibody (usually rabbit anti-human antibody) is directly conjugated to the label (peroxidase enzyme or fluorochrome). This conjugated or labeled antibody reacts with the antigen directly. This antigen may be present in tissue (histology) or smear (cytology) (Fig. 1).

Use

Demonstration of implement and immunoglobulin in frozen sections of kidney and skin biopsies.

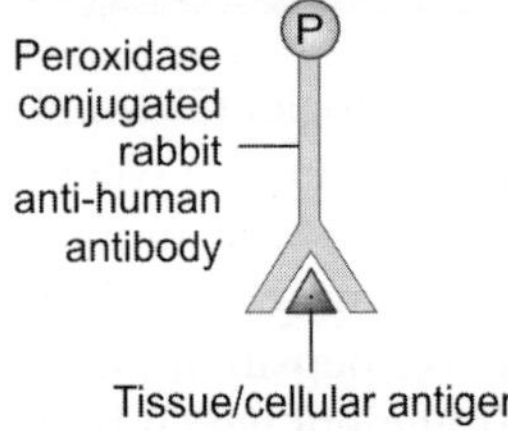

Fig. 1: Labeled direct method

Advantage

Quick and easy to use.

Disadvantages

- If there is low level of antigens in a tumor, then it would not be demonstrated.
- It is less sensitive technique and has little signal amplification.

Labeled Indirect (Two Step) Method

Here, two antibodies are used. The first one is the primary antibody which acts on particular human antigen. This primary antibody (anti-human) is prepared in another animal, like in the rabbit. The other antibody (secondary antibody) is directed against the primary antibody and is prepared in an animal other than that prepares the primary antibody, say (swine antibody against rabbit antibody). This secondary antibody is labeled or conjugated with an enzyme, commonly horseradish peroxidase together with an appropriate chromogen substrate which enables visualization (Fig. 2).

Polymer Chain Indirect Method (Two Steps)

In this method, the secondary antibody is conjugated with horseradish peroxidase labeled polymer (dextran) chain. One polymer chain may attach many enzymes and secondary antibody simultaneously. The secondary antibody may be anti-rabbit or anti-mouse in origin. It is directed against primary antibody which may be monoclonal (rabbit or mouse anti-human antibody) or polyclonal (rabbit anti-human antibody) (Fig. 3).

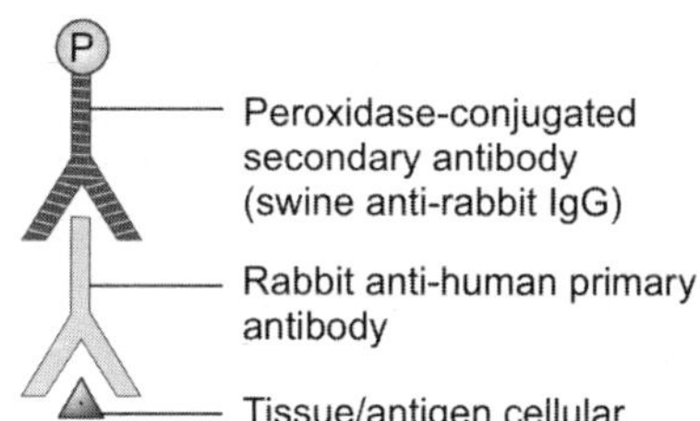

Fig. 2: Labeled indirect method

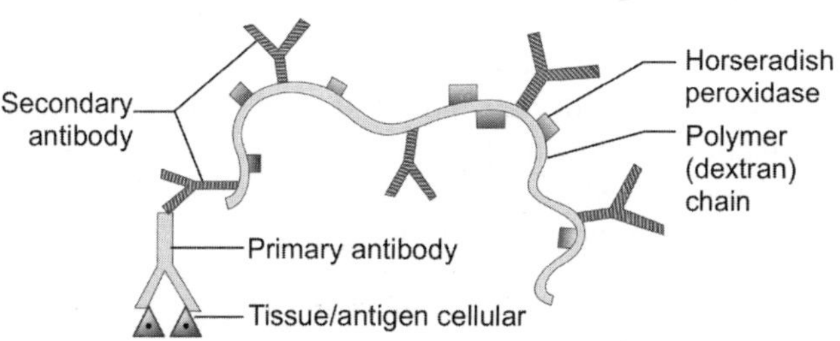

Fig. 3: Polymer chain indirect method

Use

This technique is very popular nowadays and is probably the commonest method used for IHC.

Advantages

- This method is reliable, quick and easily reproducible.
- It has high sensitivity.
- Its biotin free, so interference with endogenous biotin is absent.
- It can be used for multicolor staining.

UNLABELED ENZYME-ANTIENZYME COMPLEX METHOD (PEROXIDASE-ANTI-PEROXIDASE COMPLEX METHOD)

In this method, apart from primary antibody and secondary antibody, a third layer of enzyme-antienzyme complex is used. Commonly peroxidase-antiperoxidase complex is used as a third layer of staining. This complex is prepared by three peroxidase enzymes and two anti-peroxidase antibodies. This peroxidase-antiperoxidase (PAP) is a soluble complex and is bound to the primary antibody (rabbit anti-human antibody) with the help of a bridging secondary antibody (swine anti rabbit IgG).

Similarly, alkaline phosphatase-anti-alkaline phosphatase complex can be used as a third layer. These methods are not popular and have been replaced by streptavidin-biotin techniques (Fig. 4).

Disadvantages

- It has lower sensitivity.
- Difficulty in producing enzyme-anti-enzyme PAP complexes.

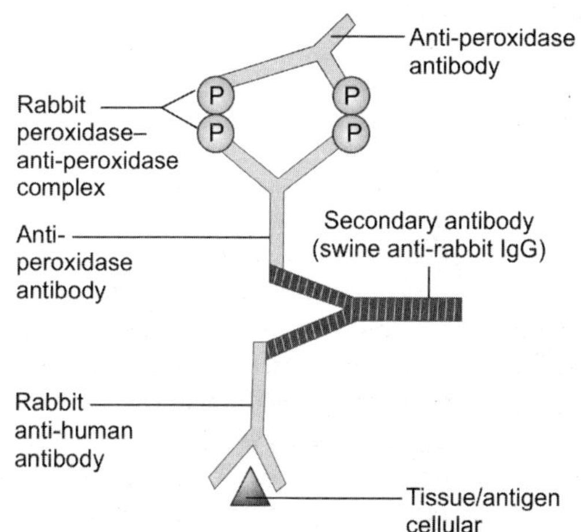

Fig. 4: Unlabeled enzyme-antienzyme complex method

(Strept) Avidin-Biotin Method

This is also a three-step technique. The first layer is formed by primary antibody (mouse anti-human antibody) and second layer is formed by secondary antibody (rabbit anti-mouse IgG). The third layer is enzyme-labeled (peroxidase or alkaline phosphatase)—avidin-biotin complex. Streptavidin can be used in place of avidin. This enzyme is used with a chromogen of choice.

Biotin (vitamin H), an egg-white protein, has an intense affinity for a low molecular weight vitamin, avidin. This binding is much stronger than many other antigen-antibody bindings and is practically irreversible. The resulting avidin-biotin-peroxidase complexes are lattice like and can deliver many active peroxidase molecules which makes this technique highly sensitive.

Streptavidin has also high affinity for biotin and has four binding sites like avidin. But due to molecular rearrangement all these four sites are not available for binding unlike avidin. This streptavidin can be prepared from the bacterium *Streptomyces avidinii.*

Biotin or vitamin H is easily conjugated with secondary antibodies and enzymes (horseradish peroxidase). As many 150 biotin molecules can be attached to a single antibody (Fig. 5).

Use

Streptavidin-biotin technique is the most widely used methodology in the IHC. Streptavidin has replaced the avidin as avidin has a tendency to react with lectins via a carbohydrate moiety which causes nonspecific staining.

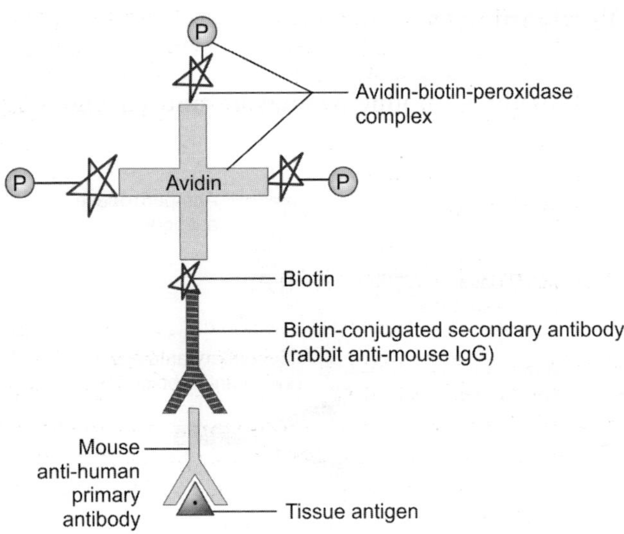

Fig. 5: Avidin-biotin method

Advantages

- It has high sensitivity compared to other techniques.
- It allows a higher dilution of the primary antibody as a large number of biotins can be attached to a single antibody.

Disadvantages

- Tissues rich in endogenous biotin will require the use of an avidin-biotin block before applying primary antibody. Liver and kidney are such organs which are rich in biotin.
- Avidin is positively charged at neutral pH, because of its high isoelectric point, so it may bind nonspecifically to some negatively charged structures like nuclei.
- Avidin reacts with lectin which causes nonspecific staining.

TECHNICAL ASPECTS OF IMMUNOHISTOCHEMISTRY

Paraffin-embedded Specimens

When tissues are fixed and processed and subsequently embedded in paraffin; the tissue antigens remain intact in the block for several years to be detected immunohistochemically and will not be decreased by prolonged storage. So, these paraffin-embedded tissues are potential sources for many retrospective studies.

Frozen Sections

With the advent of antigen retrieval systems and highly sensitive detection techniques, routine use of frozen sections for IHC has been drastically reduced. Cryostat or frozen sections were used in the past for IHC, when monoclonal antibodies were first introduced and number of antigen was low.

When frozen samples are selected for IHC, some measures should be taken immediately. A block of tissue, no longer than 1 × 1 × 0.3 cm should be promptly immersed in liquid nitrogen which is called snap-freezing. A mixture of liquid nitrogen and isopentane will result in a more uniform freezing of tissue and hence it will preserve best histomorphology. Slow freezing by placing the specimen in a freezer will result in a great loss of antigens and also poor histomorphology. Thawing and re-freezing also cause antigenic loss and negative impact on morphology. Snap-frozen fresh tissue can be stored at –70°C without appreciable antigen loss for a long time.

Plastic-embedded Tissue

Thin sections from tissues embedded in different types of plastics such as epoxy resin, araldite and methacrylate demonstrate excellent morphologic details. It is necessary to remove the resin with sodium ethoxide and re-expose the antigens by antigen retrieval (heat induction or protease digestion), when IHC is to be carried out. But still the result is unpredictable and IHC is not recommended on plastics sections.

Fixatives

- **Formalin**: Most laboratories use fixation based on formalin such as 10% neutral buffered formalin or 10% formal saline. But formalin is not the best fixative for IHC as for example it is not suitable for certain proteins like light and heavy chain immunoglobulins. Most other cytoplasmic antigens and nucleic acids are demonstrable in this fixative.
- **Alcohol containing fixative**: Alcohols and alcohol based fixatives such as Carnoy's and methacran have some advantages as they penetrate tissue rapidly. They are fixatives of choice to demonstrate intermediate filaments. But most other tissue antigens show poor results.
- **Picric-acid containing fixatives**: Tissues fixed in Bouin's solution is good for demonstration of most cytoplasmic antigens except immunoglobulin and intermediate filaments. It is also very good to demonstrate viral antigens and peptide hormones. Zamboni's solution (picric acid-paraformaldehyde) is suitable for electron microscopy.
- **Mercuric fixatives**: Zenker, Susa, B_5 are better than formalin in preserving nuclear morphology. These fixatives are considered best for IHC demonstration of immunoglobulin and most lymphoid cell markers in paraffin-embedded tissue sections. But they are not suitable for other cellular antigens. Also, they produce undesirable background staining.
- **Fixatives for frozen sections**: Cold acetone is very good fixative (5 minutes at 4°C) and preserves most cell surface antigens. Good results are also seen in frozen sections which are fixed few minutes in ethanol, formalin and Zamboli's solution (picric acid-paraformaldehyde).
- **Fixation time**: Optimal formalin fixation time for a block of tissue measuring $1 \times 1 \times 0.3$ cm is 12–18 hours. If alcohol, picric acid or mercuric chloride is used as a fixative, optimal time for fixation of $0.5 \times 0.5 \times 0.2$ cm block of tissue is 2–5 hours. Prolonged fixation will cause antigenic loss, especially in formalin. Fixation time can be reduced dramatically by use of conventional microwave oven. The use of microwave oven will reduce formalin fixation time to mere few seconds and it also preserves both stainable tissue antigens and morphology.

CYTOLOGICAL PREPARATIONS

The use of IHC on cytological preparations or smears is increasing day-by-day. For this purpose, acetone fixed smears or cytospins are often preferred as acetone allows many primary antibodies to be employed without destroying the target antigens or epitopes. Moreover, the acetone not only assists with the preservation of antigen and its morphology but also it destroys most harmful infectious agents. Most people use cold acetone for this.

ADHESIVE FOR HISTOLOGIC SECTIONS

Loss or detachment of paraffin and frozen sections from the slide during IHC is not uncommon. Chances of this loss are more when sections are undergone heat-induced antigen retrieval or protease-digestion using a microwave oven. The most efficient way to keep the sections intact is to use slides that are either poly-L-lysine coated or electrostatically charged. The second option though is more effective and convenient, but also more expensive. Amino-propyltriethoxysilane (APTES) and Vectabond of Vector laboratories are other good adhesives.

ANTIGEN RETRIEVAL TECHNIQUES

Aldehyde/formaldehyde fixative causes protein cross-linkages that may mask many tissue antigens. Removal of these cross-linkages and unmasking of the tissue antigens are important before one proceeds for IHC. Two common methodolies for unmasking tissue antigens are: (1) Proteolytic enzyme methods and (2) Heat mediated antigen retrieval.

Proteolytic Enzyme Methods

Protein digestion by proteolytic enzyme methods are suitable only for formalin fixed paraffin embedded (FFPE) sections. For this, the digestion media should be freshly prepared as the activity of proteolytic enzyme decreases with time. The ideal time for digestion should be determined by indivual laboratory as per their standardization. Again, some antigens like pan-cytokeratin require less digestion time whereas some like immunoglobulins require more digestion time.

Pepsin Method

1. Incubate the histologic sections in pre-warmed distilled water at 37°C.
2. Make a solution of 0.4% pepsin in 0.01M hydrochloric acid (pH 2) at 37°C.
3. Incubate these histologic sections in pepsin solution 0.4% for 10–60 minutes at 37°C. (individual laboratory should standardize the digestion time).
4. Wash in cold running tap water to stop further enzyme digestion for 5–10 minutes.
5. Proceed with the desired immunostaining method.

Protease Method

1. Incubate sections in pre-warmed distilled water at 37°C.
2. Make a solution of 0.1% protease in distilled water at 37°C. Ensure the pH to 7.8 with the help of 1M NaOH (sodium hydroxide).
3. Incubate the histologic sections in 0.1% protease solution for 5–6 minutes at 37°C.
4. Wash in cold running tap water for 5–10 minutes to prevent further enzyme digestion.
5. Proceed with the desired immunostaining method.

Trypsin/Chymotrypsin Method

1. Incubate histologic sections in pre-warmed distilled water at 37°C.
2. Prepare a solution of 0.1% trypsin in 0.1% calcium chloride in distilled water at 37°C. Make the solution alkaline (ph 7.8) using 0.1 M NaOH.
3. Incubate the sections in trypsin solutions for 10 minutes at 37°C.
4. Wash in cold running tap water for 5–10 minutes to prevent further digestion.
5. Proceed with the desired immunostaining method.

Points to Remember

- The most popular enzymes for enzyme digestion are protease and trypsin. Other enzymes which may be used are pepsin, pronase, chymotrypsin and proteinase K.
- During enzyme digestion, pH, temperature, other co-enzyme like calcium chloride with trypsin must be optimized to get consistent high quality IHC staining.
- A suitable alternative to trypsin is chymotrypsin. The procedure is same as outlined in C.
- Some antigens like basement membrane proteins are stained better if pepsin digestion is used.
- Demonstration of immunoglobulins, complement in FFPE sections (renal biopsies) is favored with proteolytic digestion than heat induced antigen retrieval.

HEAT MEDIATED ANTIGEN RETRIEVAL

The underlying mechanisms are not completely understood although many different theories have been suggested. Some of them are:

- **First theory**: During formalin fixation, calcium coordinated bonds are formed which prevent antibodies to combine with epitopes. The heat or high temperature breaks or weaken this bond. Simultaneous use of chelating agent like EDTA competes for these disrupted bonds and removes these calcium complexes.
- **Second theory**: During formalin fixation there is formation of methylene bridges and weak Schiff bases which are basis of cross-linkages of formalin fixative. Heat removes at least the weak Schiff bases making the cross-linkages weak.
- **Third theory**: Protein precipitating fixatives are better in preserving antigens than aldehyde fixatives like formalin which form cross-linkages. Heavy metal salts which act as protein precipitant, form insoluble complexes with polypeptides. These insoluble complexes after staining are readily visible under microscope.

Microwave Heating Method

Preparation of heat-mediated antigen retrieval fluid:

1. Citrate buffer
   - Anhydrous citric: 10.5 g
   - Distilled water: 5 liters
   - Adjust pH to 6.0 using 2M sodium hydroxide.
2. Tris-EDTA buffer
   - Tris: 14.4 g
   - EDTA: 1.44 g
   - Hydrochloric acid (1 M): 1 mL
   - Tween: 20–0.3 mL
   - Distilled water: 600 mL.

   Firstly add Tris, EDTA and hydrochloric acid into distilled water. Then adjust the pH to 10 with the hydrochloric acid. Next, add Tween 20 to the solution.

Microwave antigen retrieval method:

1. Place the sections into a plastic staining rack with a loose lid (maximum 25 sections). Pour 600 mL of 0.01 M citrate buffer pH 6.0.
2. Place the rack in microwave oven. Heat (irradiate) on high power (800 W) for 20–25 minutes.
3. Remove the plastic rack/container from microwave oven, flood with cold water.
4. Proceed with desired IHC staining protocol.

Pressure Cooker Method

1. Pour 1.5 liter antigen retrieval buffer into the pressure cooker (5 liter domestic stainless steel). Keep the

pressure cooker open (do not close the lid) and bring to boil.

2. Carefully place the slide racks (maximum three racks, each containing 25 slides) into the solution, when antigen retrieval buffer is boiling. Now, seal the lid of pressure cooker.
3. Allow the pressure cooker to reach full pressure (15 psi or 10.3 kappa) and incubate for 2–3 minutes. Practically. one whistle blow is sufficient for most antigens.
4. Now, place the hot cooker into a sink and run cold water over the lid to release the full pressure.
5. Also flood the pressure cooker with cold water to bring down the temperature. Wait until the slides are cool and remove them.
6. Proceed with desired IHC protocol.

Autoclave Method

1. Pour 250 mL of antigen retrieval buffer into the incubation chamber. Place the sections into this chamber.
2. Cover the incubation chamber with lid to prevent excess evaporation.
3. Now, place the incubation chamber into the autoclave and close the lid of autoclave.
4. Heat for 15 minutes at 120°C.
5. Release autoclave pressure. Take the incubation chamber out of the autoclave.
6. Flood the incubation chamber with cold water and wait until the slides are cold.
7. Proceed with desired IHC protocol.

Points to Remember

- Certain epitopes like Ki67, CD2, CD4, CD5, CD7 and CD8 can only be demonstrated in FFPE sections after heat pretreatment.
- Heat pretreatment allows greater dilution of the antibodies.
- Among the many antigen retrieval solutions, most popular are citrate buffer (0.01 M, pH 6.0) and EDTA buffer (0.1 mM, pH 8.0). Many ready to use commercially available antigen retrieval solutions are available which are pH calibrated and fully certified.
- Heating time is less for a 3 μm section than a 5 μm section.
- Certain nuclear antigens require more heating time for antigen retrieval.
- Pressure cooker is preferred for unmasking some nuclear antigens like p21, p23, bcl-6, estrogen and progesterone receptors.
- Autoclave is an alternative method and gives good results with nuclear antigens like p21, p53 and Mib1 (Ki67).
- Overfixed tissues require more heating time than under fixed tissues.
- Demonstration of immunoglobulins (heavy chains) is more reliable and reproducible in heat pretreatment compared to enzyme digestion.
- Do not allow the sections to dry after heat mediated antigen retrieval as it will cause loss of antigenicity.
- Poorly fixed tissues, fatty tissues and fibrous tissues may be damaged after boiling. To prevent this, APES coated or Vectabond coated slides are dipped in 10% formal saline for 1–2 minutes. This improves adhesion and now proceeds for heat pretreatment.
- For poorly/suboptimally fixed tissue, volume of buffer should be reduced to 400 mL (instead of 600 mL) in microwave oven and heating time is also reduced to 15 minutes.

PREPARATION OF PARAFFIN WAX SECTIONS FOR IHC

- Cut 3–4 μm sections from paraffin blocks.
- Place these slides either on APES (Aminopropyltriethoxysilane) or poly-lysine coated slides. Commercially available Vectabond of Vector laboratories can also be used. Electrostatically charged slides (Superfrost plus slides) are better if available.
- Dry these slides in an incubator at 37°C overnight.
- Deparaffinize the sections by putting them in xylene, followed by absolute alcohol.
- Block the endogenous peroxidase by keeping the slides in 0.5% hydrogen peroxide in methanol solution for 10–25 minutes.
- Wash well in running tap water to rehydrate.
- Proceed with preferred/required antigen retrieval system.

Points to Remember

- Instead of incubator, the slides may be dried by hot plate (10–15 minutes at 60°C). But estrogen, progesterone receptors and few other antigens loose antigenicity; hence not ideal for drying.
- For deparaffinization/dewaxing, histoclear may be used instead of xylene. Prewarmed xylene or histoclear (37°C at incubator) makes complete removal of paraffin.
- The thickness of paraffin sections should not be > 4 μm. Freshly cut sections should be used. Stored sections give poor staining quality.
- Blocking endogenous peroxidase by H_2O_2 (hydrogen peroxide) in methanol should be done in later stages (after the primary antibody addition) for some labile antigens like CD2 and CD4. Otherwise, antigenic

epitopes will be altered, resulting in poor staining quality.

IHC STAINING PROTOCOL

Preparation of buffer solutions (wash buffer):

- TBS (Tris-buffered saline, 0.5 M) buffer
  - Tris (hydroxymethyl) aminomethane: 6.05 g
  - Sodium chloride (NaCl): 8.5 g
  - Distilled water: 1000 mL.

  Mix well. Adjust pH to 7.6 with 50% hydrochloric acid.
- TBS containing bovine serum albumin (BSA) or BSA-TBS.
  - Tris (hydroxymethyl) aminomethane: 2.428 g
  - Sodium chloride: 9 g
  - Bovine serum albumin: 1 g
  - Sodium azide: 1.3 g
  - Distilled water: 1000 mL

  Mix well. Adjust pH to 8.2 by 1M hydrochloric acid.

Preparation of heat-mediated antigen retrieval fluids:

- Citrate buffer
  - Citric acid (anhydrous): 2.1 g
  - Distilled water: 1000 mL
  - Adjust pH to 6.0 by using 2 M sodium hydroxide (NaOH).
- Tris-EDTA
  - Tris: 28.8 g
  - EDTA: 2.88 g
  - Hydrochloric acid (1M): 2 mL
  - Tween 20: 0.6 mL
  - Distilled water: 1200 mL.

Firstly, add Tris, EDTA and hydrochloric acid to distilled water. Then adjust pH to 10 with the help of hydrochloric acid. Now add the Tween 20.

(Strept) Avidin-Biotin Technique

- Rinse the histologic sections with TBS buffer.
- Incubate in 10% casein solution (Vector laboratories) for 10 minutes.
- Apply optimally diluted primary antibody for 60 minutes.
- Wash the slides with TBS buffer.
- Apply secondary antibody (optimally diluted biotinylated) for 30 minutes.
- Wash the slides in TBS buffer.
- Apply streptavidin-biotin complex (optimally prepared) for 30-60 minutes.
- Wash the slides in TBS buffer.
- Apply DAB (3, 3α-diaminobenzidine tetrahydrochloride) solution [chromogen or substrate (Table 2)] for 7-10 minutes.
- Wash in running tap water.
- Counterstain the nuclei in hematoxylin for 5-10 minutes.
- Dehydrate, clear and mount.

Note:

- Instead of streptavidin-biotin complex; avidin-biotin complex may also be used.
- In peroxidase-antiperoxidase (PAP) method, peroxidase-antiperoxidase complex is applied in step 7 (instead of streptavidin-biotin complex).

Polymer Technique (Dako EnVision)

- Rinse histologic sections in TBS.
- Incubate in 10% casein solution (Vector laboratories) for 10 minutes.
- Apply optimally diluted primary monoclonal antibody for 60 minutes.
- Wash the slides in TBS buffer.
- Apply Dako EnVision polymer reagent for 30 minutes.
- Wash the slides in TBS buffer.
- Apply freshly prepared DAB solution/substrate or chromegen for 10 minutes.
- Rinse in TBS buffer, then transfer to running water.
- Counterstain nuclei in hematoxylin for 5-10 minutes.
- Dehydrate, clear and mount.

MULTIPLE STAINING

In many cases, two or more antigens have to be detected from the same tissue specimen IHC. For this, one needs

Table 2: Different chromogen substrates

Enzyme label	*Substrate/chromogen*	*End product*	*Application*
Peroxidase	3,3′-Diaminobenzidine (DAB)	Insoluble	Immunohistology Immunoblotting
	3-Amino-9-ethylcarbazole (AEC)	Insoluble	Immunohistology Immunoblotting
	4-Chloro-1-naphthol (4C1N)	Insoluble	Immunoblotting Immunohistology
	Dianisidine	Soluble	ELISA
	3,3′,5,5′-Tetramethylbenzidine (TMB)	Soluble	ELISA
	5-Aminosalicylic acid (SAS)	Soluble	ELISA
Alkaline phosphatase	P-Nitrophenyl phosphate (pNPP)	Soluble	ELISA
	5-Bromo-4-chloro-3-Indolyl phosphate/Nitro Blue Tetrazolium (BCIP/NBT)	Insoluble	Immunohistology Immunoblotting
	Fast Red/Naphthol AS-TR phosphate	Insoluble	Immunohistology Immunoblotting

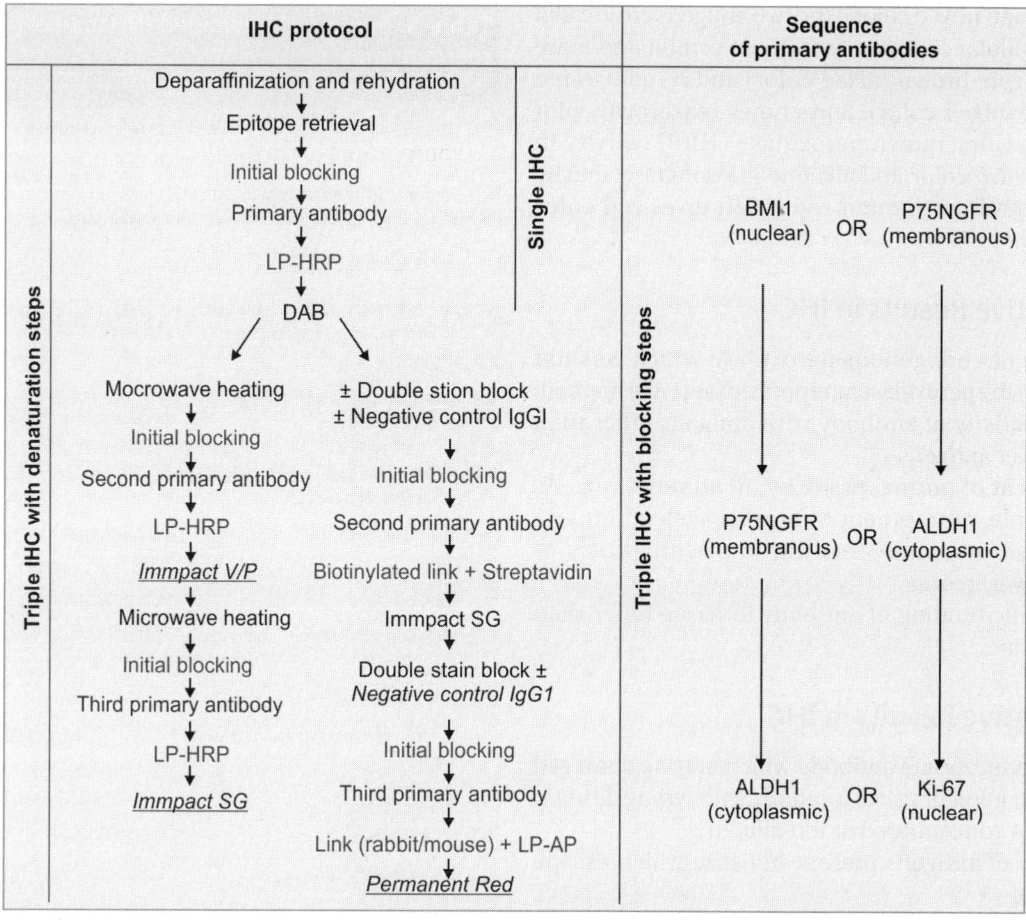

Fig. 6: IHC protocol in multiple staining

the serial sections from that tissue which is laborious and also problematic for small cell types. As for example, the diameter of small lymphocyte (3–5 µm) is close to or even smaller than tissue sections (3–4 µm). So, serial sections may fail or have inconclusive results sometimes.

In the year 1968, Nakane published a multiple-staining method, applying three indirect immunoperoxidase techniques sequentially. In this way, he demonstrated three different antigens in one tissue section by three different colored peroxidase reaction products in different cellular compartments (Fig. 6).

The study of co-localization (the presence of two antigens in one cell) is one of the main reasons for performing double staining. When two different antigens are present in the same cellular compartment, (say cytoplasm), co-localization is marked by a mixed color. But when two antigens are located in two different cellular compartments (nucleus-cytoplasm, nucleus-cell membrane, cell membrane-cytoplasm), co-localization should be observed by two separate colors.

Two major methods for multiple staining are immunofluorescence (IF) and immunoenzyme/IHC method, IF method has many drawbacks like fading of fluorescence signal after sometime, appearance of auto-fluorescence by formaldehyde fixation, quenching (initial rapid freezing) of the fluorescence signal at excitation, etc. So, many prefer IHC staining method (immunoenzyme) for this purpose.

When different antibodies are applied on serial sections to detect different antigens in a tissue, it is sometimes difficult to understand which cell type is positive. As for example, when observing a few positive nuclei with Mib1/Ki67 proliferation marker, it is not well understood always which cell type is actually proliferating. But in a double-staining method, the antibody of interest (say Mib1/Ki67) is mixed with an antibody against a structural marker for detecting epithelial cell (cytokeratin), smooth muscle cell (SMA), lymphocyte (LCA), plasma cell (CD 38 or CD138) or endothelial cell (CD 31 or CD34), etc. This double-staining pin point which type of cell is actually proliferating.

During the history of IHC, many different chromogen combinations for double staining have been proposed (van der Loos 1999). Among them only tow combinations are suitable for direct visual observation of two different chromogens and mixed color if the two antigens are located in the same cellular compartment. These combinations are red-blue (purple-brown mixed color) and turquoise-red (purple-blue mixed color). Sometimes red-brown color is also used. Horseradish peroxidase (HRP) activity in DAB gives brown color and alkaline phosphatase activity in Dako's liquid permanent red (LPR) gives red color (Figs 7 and 8).

False-positive Results in IHC

- Presence of endogenous peroxidase which was not blocked in the peroxidase-antiperoxidase (PAP) method.
- Cross reactivity of antibody with antigens other than sought after antigens.
- Entrapment of normal tissue by the tumor tissue. As for example, entrapment of normal skeletal muscle by soft tissue tumor leading to misdiagnosis of rhabdomyosarcoma.
- Nonspecific binding of antibody to tissue other than target tissue.

False-negative Results in IHC

- Use of inappropriate antibody which may be damaged by denaturation or use of antibody with wrong dilution (either too concentrated or too diluted).
- Low level of antigens present in tissue which escape detection.
- Loss of antigen due to diffusion or autolysis, to prevent this do not keep the tissue in formalin for a prolonged period (over fixation) which cause leak of antigens even after fixation by diffusion. Again, if the tissue is not fixed with a fixative, the tissue will be autolyzed.

Use of Controls

- **Positive control**: A positive control is a histologic section which is known to contain the antigen under detection. For a negative reaction to be considered truly negative, the known positive slide must show positive staining. Practically, intermediate intensity is good for positive control, as they become negative if the sensitivity of that immunomarker is reduced. On the other hand, a strongly positive control will still be positive when the test slide is negative (Table 3).
- **Negative (antibody) control**: An antibody control should also be included in IHC. Its negativity validates positive result. As the primary antibody is costly, many use either nonimmune serum or another antibody with a different specificity. But use of buffer solution as a substitute of primary antibody is not recommended.

Table 3: Some recommended IHC markers to diagnose specific tumor

Tumor type	*IHC markers/ immunomarkers*
1. Carcinoma	Pancytokeratin (CK), epithelial membrame antigen (EMA)
2. Sarcoma (mesenchymal tumors)	Vimentin, desmin, smooth muscle actin (SMA)
3. a. Hodgkin lymphoma, classic type b. Hodgkin lymphoma, nodular lymphocyte predominant type (NLPHD)	CD45-, CD15, CD20, CD30, MUM1 and PAX-5 in nodular sclerosis CD 45+, CD 20, CD15-, CD20-, MUM1-
4. Non-Hodgkin lymphoma (NHL) a. B-cell type b. T-cell type c. Anaplastic large cell lymphoma (ALCL)	 CD45, CD19, CD20 CD45, CD3, CD5 CD30, EMA, ALK-1, CD 45+
5. Mesothelioma	Calretinin, WT-1, D2-40
6. Neuroendocrine tumor (carcinoid)	NSE, Synaptophysin, Chromogranin
7. Melanoma/malignant melanoma	HMB-45,S-100, Vimentin, Mart-1/ Melan-A
8. Langerhans cell histiocytosis	CD1a, Langerin, S-100
9. Gastrointestinal stromal tumor (GIST)	CD117/C-kit, CD 34, SMA
10. Ewing's sarcoma	CD 99/ Mic-2 (also PAS positive)
11. Rhabdomyosarcoma	Myo-D1, Desmin, Actin
12. Thyroid carcinoma	Thyroglobulin, TTF-1 (also in lung cancer)
13. Breast carcinoma	ER, PR, Her-2 –neu /Cerb-2
14. Urinary bladder cancer	Uroplakin, Thrombomodulin
15. Prostate cancer	PAP (Prostatic acid phosphatase), prostate specific antigen (PSA)
16. Germ cell tumor	Placental alkaline phosphatase (PLAP)
17. Granulosa cell tumor	Inhibin
18. Wilms' tumor	WT-1
19. Angiosarcoma/Kaposi's sarcoma	CD31, CD34, Factor VIII
20. Multiple myeloma	CD38, CD 138

Perhaps the most reliable controls in IHC are internal (built-in) positive and negative controls. These represent different components of the tissue under study which are expected to react either positively or negatively with the antibody used.

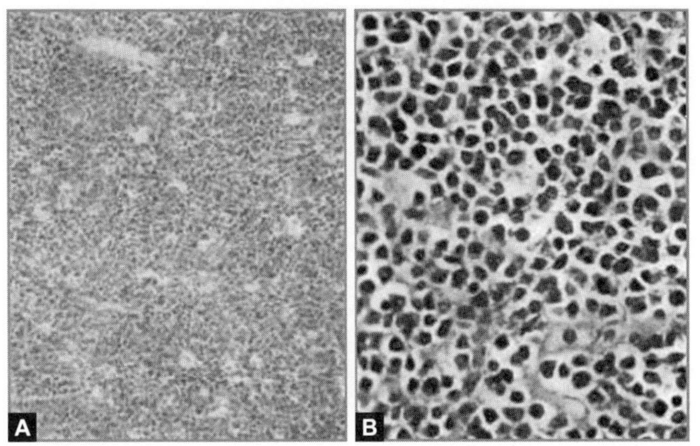

Figs 7A and B: Photomicrograph showing a tumor composed of monomorphic round cells arranged in diffuse sheets in Burkitt's lymphoma. (A) Characteristic starry sky pattern is evident (Hematoxylin and Eosin, ×100); (B) Photomicrograph showing small to intermediate sized cells having round nuclei with clumped chromatin (Hematoxylin and Eosin, ×400) *(For color version, see Plate 6)*

Use of CK7 and CK20 to Diagnose Different Carcinomas

- **$CK7^+$/$CK20^+$:** Most of the pancreatic, renal pelvis, urinary bladder, and bile duct carcinomas. Some gastric carcinomas (30–35%).
- **$CK7^+$/CK20:** Carcinomas of breast, lung, ovary, thyroid, mesothelioma, endometrium and salivary gland.
- **$CK7^-$/$CK20^+$:** Merkel cell carcinoma and large bowel carcinoma. One-third of gastric carcinomas.
- **$CK7^+$/CK20:** Carcinomas of prostrate, liver, kidney, adrenal cortex and adrenal gland.

Reporting of ER and PR in Breast Carcinoma

There are two scoring systems—one is H-score and another is Quick score. Both of these scoring systems combine intensity and proportion of cells reactivity (Figs 9 and 10).

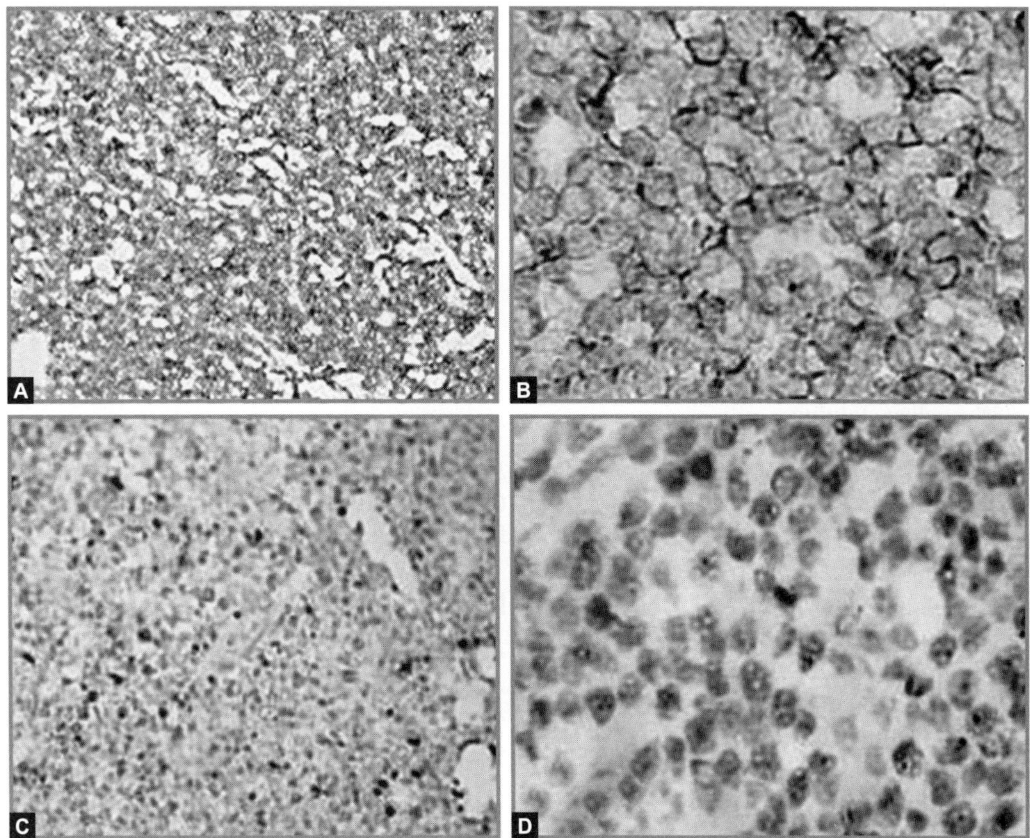

Figs 8A to D: (A) Tumor cells of Burkitt's lymphoma showing strong membrane positivity for leukocyte common antigen (LCA) [×100]; (B) Tumor cells showing strong membrane positivity for B-cell marker CD20 [×400]; (C) Tumor cells showing strong nuclear positivity for Ki-67 [×100]; (D) Tumor cells showing membrane negativity for T-cell marker CD3 [×400] *(For color version, see Plate 6)*

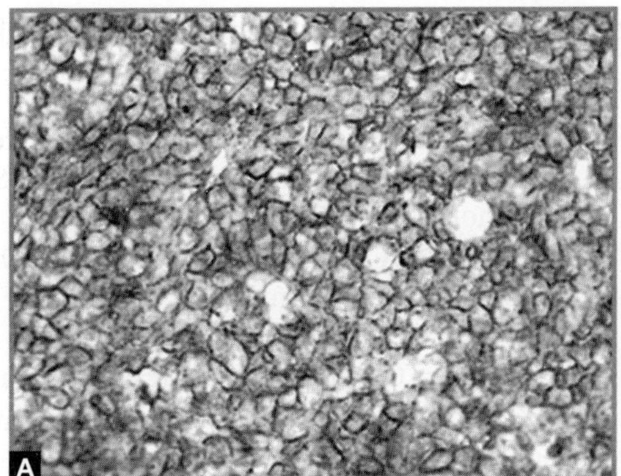
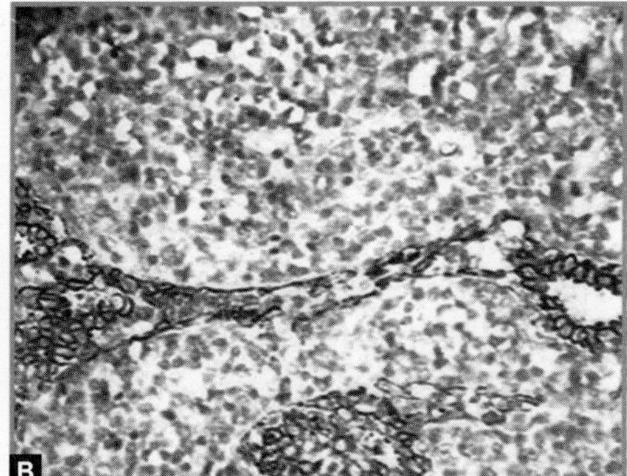

Figs 9A and B: (A) Immunohistochemistry showing diffuse cytoplasmic membrane staining of CD20 in the tumor cells of diffuse large B-cell lymphoma (DLBCL) in breast [×400]; (B) Immunohistochemistry showing negative expression of cytokeratin antigen by the tumor/lymphoma cells, while the entrapped ductal epithelial cells are positive for cytokeratin [×100] *(For color version, see Plate 7)*

- **H-score:** This is based on a summation of the proportion of tumor cells showing different degrees of reactivity (nuclear positivity).
  - No reactivity = 0
  - Weak reactivity = 1
  - Moderate reactivity = 2
  - Strong reactivity = 3

  This gives a maximum total score of 300, assuming 100% of tumor cells show strong reactivity. If 50% of cells show moderate reactivity, then the score will be 50 × 2 = 100.
- **Quick score:**

  Scores for proportion
  - 0 = no staining
  - 1 = <1% nuclear staining
  - 2 = 1–10% nuclear staining
  - 3 = 11–33% nuclear staining
  - 4 = 34–66% nuclear staining
  - 5 = 67–100% nuclear staining

  Scores for intensity
  - 0 = no staining
  - 1 = weak staining
  - 2 = moderate staining
  - 3 = strong staining

  The scores are summed to give a maximum score of 8. If 50% of the nuclei show moderate staining then the score will be 4 + 2 = 6 out of 8. Tumors scoring 2 or less are considered negative. Many laboratories now prefer this scoring system.

Note: Some laboratories use water bath (95–98°C) during antigen retrieval for Her-2-neu immunomarker, e.g. Dako Hercept test. It has the advantage of being gentler to the tissue compared to other antigen retrieval techniques, because the temperature is set below boiling point (100°C). Also, the antigen retrieval solution does not evaporate with this temperature, which constitutes another advantage (cost friendly) (Tables 4 and 5).

Table 4: Her-2-neu/Cerb-2 IHC reporting in breast carcinoma

Score to report	*Her2-neu overexpression assessment*	*Staining pattern*
0	Negative	No staining is observed, or cytoplasmic membrane staining is <10% tumor cells
1+	Negative	A faint cytoplasmic membrane staining is observed in >10 % of tumor cells but it stains only part of the membrane not entire membrane
2+	Borderline or weakly positive	A weak to moderate complete membrane staining is noted in >10% of the tumor cells
3+	Positive/strongly positive	A strong complete membrane staining is observed in >30% (formerly 10%) of the tumor cells

IHC on Frozen Section

- Cut 6 µm section and placed on adhesive coated slides (poly-L lysine, APES, etc).
- Keep the sections at room temperature for air drying.
- Fix the sections in absolute acetone (some prefer cold acetone) for 20 minutes at room temperature. Make the sections air dried.
- Wash the slides in TBS buffer for rehydration.
- Apply optimally diluted primary antibody (dilution should be made by use of TBS). Don't use detergents like Tween 20 or Triton.
- Skip the blocking endogenous peroxidase step.

Table 5: Malignant round cell tumors and IHC

Tumor	*VIM*	*DES*	*CK*	*Chromogranin*	*WT-1*	*CD99 (Mic-2)*	*CD45*	*TdT*	*CD68/MPX*
EWS/PNET	+	–	±	±	–	+	–	–	–
Rhabdomyosarcoma	+	+	–	–	–	–	–	–	–
Neuroblastoma	±	–	–	+	–	–	–	–	+
Lymphoma/leukemia	+	–	–	–	–	+*	+	–	±**
Wilms' tumor (blastemal)	+	±	–	–	+	–	–	–	–
Neuroendocrine carcinoma	–	–	+	+	–	–	–	–	–
DSRCT	+	+	+	±	+	±	–	–	–

Abbreviations: EWS/PNET, Ewing sarcoma/primitive neuroectodermal tumor; DSRCT, desmoplastic small round cell tumor; VIM, vimentin; DES, desmin; CK, cytokeratin (PAN); WT, Wilms' tumor; MPX, myeloperoxidase; (*) CD99, expressed in lymphoblastic luekemia or lymphoma; (**), CD68 is expressed in acute monocytic leukemia (M5); MPX is expressed in acute myeloid leukemia (M1, M2 Aml)

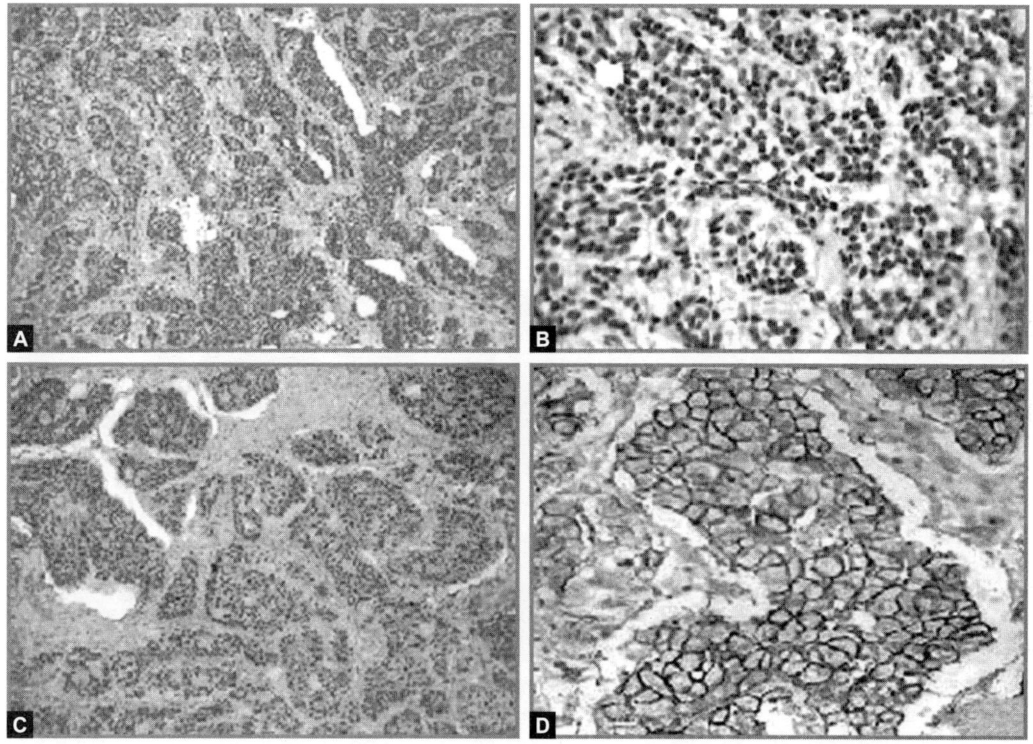

Figs 10A to D: (A) Microphotograph showing ER positivity (nuclear) in breast carcinoma (IHC, ×100); (B) Microphotograph showing strong ER positivity (nuclear) in breast carcinoma (IHC, ×400); (C) Microphotograph showing PR positivity (nuclear) in breast carcinoma (IHC, ×100); (D) Microphotograph showing Her-2/neu positivity (complete cytoplasmic membrane staining in >30% of tumor cells) in breast carcinoma (IHC, ×400) *(For color version, see Plate 7)*

- Proceed for preferred antigen retrieval system and subsequent IHC staining technique.

Note: Frozen sections are often associated with poor morphology. Frozen sections dried both before and after acetone fixation, improve the morphology. Moreover, acetone destroys most harmful agents.

IHC on Nongynecological Cytology/FNAC Smears

Cytology smears, FNAC smears, cytospins, imprints, etc. should be air dried for 1–3 hours. Then fix the smears in absolute acetone (some prefer cold acetone) for 20–30 minutes at room temperature. Make the smears air dried again. Then proceed as outlined in frozen section IHC (from step 4 onwards) (Figs 11A to D).

Storage (for Future Application) of Frozen Sections and Smear

The frozen sections or smears can be stored after fixation in acetone. Wrap the slides with foil and place them in the freezer at –20°C. When required, take the sections/smears out of the freeze and bring them in room temperature before unwrapping. Then, proceed as per the desired protocol.

Automation in Immunohistochemistry

These instruments have well defined steps and standardized variables such as volume, temperature and time. The greatest advantage is improved intra and inter laboratory reproducibility of assays. Although cost saving is not significant compared to manual methods, but it is capable of completing significant larger workloads in considerably shorter times. A summary of IHC protocol in brief is being presented in Figure 12.

Some Common Problems and Their Solutions in IHC

1. Problem: Everything Looks Blue; No Brown Staining on Slide.

Possible solutions:

- Is the IHC reagent fresh? Reagent should be stored according to the manufacturer's instructions. It means reagents should be either at 4°C in a fridge, or at –20°C in a freezer. Avoid leaving things out on bench for longer than necessary, and minimise any freeze-thaw problems by aliquoting reagents out the first time you use them.
- **Problems with primary antibody**:
  - Are you using the appropriate concentration? If the primary antibody is too dilute you would not get much (or any!) color. You may try a range of concentrations (e.g. 1:10, 1:100, 1:1000 dilution series) to optimize the protocol. Similarly, incubating the antibody on the slide for longer time may also be tried.

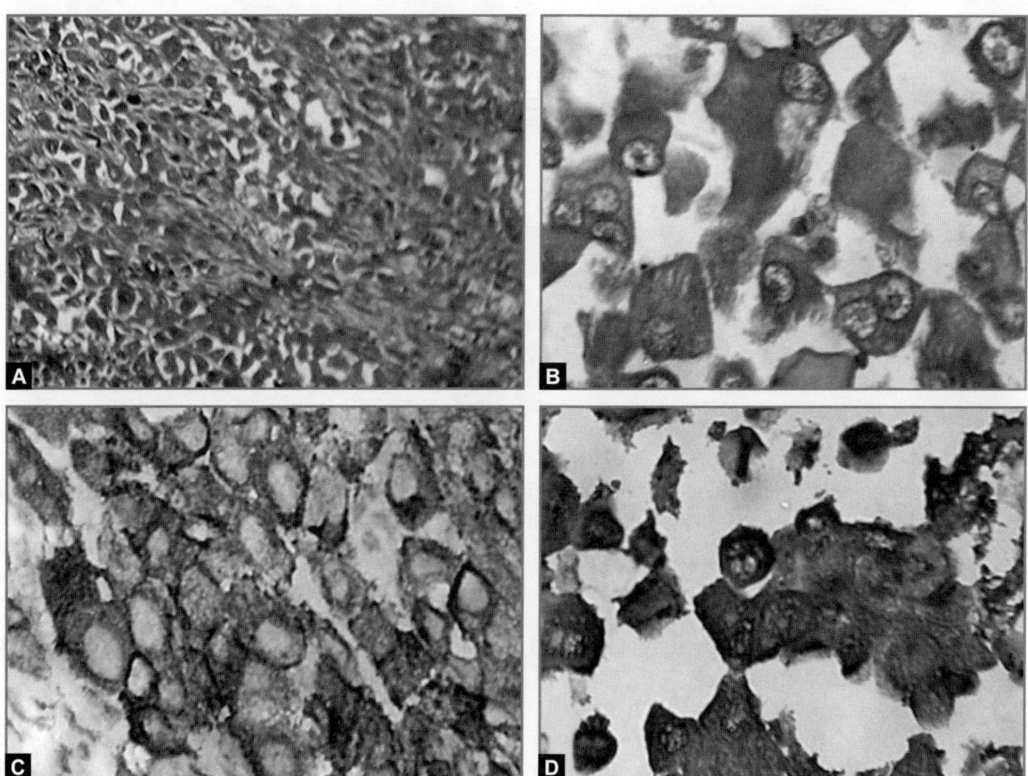

Figs 11A to D: Amelanotic melanoma (epithelioid type). (A) Microphotograph showing melanoma cells in paraffin section (H and E × 100); (B) High power view showing prominent nucleoli in melanoma cells and binucleated tumor cells (H and E × 400); (C) Immunocytochemistry on FNAC smears showing Melan A/Mart-1 positivity (cytoplasmic) in many melanoma cells; (D) Immunocytochemistry on FNAC smears showing S100 positivity (both nuclear and cytoplasmic) among tumor cells *(For color version, see Plate 8)*

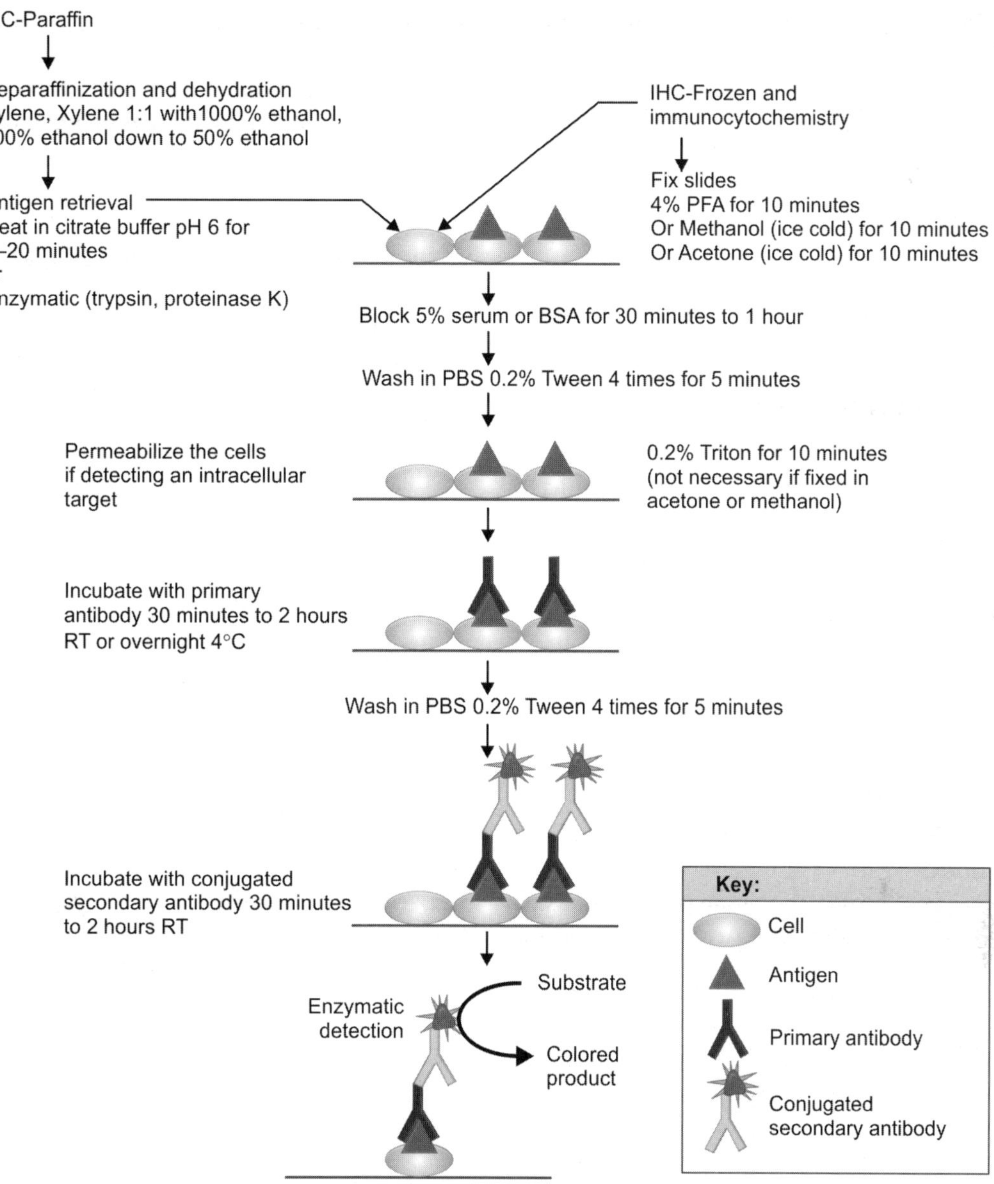
IHC-Paraffin
Deparaffinization and dehydration
Xylene, Xylene 1:1 with1000% ethanol,
100% ethanol down to 50% ethanol
Antigen retrieval
Heat in citrate buffer pH 6 for
5–20 minutes
or
Enzymatic (trypsin, proteinase K)
IHC-Frozen and
immunocytochemistry
Fix slides
4% PFA for 10 minutes
Or Methanol (ice cold) for 10 minutes
Or Acetone (ice cold) for 10 minutes
Block 5% serum or BSA for 30 minutes to 1 hour
Wash in PBS 0.2% Tween 4 times for 5 minutes
Permeabilize the cells
if detecting an intracellular
target
0.2% Triton for 10 minutes
(not necessary if fixed in
acetone or methanol)
Incubate with primary
antibody 30 minutes to 2 hours
RT or overnight 4°C
Wash in PBS 0.2% Tween 4 times for 5 minutes
Incubate with conjugated
secondary antibody 30 minutes
to 2 hours RT
Key:
Cell
Antigen
Primary antibody
Conjugated
secondary antibody
Substrate
Enzymatic
detection
Colored
product

Fig. 12: IHC protocol summary

- Keep the antibodies in cold temperature, even you are not working on a particular day. Antibodies are susceptible to temperature change. Try adjusting your thermostat (if you have one), finding a constant temperature room, or borrow it for few hours.
- Is the antibody suitable for IHC? Some work better on blots than stains, but some are good all-rounders. The antibody must be indicated for IHC.

❖ **Problems with secondary antibody:** Please double-check to make sure you are using the right secondary antibody for the species your primary antibody was raised in!

❖ **Problems in dewaxing:** Check the melting point of paraffin wax as some of them have higher melting point.

❖ **Problems in hydrogen peroxide step:** Sometimes the hydrogen peroxide step to block endogenous peroxidase activity may damage the antigen. In this situation, incubate with primary antibody first, followed by the hydrogen peroxide.

❖ **Problem with antigen masking:** Fixativess used in the fixation process (particularly formalin) can cause proteins to cross-link or lose their solubility sometimes and it makes antibody binding difficult (Fig. 13). A simple step to overcome this is to (after having passed the slide through the first series of clearing agent and ethanol and washed it) submerge the slide in citrate buffer (10 mM citric acid in 1 liter of distilled water, pH 6) in a Coplin jar, and heat on high temperature in a

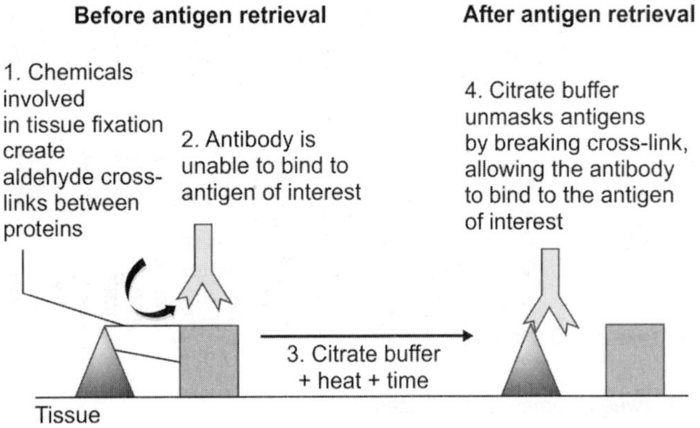

Before antigen retrieval

After antigen retrieval

1. Chemicals involved in tissue fixation create aldehyde cross-links between proteins

2. Antibody is unable to bind to antigen of interest

3. Citrate buffer + heat + time

4. Citrate buffer unmasks antigens by breaking cross-link, allowing the antibody to bind to the antigen of interest

Tissue

Fig. 13: Antigen masking and retrieval with citrate buffer to improve antibody binding

microwave for 5 minutes (if it boils do not be panic, it's normal!). Top up the citrate buffer and heat on high for 5 minutes again. Then leave the slide to cool for about 20 minutes and wash twice in 1X PBS. Continue with the protocol as normal after that.

- If someone tries all these solutions to problems and still gets nothing, then maybe fixed tissue simply does not express this protein much.

2. Problem: Everything is Brown, No Blue/Other Color!

Possible Solutions

When everything goes brown, the tissue is called 'toasted'. This is basically giving you too strong a background signal, so you need to try and improve desire signal (brown) to noise (blue hematoxylin) ratio.

- Primary antibody problem:
  - Excess primary antibody (above than required concentration). This is the most common cause of toasted slides. Diluting it as per instruction.
  - Are you incubating for too long? Or is the laboratory very hot? Adjust the incubation time and the room temperature.
- **Blocking the slide as you incubate with the primary:** Blocking with 1% BSA in PBS will help to reduce non-specific background binding. If this still is not helping, perhaps introduce a separate blocking step where you incubate with 5% BSA for an hour before adding the primary.
- **Has the hydrogen peroxide step been carried out?:** This is really important. The hydrogen peroxide block any peroxidase enzyme that is naturally found in the tissue which would otherwise react with the DAB chromagen at the end stages of the protocol and give a false-positive (Fig. 14).

Reduce incubation times for your secondary antibody and streptavidin-HRP complex.

Most of the kits only specify 20–30 minute incubations, so anything longer than this might be causing problems.

- Problem: Tissue looks cracked/glassy and trouble focusing it under the microscope.

Possible solutions: This is usually due to poor tissue preparation. Try to stick to the right tissue preparation protocol. The problem may be due to thicker sections, sliding of the coverslip on top of the tissue or drying out the tissue. Fix the problem as the case may be.

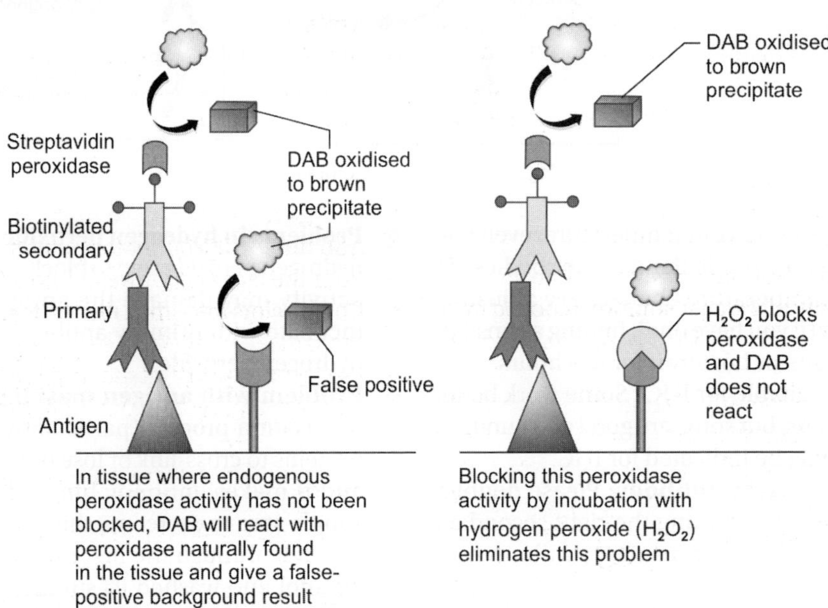
Streptavidin peroxidase
Biotinylated secondary
Primary
Antigen
DAB oxidised to brown precipitate
False positive
In tissue where endogenous peroxidase activity has not been blocked, DAB will react with peroxidase naturally found in the tissue and give a false-positive background result
DAB oxidised to brown precipitate
H_2O_2 blocks peroxidase and DAB does not react
Blocking this peroxidase activity by incubation with hydrogen peroxide (H_2O_2) eliminates this problem

Fig. 14: Blocking endogenous peroxidase activity with hydrogen peroxide helps eliminate background staining

CHAPTER 16

Cell Block and Diagnostic Cytopathology

INTRODUCTION

Cell blocks (CB) can be prepared from fluid specimen of all types like effusions, fine needle washings, endometrial aspirates and brush sample.

PREPARATION OF CELL BLOCK USING AGAR

Firstly, prepare 2% agar (12 g powdered agar dissolved in 100 mL of distilled water). Then proceed for the following steps:

- Keep the specimen (fluid, washings, aspirates) in a conical tube for centrifugation and obtain cell button.
- Centrifuge the sample for 5–10 minutes at 2000 rpm.
- Decant supernatant and resuspends cells in normal saline.
- Recentrifuge for 5 minutes at 2500 rpm.
- Decant the supernatant and invert the conical tube to drain.
- Warm the tube under hot water/water bath to 45°C.
- Add an equal quantity of 2% agar solution (cooked from boiling to 50°C) to the cell deposit. Agitate and mix them thoroughly.
- Centrifuge for 2–3 mintues at 1000 rpm. The agar should be solidified (if not, then wait until it solidifies).
- Cool the tube in cold water for 10–15 minutes. The solidified agar mixture will contract. Take it out. Alternatively, agar cone may be teased out by wooden orange stick.
- Place the agar cone into 10% formol-saline. Wait for 60–90 minutes, so that the agar transform into irreversible gel.
- Proceed for section by microtome (after paraffin embedding).

PREPARATION OF CELL BLOCK USING THROMBIN AND PLASMA

- Prepare supernatant by centrifuging the sample for 5–10 mintues at 2000 rpm.
- Decant supernatant and resuspends cells in normal saline.
- Recentrifuge for 5 minutes at 2500 rpm.
- Decant the supernatant and invert the conical tube to drain.
- Add 2–3 drops of plasma to the sediment. Mix the two together (Plasma is collected from blood bank or may be collected individually).
- Add 3–4 drops of thrombin solution to the mixture. Mix again.
- Leave the mixture to clot (take only few seconds).
- Add tinted 10% buffer formalin to the clot.
- Pour the clot and formalin into a Petri dish.
- Cut the clots into small pieces by small scissor and allow them to fix in 10% buffer formalin for 30–40 minutes.
- Process the clot as tissue fragments and cut sections by microtome after paraffin embedding (Figs 1A and B).

POINTS TO REMEMBER

- Sometime the fluid, aspirate or other specimen contain a voluminous clot unless it is anticoagulated. The neoplastic cells may get entrapped within this clot. Consequently smears prepared from the remaining

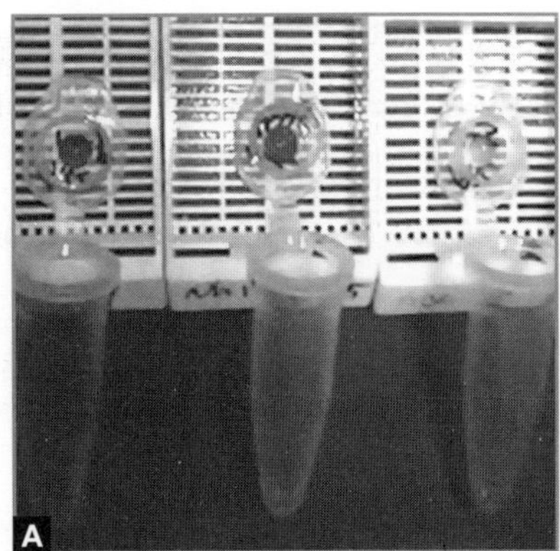

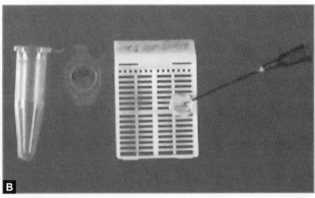

Figs 1A and B: (A) Specimens are taken into eppendorf tube for centrifugation; (B) After centrifugation and fixation, materials are placed into a cassette for paraffin embedding and processing

fluid may be devoid of neoplastic cells of interest. On the contrary the spontaneously formed clot frequently revealed numerous, obvious neoplastic cells. So, use of this clot in cell block has diagnostic value.

- The discrepancy between positive cell block and negative smears is explained by the fluid's spontaneously and rapidly clotting before the specimen was processed resulting in entrapment of neoplastic cells in clot. Such spontaneously formed clot when processed in cell blocks appears as dense, deep magenta and often containing laminated fibrin. But the induced clot of the sediment obtained after centrifugation has delicate fibrin thread.
- The fibrin if spontaneously formed clot had enough time to form and contract, hence become dense. But the fibrin in induced clot does not get enough time as it is fixed within few seconds or minutes in formalin.
- The formalin used to fix the cell block should be tinted by adding small amount of eosin. It will give pink orange color to the fixed tissue. When it is embedded in paraffin, then the task become easier for the histotechnologist to cut paraffin sections.

USE OF CELL BLOCK

- Cell block (CB) technique has several advantages compared to the cytologic routine smear: preservation of cell architecture, achievement of routine hematoxylin-eosin (H and E) staining equivalent to that surgical samples.
- CB allows the availability of an adequate number of serial sections, with increased possibility to detect malignant cells, reactive non-neoplastic elements, other diagnostic cells or even pathogenic organisms.
- Cell block often reveals patterns of neoplastic cells like papillary pattern, acinar pattern, duct like formations, etc. Psammoma bodies and other calcific concretions are also well demonstrated in cell block which are difficult/impossible to find in the permanent smear.
- Cell block may reveal other tissue materials which are extremely rare on permanent smears, like cholesterol clefts, granulation tissue, etc.
- Cell blocks also offer materials for IHC, histochemical stains, in situ hybridization studies and molecular studies.

NORMAL SALINE RINSE METHOD

It is one of the commonly used methods for cell block (CB) preparation. Rinse the fine needle aspirates in 20–30 mL of normal saline and centrifuged immediately (or may be preserved in RPMI or Rosewell Park Medical Institute for future use). Then processing is done as for a tissue biopsy.

Alternatively, the aspirates or fluid may be rinsed directly in 10 mL of 50% ethanol or in 10 mL of formation or paraformaldehyde.

FIFTY PERCENT ETHANOL RINSE METHOD

The needles and syringes are rinsed in 10 mL of 50% ethanol into a special container. Then the content is centrifuged in a 10 mL disposable centrifuge tube at 4000 rpm for 6 minutes to create 1–2 cell pellets. The supernatant fluid is decanted and the pelleted material obtained by sedimentation is immediately fixed in a freshly prepared solution of 4% neutral buffered formalin for 45 minutes. After that, the cell pellets are placed in a cassette and stored at 80% ethanol until they are processed (automatic tissue processor/manual).

TISSUE COAGULUM CLOT METHOD

In this method, there is no saline or ethanol rinse. It allows the blood and clot of tissue within the lumen of the needle to form the coagulum. When the coagulum comes out from

Table 1: Comparison of commonly used methods in cell block (CB)

Name of the method	*Advantage(s) of the method*	*Disadvantage(s) of the method*	*Use(s)*	*IHC and molecular studies*
1. Agar method	• Cheap • Better orientation of CB	• Heat-related artifacts if not properly cooled (shrunken cells, dense/frayed cytoplasm, large vacuoles)	Any fluid or FNA specimen	IHC: Optimal result. Molecular studies: suitable
2. Plasma-thrombin method	• Optimal morphology • Simple and cheap • Cleaner background for ancillary studies	• Uneven cell concentration • Cross-contamination	Good for FNAs, serous fluid, LBC, washings and cell suspension without formalin fixation	IHC: Optimal result. Molecular studies: Optimal result
3. Normal saline needle rinse method	• Rapid and easy method	• Cellular yield variable	Any type of FNAs	IHC: Suitable before agar or plasma-thrombin CB Molecular studies: Commonly used and recommended
4. Ethanol rinse method	• Simple and easy technique	• Cellular yield variable	Any type FNAs	Suitable
5. Tissue coagulum	• Minimally diluted and disrupted tissue clot	• Variable cellularity	FNAs with smaller amount of material	IHC and molecular studies: Satisfactory
6. Cellienttm automated method	• Good nuclear and cellular morphology • High cellular yield • Even distribution of cells at face of CB • No cross-contamination • Lesser time required	• High cost of machine and other reagents • Trained stuffs to make thin blocks • Poor hormone receptors (ER, PR, HER2) and Mib1 staining in IHC	• Cervical LBC • Specimen with low-cellularity	IHC: Not suitable for all molecular studies: Excellent as it provides high quality DNA and RNA
7. Shandon cytoblock method	• Small/tiny fragments of tissue can be processed	• High cost	• FNAs, curettages, body fluid with less cellular yield	IHC: Suitable. Molecular study: Not known because of limited data

Abbreviations: FNA, fine needle aspirate; LBC, liquid-based cytology; IHC, immunohistochemistry.

the needle tip, it is collected onto a filter paper. Now, the coagulum is air-dried slightly to preserve cell morphology and not to be fully air-dried. The tissue coagulum is placed into a formalin container and processed as for a tissue biopsy. The most commonly used methods in cell block are compared in Table 1.

CELLIENT™ AUTOMATED CELL BLOCK SYSTEM

This automated technique allows achieving higher cellularity and better cellular presentation in terms of architecture and details. Also, it is faster and more reliable due to operator dependency. Gorman and Coll, showed that Cellient cell block gives an adequate cellularity in all analyzed cases but formalin and thrombin CBs show a progressively decreasing adequacy. The main drawback of Cellient system is its methanol-based fixation, which has a negative effect on immunohistochemistry (IHC). In fact a weaker IHC staining pattern is noted for ER, PR, HER2 and Mib1/Ki-67. To overcome this problem, formalin pre-fixation prior to Cellient technique may be tried. Thirty minutes prefixation is preferred than longer fixation to obtain good morphology.

SHANDON CYTOBLOCK METHOD

In this method, the cells are concentrated by centrifugation in a Thermo Shandon Cytospin using Cytoblock cassette and reagents which are provided along with the kit.

FIXATIVES USED IN CBS

- **Formalin fixative:** Formalin has been used to fix FNA rinses and is considered as 'the poor man's CB' as it does not require special reagent or equipment. Alternatively, body fluid or FNA rinses may be cetrifused to obtain cell pellet, then the pellet is mixed with an equal mixture of 10% formalin and 95% ethanol. Again, it is recentrifuged to get cell button. Formalin is widely used as an universal fixative. It is good for morphology as well as IHC. But 4% neutral buffered formalin fixation for 45 minutes is better choice. It is suitable for certain immunomarkers like hormone receptors, and other nuclear antigens such as Ki-67, PCNA and p53.
- **Alcohol fixative:** An 80% ethanol is good storage of cell pellets until processing is done. ThinPrep LBC uses 50% methanol whereas the Cellient system uses methanol as

a fixative. SurePath uses 21.7% ethanol, 1.2% methanol and 1.1% isopropanol as fixative. Alcohol gives good morphology but inhibits S-100 and hormone receptor markers in IHC (Figs 2A and B).

- **Microwave fixation:** Limited data is available regarding the use of it in CB preparation. It can expedite the overall process of CB preparation and can reduce the turnaround time significantly. It gives good morphology and satisfactory IHC results (Figs 3A to D).
- **Heavy metal fixatives (Zenker's, B5):** They give optimal morphological characterization but are hazardous. Rarely, used nowadays. Zenker's fluid is ideal for

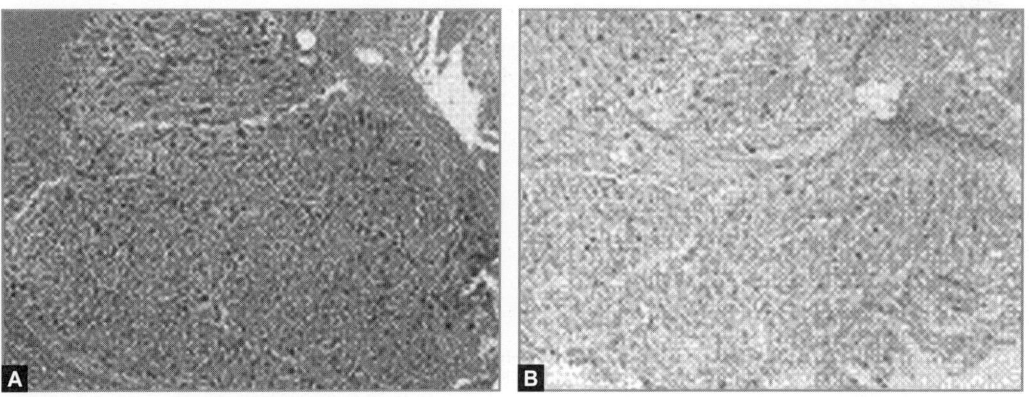

Figs 2A and B: (A) Cell block showing fascicles of spindle cell proliferation in GIST (hematoxylin and eosin stain, 100x magnification); (B) Immunohistochemistry of cell block demonstrating c-kit/CD117 positivity (100x magnification) *(For color version, see Plate 9)*

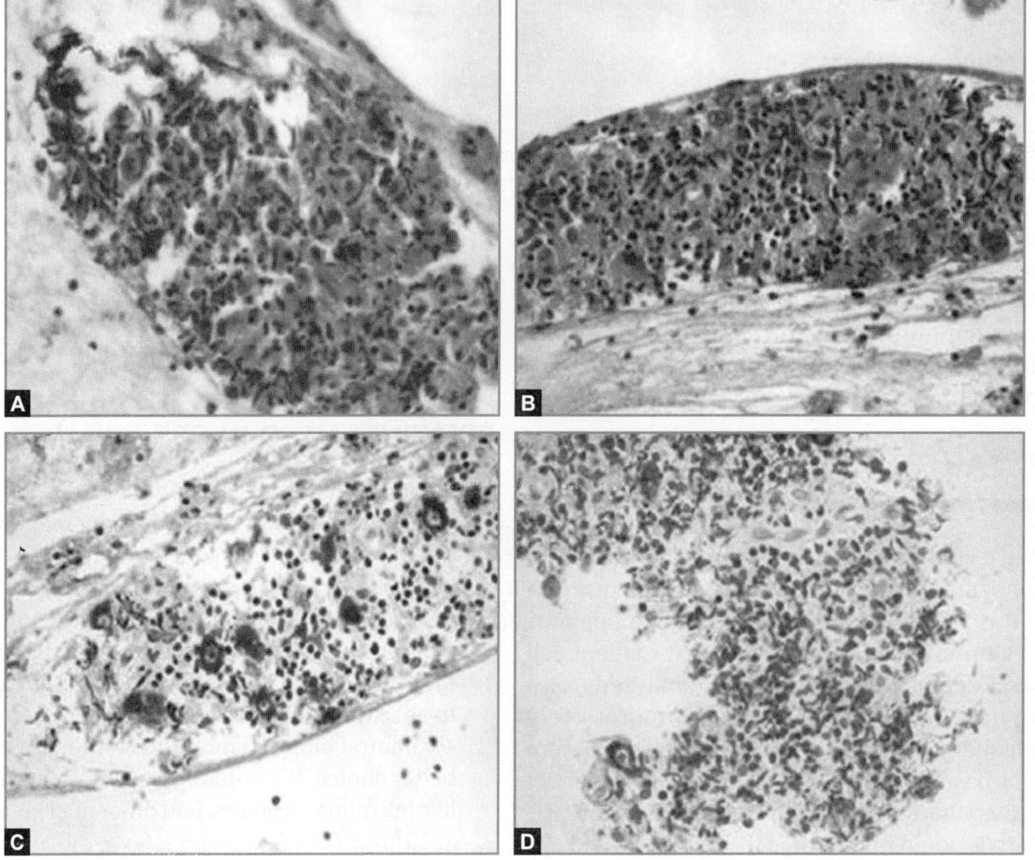

Figs 3A to D: A case of Hodgkin's lymphoma that was diagnosed by FNA. (A and B) showing the cell block of this case that contains few Reed-Sternberg (RS) cells. The cells were immunoreactive for CD 15 (C) and CD 30 (D) and were negative for CD 45 and CD 20, confirming the diagnosis *(For color version, see Plate 9)*

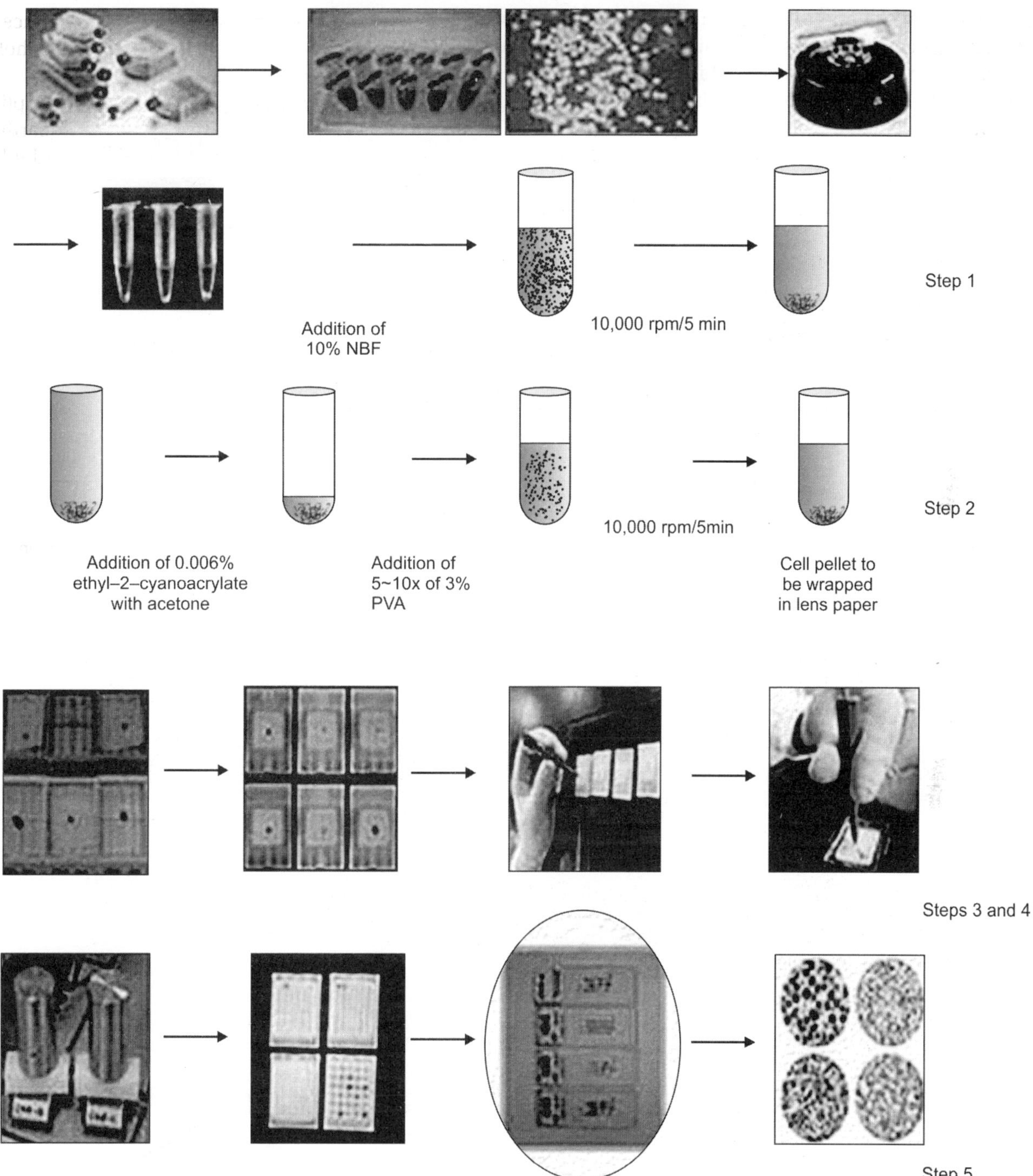

Fig. 4: The method for preparing paraffin block, wherein the spontaneous infiltration process is performed by treating the aggregated sample sediment wrapped by paper with alcohol, xylene, and paraffin sequentially

hemorrhagic specimens. B5 is considered fixative of choice for IHC.

- **Nathan alcohol formalin substitute (NAFS):** NAFS consisting of 9 parts of 100% ethanol and 1 part of 40% formaldehyde or formalin. Fresh working solution of formalin is desired as formalin is capable of oxidizing to formic acid after exposure to air and reacting with blood to form acid hematin pigment artifacts. The fixed cell pellets, at the end of 45 minutes' fixation, were recentrifuged at 4000 rpm for 6 minutes. These pellets should detach themselves or can be taken out easily with a disposable Pasteur pipette following centrifugation. The cell pellets were wrapped in crayon paper and placed in a cassette. It is stored in 80% ethanol until ready for processing. The cell pellets are processed with paraffin to obtain good cytomorphology with less toxicity (Fig. 4).

EMBEDDING AND PARAFFIN SECTIONS

After fixation, whatever is the method; clots and/or precipitates are embedded in paraffin at 56°C to realize cell blocks which are cut at 3 μm thickness. These sections are routinely stained with H and E or mounted on poly-L-lysine coated glasses for IHC.

SHORT SCHEDULE FOR AUTOMATIC TISSUE PROCESSING FOR CELL BLOCKS (13 HOURS)

- 80% ethanol with one change: 2.5 hours
- 95% ethanol: 1 hour
- 100% ethanol, four changes: 4 hours (1 hour each)
- 1:1 ethanol/xylene: 1 hour
- Xylene, three changes: 3 hours (1 hour each)
- Paraffin wax at 60°C: 1 hour
- Paraffin wax at 60°C
- Vacuum impregnation at 20 pounds: 0.5 hour.

CHAPTER 17

Plastic/Resin Embedding Media

INTRODUCTION

Paraffin wax is the most common embedding media used in histopathology. They are useful for embedding most surgical specimens and section thickness of 4–5 μm is easily cut. But there are few areas where paraffin is unsuitable as embedding medium and use of plastic/resin offers significant advantages:

- Some substances are labile, e.g. enzymes which are destroyed easily during paraffin embedding. In these cases, plastic or resin embedding media offers great help.
- Paraffin wax does not support if sections are required to cut at 1–2 μm thickness. In fact, paraffin embedded tissues cannot be sectioned at a <2 μm thickness. Practically, even with experts' hand a thickness of 3 μm can be sectioned.
- For some tissues, e.g. extremely hard tissue is unsuitable for embedding media and paraffin does not offer sufficient support during microtome sectioning.

So, in order to cut semi-thin (2–3 μm) and ultrathin (30–80 nm) sections, it is necessary to embed the tissues in plastic/resins. There are three main areas where plastic/resins are used.

1. Electron (Ultrastructural) microscopy: Paraffin and other standard waxes are unsuitable for ultrastructural (electron-microscopic) studies, because they are unable to withstand the high energy electron beams which passes through the sections in electron microscope. Moreover, they cannot cut ultra-thin sections (approximately 30–80 mm) which are required for electron microscope examinations. The use of plastic/resins for ultrastructural studies was advocated by Nunn (1970) and Glauert (1987).

2. High resolution light microscopy: Some tissues need to be cut at 2–3 μm thickness to detect certain histological or cytological changes, e.g. kidney, bone marrow/trephine and lymph node biopsies. These semi-thin plastic/resin sections (2 μm thickness) when seen under light microscope using high quality optics, can reveal subtle changes. The high-resolution light microscopy can detect certain nuclear and cytoplasmic characteristics which are usually obscured in thicker sections (usual 4–5 μm paraffin sections). More thinner sections (0.5–1 μm) when seen under these high resolution light microscopy, will be very useful to find certain features which are undetected in conventional paraffin sections. In fact, high resolution light microscopy of these thinner (0.5–1 μm) sections has diagnostic value and is very common practice prior to ultra-thin (30–80 nm) sectioning for electron microscopic examination.

3. Very hard tissues: When dealing with very hard tissue, e.g. undecalcified bone, sectioning is practically impossible using paraffin wax embedding medium. Because the hardness of paraffin wax is lesser than the undecalcified (cortical) bone. Hence, paraffin cannot provide adequate support during sectioning. Sectioning of these very hard tissues (without decalcification) is possible using a harder embedding medium, i.e. plastic/resin embedding medium. Sectioning of these extremely hard tissues can be done in two ways:

- **Motorized microtome:** Instead of conventional rotary microtome a special motorized microtome is used.
- **Ground section:** Here slices of embedded tissues are taken firstly. Then thinner sections of required thickness (ground sections) are made from slices. These ground

sections are needed if some inorganic materials like stent or teeth are to be cut.

CLASSIFICATION OF PLASTIC MEDIA

Plastics are classified in three groups:

1. Epoxy resin
2. Acrylic resin
3. Polyester.

Composition

Plastics are basically macromolecules called polymers. These polymers are made up of several monomers (small units). Apart from polymer (monomers) many different ingredients are present in plastics to make these plastics suitable as an embedding media. The process of joining different molecules to produce these complex macromolecules is called polymerization. This transforms the physical state of the embedding medium from liquid to solid.

EPOXY RESINS/PLASTICS

The name epoxy comes from the epoxide (oxirane) groups which are present in these plastics. These active groups can join in single or multifunctional conformations to infinite number in a chemical structure. These epoxy plastics when polymerized are hard enough to cut sections as thin as 30–40 nm. Epoxy embedding plastics are a balanced mixture of epoxy plastic, accelerator and catalyst. Anhydride/amine type is used as catalyst and they cause curing (treatment of tissue) of the resin to form ester cross-links and polymers. Mono or poly functional amines are used as accelerators. Presently, three types of epoxy plastics are in use:

1. Glycerol (Epon)
2. Bisphenol A (Araldite)
3. Cyclohexene dioxide (Spurr).

The glycerol (Epon) plastics have lower viscosity while cyclohexane dioxide (Spurr) plastics infiltrate fastest when used as embedding media.

Use of Temperature

Infiltration of plastics into tissue can be augmented by application of heat or curing (treatment of tissue). Rapid curing at 120°C for 1 hour cause numerous cross links required for polymerization. But it also makes tissue fragmented and brittle. Tissue if cured at 60°C for 18 hours makes tougher blocks which are good for sectioning and subsequent microscopy. If cured tissue/block is very hard, then sodium methoxide can be used to soften it (it reduces the cross-links by transesterifying the already formed ester cross-links).

Disadvantages of Epoxy Plastics

Many epoxy plastics contain harmful ingredient which are toxic. Some of them like vinyl cyclohexane dioxide (VCD) are even carcinogenic.

Epoxide group anhydrides present in these plastics can react with proteins which may cause reduction in antigenecity. Epoxy plastics are hydrophic (insoluble in water). So, subsequent application of peroxide to correct this (by oxidation) may result in tissue damage.

Section Cutting

Thinner sections of 0.5–1 μm thickness cannot be cut on a standard (rotary) microtome using steel knife. These semi-thin (2 μm) or thinner sections (0.5–1 μm) are cut on a motorised microtome using diamond or glass knife.

Staining

Toluidine blue: It is the most useful and informative stain for epoxy-embedded tissue sections. The rate of penetration of this stain can be increased using high alkaline pH or heat. The staining intensity depends on the electron densities of different tissue components; hence it can predict the subsequent electron microscopic examinations.

Paragon and other polychromatic stains: It resembles hematoxylin and eosin stain, used in paraffin embedded sections. Pretreatment with alcoholic sodium-hydroxide (etching) and oxidizing osmium tetroxide fixed tissue without etching have been suggested by some to get consistent staining. Jane (1979) advocated successful staining of 1–2 μm spurr resin sections following etching by hematoxylin and phloxine, inter alia, geulgen, PAS, phloxine, tartrazine, etc.

ACRYLIC RESINS/PLASTICS

These are made up of either esters of acrylic acid or more commonly methacrylic acid, which are known as acrylates and methacrylates respectively.

Many mixes are made to alter the properties of the acrylic plastics and is used for different reasons. Methyl, butyl, glycol methacrylate were mixed in the past for electron microscopy. But as the plastics/resins disrupt electron beam they are not used nowadays. To prevent premature polymerization, hydroquine is added. Formation of radicals occurs in light and temperature, so acrylic plastics should be stored in dark bottles.

Many catalysts are used, e.g. benzoyl peroxide, Perkadox 16 and azobisisobutyronitrile. Also, some amines and other activators or accelators are also added like sulfonic acid and barbiturates. Softner or plasticizers are added to make sectioning easier, e.g. 2-butoxyethanol, polyethylene glycol, dibutyl phthalate and 2-isopropoxyethanol. Nevertheless, all polymers of acrylic plastics contain monomer 2-hydroxyethyl methacrylate (HEMA).

To make acrylic plastics, it is first cured. Then the monomer is exposed to a catalyst (usually benzoyl peroxide) to produce radicals from its breakdown products. This radical is decomposed to form phenyl radical which breaks down the double bond of monomer. This behaves as an active site and monomers join one after another to form a large chain of polymer. Finally, a phenyl radical is attached to stop it and complete the polymerization process.

Poly Glycol methacrylate (GMA) or 2-hydroxyethyl methacrylate is a very popular medium for light microscopy. Because it is tough enough to make good sections after dehydration and also it allows many tinctorial staining methods as it is hydrophilic (water soluble). For undecalcified bone, stents or implants and other tissues, methyl methacrylate (MMA) is most popular. Because MMA provides enough support as an embedding medium and MMA itself is very hard.

APPLICATION OF ACRYLIC PLASTICS

Acrylic plastics can be used as embedding medium for both light microscopy and electron microscopy. As for example, LR white and unicryl can be used for both light and electron microscopy.

Some plastics like GMA and LR white are hydrophilic and allow sections to be stained without removal of the plastic embedding medium.

Tinctorial Staining

As already stated, GMA, LR white and other hydrophilic acrylics can be used for staining without removing the plastics. Many histologic stains can be applied to these sections, like H and E, PAS, reticulin stain, Van Gieson, Alcian blue, Giemsa, Perls' stain, etc. But not only the embedded tissues but also the plastic embedding medium may also become stained. To overcome this problem, various washing procedures are followed.

The plastic MMA can be removed before staining by some similar procedures used routinely to dewax the paraffin sections. But it needs slightly more time than paraffin dewaxing.

Enzyme Histochemistry

As some acrylic plastics can be processed, embedded and polymerized at low temperature, it allows many enzymes to retain its activity and to be stained in tissue sections. Many enzymes can be demonstrated like acid phosphatise, succinate dehydrogenase, NADH, alkaline phosphatase, lactate dehydrogenase, nonspecific esterase, sucrase, peroxidase, glucose-6-phosphatase, adenosine triphosphate, etc.

Prior to histochemical staining, fixation, processing and polymerization are done at 4°C. Sections are dried on to a slide or cover glass at room temperature rather than at 60°C. As fixative, 10% formal calcium is very good. Subsequent washing in 3% buffered sucrose solution at 4°C improves the staining quality.

Immunohistochemistry

Although immunohistochemistry (IHC) has been tried and more than 100 antibodies have been demonstrated, IHC staining in plastic sections is a controversial topic. Many of these results are unreliable. The reasons are:

- Many of the acrylics are insoluble in polymerized form.
- Low density of the optical density of the chromogen DAB 3, 3-diaminobenzide.
- Inconsistencies in processing time and temperature.

An alternative method using MMA plastic has been accepted. Here, the acrylic MMA is water-soluble when it is polymerized. It can be removed prior to staining during IHC procedure.

POLYESTER PLASTICS

It is rarely used nowadays and has been replaced by superior epoxy resins/plastics. Polyester plastics were used in the mid-1950 for electron microscopy.

PROCESSING AND EMBEDDING FOR METHYL METHACRYLATE

Reagents (Solution)

- Methyl methacrylate monomer: 75 mL
- Dibutyl phthalate: 25 mL
- Dried benzoyl peroxide: 5g

Fixative: 10% formal-calcium, 10% formalin or 10% formal-saline for 1–2 days.

Processing and Embedding Process

- Dehydrate in ascending alcohol, 50%, 70% and 90% alcohol each 1 hour duration. (average block size of 10 × 5 × 2 mm).
- Dehydrate in 100% or absolute alcohol, two changes of 1 hour duration.
- Immerse in reagent (solution) for 1 hour, two changes.

- Immerse in the solution and keep it overnight.
- Now, embed this tissue to mixture which contains 10 mL of reagent (solution) and 125 µl of N, N-dimethylaniline. Polymerization of the MMA will be completed within 3–4 hours.
- Now, embed this tissue to mixture which contains 10 mL of reagent (solution) and 125 µl of N-N-dimethylaniline. Polymerization of the MMA will be completed within 3–4 hours.

PROCESSING AND EMBEDDING FOR LR WHITE

LR white is commercially supplied as hard, medium and soft. One has to choose depending on the hardness of the tissue to be processed.

Fixative

Formalin (10% formalin saline, 10% neutral buffered) or buffered paraformaldehyde.

Processing and Embedding

- Dehydrate through ascending grade alcohol, 70%, 90% and 100%, two changes in each solution and duration of each 15–20 minutes.
- Infiltrate in LR white overnight or 3 changes each 60–90 minutes (depending upon the hardness of tissue, i.e. hard tissue needs overnight infiltration).
- Polymerize using curing, either by heat or by cold. For heat curing place the moulds at 55–60°C for 20–24 hours in an incubator. For cold curing, add 1 mL of accelator to 10 mL of plastic. Usually, polymerization is complete within 15–20 minutes.

PROCESSING AND EMBEDDING FOR GLYCOL METHACRYLATE

Fixative

A 10% neutral buffered formalin, 10% formal saline or buffered paraformaldehyde.

Reagents

- Solution a:
  - 2- hydroxyethyl (glycol) methacrylate: 40 mL
  - 2- butoxyethanol: 8 mL
  - Benzoyl peroxide (dried): 135 mg
- Solution b:
  - N,N-dimethylaniline: 1 part
  - Polyethylene glycol 400: 15 parts.

Processing and Embedding

- Rinse in appropriate buffer (e.g. phosphate buffer) if necessary for 10–15 minutes.
- Dehydrate through graded alcohol, 70%, 90% and 100% ethanol, two changes each 15–20 minutes duration (average block size 10 × 5 × 2 mm).
- Infiltrate in solution a, two changes each for 1 hour.
- Embed in the mixture of solution a and solution b in the ratio of 42:1.
- Leave it at room temperature to polymerize. Standing the mould in cold water will make it cool (heat is generated by the reaction). Polymerization is completed within 2–4 hours.

Points to Remember for All the above Embedding Processes

- The reagents/solutions are prepared in the quantity required. After use, waste solutions should be properly discarded.
- Processing is best done, if the specimens are continuously agitated on a rolling mixture.
- Care should be taken during handling of benzoyl peroxide, which is an explosive. The dry powder should be dissolved in the solution within 30 minutes.
- For good polymerization , the moulds should be placed in oxygen-free environment. It is best done by placing the moulds inside glass dessicator and filling the chamber with oxygen-free nitrogen which creates an oxygen free environment.

SECTIONING CUTTING OF ACRYLIC RESIN/ PLASTIC EMBEDDED SPECIMENS

- Semi-thin sections (2–3 µm) of Glycol methacrylate (GMA), Methyl methacrylate (MMA) and LR white of better quality can be achieved using a glass knife on a motorized microtome. Steel knife on a rotary microtome cannot produce good quality sections.
- GMA sections are flattened by just floating on water at room temperature. MMA sections are flattened by placing the section on a water-bath at 65–70°C. LR white sections are placed on a hot plate at 60°C or they may be floated out on 70% alcohol.
- For plastic sections, 2% APES is a very good adhesive.

STAINING OF ACRYLIC RESIN/PLASTIC SECTIONS

GMA and LR white sections can be stained without removing the plastics. But MMA sections need removal of plastic embedding medium before staining. This is done by placing the slides in xylene for 10–20 minutes at 37°C. H and E stain is good for these sections.

H and E Staining Protocols

- Stain the slides in Harris or alum hematoxylin for 10–20 minutes.
- Wash in tap water for 1–5 minutes.
- Differentiate in 1% acid alcohol (hydrochloric acid) just few dips.
- Blueing in tap water for 5–10 minutes
- Wash in water for 10–15 minutes.
- Counterstain in eosin solution (1% aqueous eosin in 1% calcium-chloride) for 3–5 minutes.
- Rinse in tap water for 30 seconds.
- Blot and make the slides dry.
- Rinse in ethanol for 20–30 seconds.
- Rinse in xylene and mount in DPX.

Note:

- For MMA sections, stain the slides in hematoxylin for 30–40 minutes and in 1% buffered eosin for 5 minutes.
- For LR white sections, omit steps 3 to 9.

BASIC TECHNIQUES FOR EMBEDDING AND SECTIONING PLASTICS/RESINS

Though most techniques need to be embedded in plastics for semi-thin sections, few specimens may not require it. If the specimen is stable enough and a direct clamping device is available, the specimens can be placed in the specimen holder without plastic embedding. This is called **foil clamping system**. If the specimen is not stable enough then it has to be embedded to increase the overall stability.

In most cases, average size of sample would be 1 × 0.5 × 0.2 cm, though sample of maximum length of 1.5 cm can be processed. Larger size specimen may be cut by a rotary microtome. But sectioning of hard tissue is not possible by a rotary microtome. In this case, a heavy duty microtome for hard and large sections can be used. These microtomes have high cutting forces and special knife holders designed to achieve maximum stability. Still the hardness of MMA embedded specimens allows a rotary microtome to make sections.

For sectioning hard materials, knives with a large wedge angle are suitable. For soft materials, it is just the opposite. Majority of plastic embedded tissues can be cut best at knife angles between 20–45°. The clearance angle on knife holder should be around 5–10° which must be tested prior to serial sectioning.

Tungsten carbide knives or Tungsten carbide disposable blades are used successfully for plastic sectioning in most of the cases. For very small samples/specimens, glass knives are suitable as they produce higher quality sections when cutting <1 μm thick sections. But diamond knife offers an even better quality sections.

After sectioning, taking out the sections from knife is problematic. Because these sections tend to curl during sectioning. The sections may be collected using a small brush or carefully with forceps or with a needle. In some cases, the tap method is extremely useful and it prevents sections from rolling.

In the *tape method*, a tape is applied directly on to the plastic embedded block. After sectioning, the sections stick on the tape and they do not roll over the knife. But remember one has to use a special tape to avoid intensive colors of the tape itself in polarized light. The cutting temperature should be optimal. Some sections are to be cut at very low temperature (–100°C), e.g. elastomers and thermoplasts. In these cases liquid nitrogen is used.

CHAPTER 18

Electron Microscopy

INTRODUCTION

Electron microscopy (EM) is still an invaluable tool for the diagnosis of a wide range of diseases in various organ systems. With the advent and expansion of immunohistochemical techniques in the field of surgical pathology, the role in diagnostic pathology has became selective.

The IHC has several advantages over EM. IHC is more accessible through the use of commercially available kits. There is no requirement of very costly instrument and the stains are easily compared with hematoxylin-eosin sections. Also, IHC can examine many more cells then are usually studied in EM.

Recently, EM has been combined with IHC and in situ hybridization techniques. This technique allows antigen detection and localization at the subcellular level. But these methods need special fixation and processing protocols. Although immunoelectron microscopy is not routinely used in diagnostic surgical pathology and is primarily used for research laboratories; it throws a ray of hope in oncological surgical pathology. It is very promising for the identification and localization of targets for gene therapy.

TYPES OF ELECTRON MICROSCOPES

There are three types:

1. Transmission electron microscope (TEM)
2. Scanning electron microscope (SEM)
3. Analytical electron microscope (AEM).

Transmission Electron Microscope (Figs 1A and B)

This instrument relies on the passage of a beam of electrons through ultrathin sections of tissues. During staining, the sections have been impregnated with heavy metal atoms (such as uranium and osmium) which bind to different subcellular organelles. The resolution of TEMs can be as fine as 0.2 nm, but it requires a relatively low magnification, which ranges from 2,000X to 10,000X for most electron microscopic diagnoses.

Scanning Electron Microscope (Figs 2A and B)

It provides a three-dimensional view of tissues but it provides mainly views of surface component. Resolution of SEM is inferior to that of the TEM. The SEM provides excellent images of cell surface as well as topographical relationships of components of tissues. It can detect podocytes with their foot processes ensheathing capillaries in renal glomeruli.

Analytical Electron Microscope (Fig. 3)

This instrument provides information on the elemental composition of material within tissues. Many exogenous substance will incite inflammation (e.g. granulomas) or be linked to human diseases etiologically (such as silicosis, asbestosis). These substances have characteristic emission spectra which will be detected by AEM.

In diagnostic pathology, TEM is most commonly used followed by SEM. Indications for the use of TEM for pathologic diagnoses fall into following categories:

- Renal diseases
- Neoplasms
- Metabolic diseases
- Infectious diseases
- Genetic diseases
- Skeletal muscle and peripheral nerve biopsy
- Diseases of obscure nature or unknown etiology.

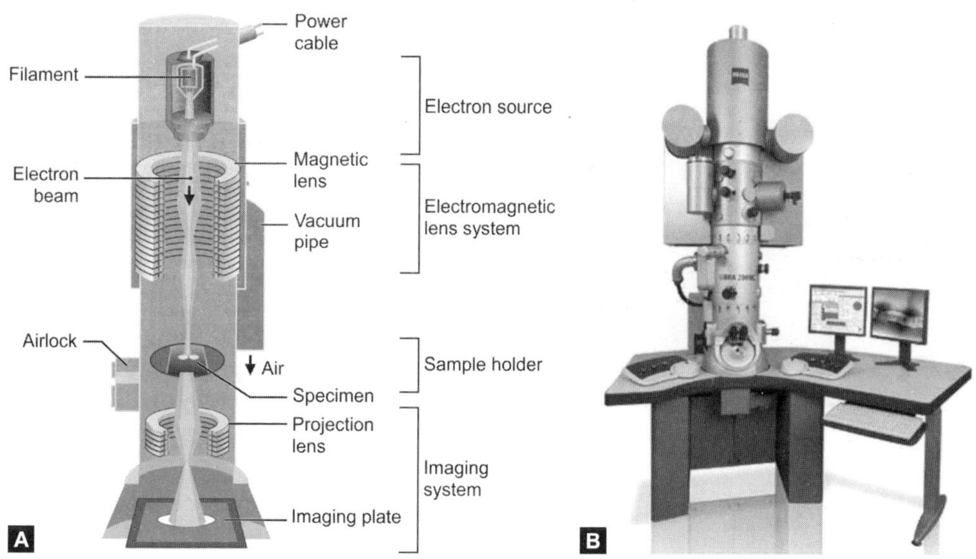

Figs 1A and B: (A) Transmission electron microscope (schematic); (B) Transmission electron microscope

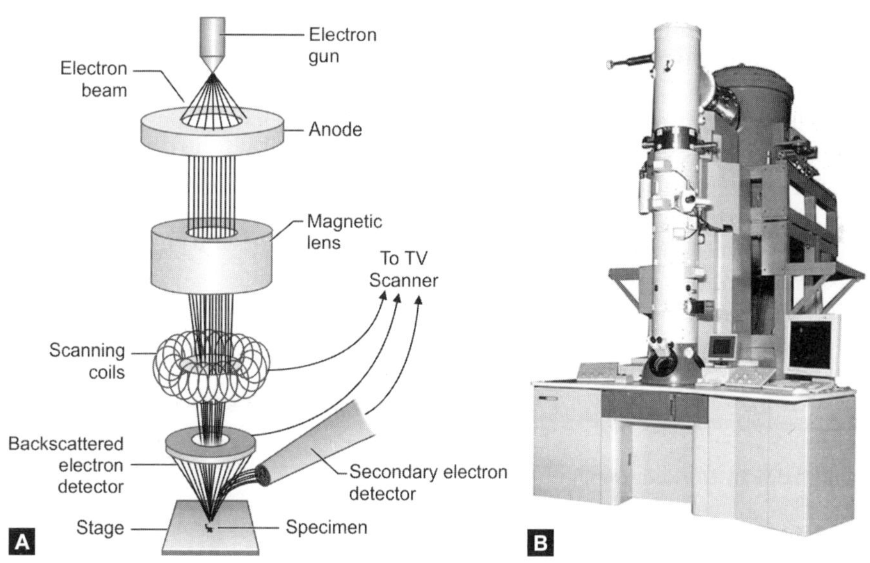

Figs 2A and B: (A) Scanning electron microscope (schematic); (B) Scanning electron microscope

RENAL DISEASES

The role of TEM in diagnosis of renal diseases is well documented. In many renal diseases, a diagnosis can not be made without use of TEM. In other instances, TEM contributes to refinement of the diagnosis (e.g. sub-classification or staging of SLE nephritis or systemic lupus nephritis) or provides crucial corroborative information. Examination of a single glomerulus by TEM may be sufficient to make a definitive disease of kidney. So, TEM examination can be ideal where there is low yield of tissue, as for example analysis of percutaneous renal biopsies.

TEM allows direct visualization and precise localization of a wide variety of primary and secondary abnormalities affecting the renal glomeruli and other component of renal parenchyma. These include:

- Immune complexes (seen as electron dense deposits).
- Intrinsic and acquired glomerular basement membrane abnormalities.
- Proteinaceous deposits.
- Subendothelial granular deposits in kappa light chain diseases.
- Amyloid fibrils in amyloidosis.

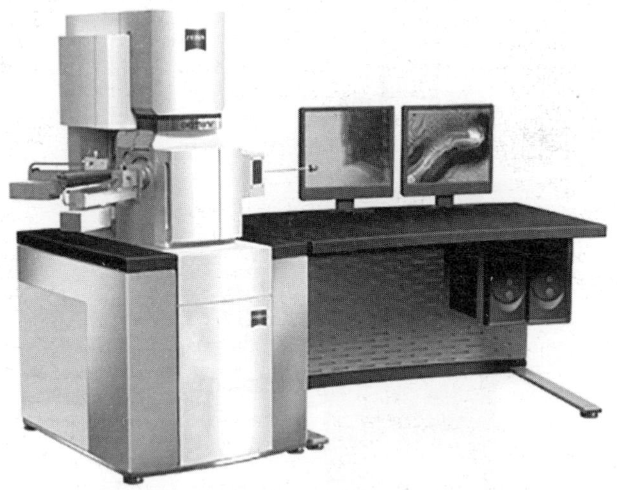

Fig. 3: Analytical electron microscope

- Cryoglobulins and other fibrillary deposits (non-amyloidotic).
- Diabetic nephropathy. Dense deposits in membrano-proliferative glomerulonephritis, type II.
- Minimal change disease.
- Hereditary nephritis/Alport's syndrome.
- Focal segmental glomerulosclerosis.
- Damage to endothelial cells (e.g. thrombotic micro-angiopathies).
- Tubuloreticular structures (most common in HIV and lupus nephritis).
- Crystals (e.g. cystine crystals in cystinosis).
- Zebra bodies (Fabry's diseases).

NEOPLASMS

Indications for the use of TEM in the diagnosis of tumors include:

- Differential diagnosis between adenocarcinoma and mesothelioma.
- Differential diagnosis between carcinoma, melanoma and sarcoma.
- Differential diagnosis of small round cell tumors of infancy which include neuroblastoma, Ewing's sarcoma/PNET, lymphoma/leukemia, Wilms' tumor, rhabdomyosarcoma, etc.
- Differential diagnosis of anterior mediastial tumors between thymoma, lymphoma, thymic carcinoid and seminoma.
- Differential diagnosis of endocrine and nonendocrine tumors.
- Poorly differentiated spindle cell neoplasms with differential diagnosis of spindle cell carcinoma, spindle cell sarcoma and spindle cell melanoma.

METABOLIC DISEASES

When metabolic storage disorders are suspected, EM may have significant role in the final diagnosis. Usually samples of liver and/or muscle and occasionally nerve are sent.

- **Glycogen storage disorders:** Excess free cytoplamic or membrane-bound glycogen may be detected within cells.
- **Neural ceroid lipofuscinosis:** Distinct inclusions are found. As for example, in the late infantile form dense curvilinear lamellar inclusions are found whereas typical finger print profiles are seen in the juvenile form.
- **Mucopolysaccharidoses:** Different types of fibro-granular and lamellar inclusions are found.

INFECTIOUS DISEASE

TEM has valuable role in the diagnosis of some viruses and other microorganisms. As for example, EM can detect intestinal cryptosporidia. Surgical specimens and paraffin sections are very rare samples for TEM. On the contrary, negative staining of fluid specimens is a rapid method to detect and structure of viruses in fluid, secretion and feces (e.g. viral capsid in the nucleus of a varicella-zoster-infected cell from pleural fluid). TEM played a pivotal role in the initial classification of human immunodeficiency virus and Hanta virus outbreak. To diagnose a viral infection, concentration of viral particles should be high (>10^5 to 10^6/mL).

GENETIC DISEASES

Here is the list of some genetic diseases.

Cell/Tissue type	*Subcellular feature*	*Use*
1. Epithelial cells	Cilia	Primary ciliary dyskinesia
2. Liver and kidney	Peroxisomes	Absence in neonatal adrenoleukodystrophy and Zellweger syndrome
3. Neurones	Lysosomes	Several types of mucopoly-saccharidoses and lipidosis
4. Hepatocytes	Lysosomes	Identification of several types of mucopolysaccharidoses

TEM is the only means to establish the presence of ciliary dysmorphology. It can also differentiate between acquired and congenital ciliary defects. The following three points should be remembered.

1. Genetic or congenital ciliary abnormality affects all cilia at all sites (diffuse involvement).
2. Acquired ciliary abnormalities are temporary and focal.
3. Some genetic ciliary abnormalities probably do not have any structural defect.

Specific ciliary defects, seen in genetic diseases include complete lack of dynein arms, defective outer dynein arm and defective ciliary spokes.

Dynein: An ATP-splitting enzyme essential to the motility of cilia and flagella because of its interactions with microtubules.

SKELETAL MUSCLE BIOPSY

Ultrastructurally, there may be nonspecific or specific changes in many muscle disorders. Nonspecific changes include myofibril loss or disarray, external lamina reduplication and Z-band streaming. Some specific changes are seen in some muscle disorder.

- **Mitochondrial myopathy**: Abnormal mitochondria (increased mitochondria size and number, crystalloids) and presence of ragged red muscle fibers (seen in modified trichrome stain).
- **Myopathy with tubular aggregates**: Presence of large number of tubular aggregates which are located in the subsarcolemmal region.
- **Inflammatory myopathy**: Undulating tubules within the endothelial cells are present apart from nonspecific myofibrilar changes.
- **Dermatomyositis**: Exocytosis of dark bodies.
- **Polymyositis**: Exocytosis of dark bodies, presence of plasma cells beneath the basement membrane of muscle fibers, lymphocytic infiltration into muscle fibers and reduplication of basal lumina (often with multiple layers).
- **Inclusion body myositis**: Characteristic abnormal filaments are present.
- **Nemaline rod myopathy**: Presence of Nemaline bodies.

PERIPHERAL NERVE BIOPSY

- **Axonal degeneration or atrophy**: Formation of columns of Schwann cells with their foot processes enclosed by basal lamina (Bands of Büngner).
- **Segmental demyelination**: Formation of 'onion bulb' which are composed of concentric layers of Schwann cells, basal lamina and collagen fibrils surrounding demyelinated and remyelinated axonal processes.
- **Krabbe's disease**: Schwann cells and endoneural macrophages contain pleomorphic electron-lucent lipid droplets.

DISEASES OF OBSCURE NATURES

Use of TEM is indicated in the study of tissues having diseases of obscure nature and/or unknown causes.

Fixatives

About 2–4% glutaraldehyde (buffered) or Karnovsky fluid (glutaraldehyde + formaldehyde). This formaldehyde or Kornovsky fluid is prepared from paraformaldehyde.

Embedding Medium

Plastic or resin like glycol methacrylate (GMA), methyl methacrylate (MMA) or epoxy resin.

Section Cutting and Staining

Refer to previous chapter of plastic/resin embedding media.

LIMITATIONS OF ELECTRON MICROSCOPY

- A very small number of cells or tissues have characteristic ultrastructural features which are unique to that cell or tissue. This paucity of specific ultrastructural features is a drawback for electron microscopic diagnosis.
- Tissue sample taken for electron microscopy is small compared to histologic examination. So, a diagnosis of neoplasm can be missed.
- If there is non-neoplastic element among neoplastic tissues and the sample is taken from this non-neoplastic element, then there will be misinterpretation under electron microscopy.

CHAPTER 19

Immunofluorescence Techniques

DEFINITION

Immunofluorescence is the laboratory technique whereby specific antibodies detect antigens, when these antibodies are directly conjugated to already identifiable fluorescent label.

FLUORESCENCE

When a light of particular wavelength is absorbed by an atom or molecule, an electron become excited and moves to higher energy level. When this displaced electron returns to its original state i.e. unexcited state, it may emit light of different wavelengths. If this light is emitted only during the time of exposure or just after exposure (9–10 seconds) then it is called **fluorescence.** But if the emission persists even after the exciting light is cut off, then it is called **phosphorescence**.

BRIEF HISTORY

Stokes first used the word 'fluorescence' in 1852, to explain the reaction of fluorspar to ultraviolet light. In 1903, RW Wood invented a filter which would absorb visible light and transmits ultraviolet light only. Subsequently, Lehmann in 1911 invented fluorescent microscope. In the year 1935, Max Haitinger described a technique using fluorescent dyes on histologic sections and smears. In 1937, Hagemann applied this technique to detect microorganism (acid fast bacilli). The present technique was first described by Coons, Creech and Jones in 1941. They described a technique for labeling protein with a fluorescent dye or fluorescent antibody staining.

Table 1: Commonly used fluorochromes and observed color (emitted light)

Fluorochome	*Wavelength of absorbing light (nm)*	*Wavelength of emitted light (nm)*	*Observed color*
1. Fluorescein isthoio cyanate (FITC)	494	518	Green
2. Tetramethyl rhodamine isothiocyanate (TRITC)	550	580	Red
3. R-phycoerythrin (PE)	565	575	Orange/red
4. Texas red	595	615	Red

The fluorochrome conjugated to antibody absorbs light of a particular wavelength to reach an unstable excited state after its electrons gain energy (Table 1). When this excited electron returns to the ground state, the fluorochrome emits light of a different, usually longer wavelength compared to excitation light. Two common fluorochromes are fluoroscein isothiocyanate (FITC) and tetramethyl rhodamine isothiocyanate (TRITC). The original work of Coons and others was an example of direct immunofluorescence (IF) technique wherein the specific primary antibody is conjugated directly with the fluorochrome and viewed under a fluorescent microscope. Weller and Coons in 1954 described the indirect technique where a specific primary antibody (unlabeled) is detected by a fluorochrome-labeled antibody (secondary antibody) in the second stage.

TECHNICAL ASPECTS

Tissue antigens which can be demonstrated by immunofluorescence (IF) are plasma proteins, enzymes, hormones, cell constituents, bacteria, protozoa and viruses. To be detected, these antigens should be insoluble in situ and they should not be denatured during procedure.

Unfixed cryostat fresh sections are preferred for this technique. If the antigens are known to be soluble, then they should be fixed with 10% cold neutral buffered formalin. Ethanol or acetone can be used as alternative fixative but they distort tissue morphology. Michel transport medium, pH 7.0 should be used for transport of biopsy tissue material.

Frozen tissue sections should be cut from unfixed fresh tissue for best result. The tissue should be snap frozen because slow freezing will cause formation of ice crystals that distort antigenic structure and tissue morphology. Frozen sections should be cut at 5–6 μm thickness. If there is a delay in section cutting then tissue should be wrapped in aluminum foil and stored at -20°C.

PROCEDURE FOR FROZEN TISSUE SECTIONS

- Place the unfixed fresh tissue on metal chuck (a small amount of OCT is already placed on it) which has been cooled to -25°C. More OCT is added on its surface before the already placed OCT and tissue freeze.
- Now the OCT and biopsy tissue is kept at -25°C for 30 minutes.
- The covering OCT is removed by sectioning 10–15 μm and the tissue material (frozen) is exposed.
- This tissue should be cut at 5 μm.
- Sections are attached to clean glass slides.
- These sections should be air-dried for 30 minutes and examined under light microscope. Check for appropriate tissue material for.

Points to Remember

- The slides can be wrapped in aluminum foil and stored at -20°C, if there is a delay in IF staining.
- For renal biopsies, sections are checked at regular intervals by staining with toluidine blue to detect the presence of glomeruli.
- For skin biopsy, sections are checked for presence of epidermal layer.

DIRECT IMMUNOFLUORESCENCE STAINING METHOD (FIG. 1A)

1. Wash sections (frozen) in 0.1 M phosphate buffered saline or PBS (three changes, 10 minutes each).
2. Drain off excess PBS and remove residual PBS by tapping the edge of the slide against a tissue paper pad.
3. Apply diluted or working strength antibody (conjugated antibody or conjugate) and incubate for 30 minutes at room temperature.
4. Drain off conjugate and wash with three changes of PBS (10 minutes each).
5. Excess PBS is drained off and removed residual PBS by tapping the edge of the slide against a pad of tissue paper.
6. The slides are mounted in buffered glycerol using cover-slips.
7. The edges of the cover slip are then sealed using nail varnish.
8. Examine the slides on a fluorescent microscope as soon as possible. The slides can be stored at 4°C. Always avoid direct sunlight.

Points to Remember

- The sections must be kept moist until they are mounted after the staining of first wash with PBS. Drying out must be avoided.
- As an alternative mountant to buffered glycol, DABCO solution or PBS may be used.

INDIRECT IMMUNOFLUORESCENCE STAINING METHOD (FIG. 1B)

1. Wash the sections (slides) in PBS for 5–10 minutes.
2. Drain off the excess PBS and remove residual PBS by tapping the edge of the slide against a pad of tissue paper.
3. Flood the section with working strength antibody (primary antibody) and keep for 30 minutes.
4. Wash the slides in PBS for 10–15 minutes.
5. Drain off excess PBS and remove residual PBS by tapping the edge of the slide against a pad of tissue paper.
6. Flood the section with second stage conjugated antibody (secondary antibody) and incubate for 30 minutes.
7. Wash the slides in PBS for 10–15 minutes.
8. Mount the slides in buffered glycol using cover slips.
9. Examine the slides on a fluorescent microscope as soon as possible.
10. For future examination, the slides can be stored at 4°C.

FLUORESCENT MICROSCOPE

The fluorescent microscope delivers light of a specific wavelength which causes excitation of fluorochrome. This fluorochrome emits light of different wavelength, which is viewed through the eyepiece of fluorescent microscope. The light source and filters are two important factors for immunoflurescence microscopy.

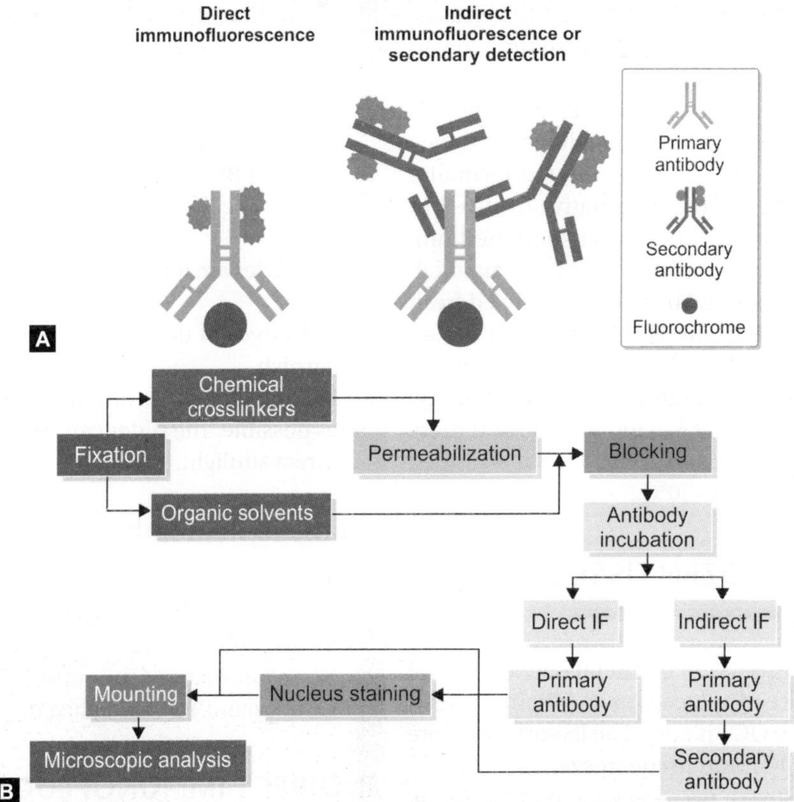

Figs 1A and B: Direct and indirect immunofluorescence *(For color version, see Plate 10)*

The light source should be capable of delivering sufficient excitation wavelength photons to make visible IF. Previously, mercury vapor or xenon was used as light source. Nowadays LED (light-emitting diode) is used.

It has **several advantages**:

- They are capable of producing high intensity monochromatic light.
- They do not have warm-up or cool-down times (regarded as waste of time).
- They do not require bulb realignment.
- They don't have explosion risk.
- They have a longer life time of 8,000–10,000 hours.

Two types of filters are used—excitation and emission filters. These excitation and emission filters act complementary to each other. They have transmission ranges of wavelengths of light that are ideal for the particular fluorochrome being used. In the past colored glass filters were used. Recently, broad or narrow band interference filters are being used.

Limitations of IF: Fluorescence fades away over time, especially, if it is exposed to the exciting light for longer period. So, the slides can not be kept for permanent record or future reference.

DIAGNOSTIC USE OF IMMUNOFLUORESCENCE

Immunofluorescence techniques are extensively used to detect different antibodies present in serum. Frozen sections are usually required for IF. But Mera et al (1980) described successful application of IF to paraffin embedded sections of skin following trypsinization (Tables 2 and 3).

Table 2: Immunofluorescene pattern in different skin diseases

Skin disease	*Substance present*	*Location of deposit*	*Pattern of deposit*
Pemphigus	IgG, C3	Intercellular squamous region	Lacelike
Pemphigoid (bullous)	C3, IgG	EBMZ	Linear
Cicatrial pemphigoid	C3, IgG	EBMZ	Linear
Bullous systemic lupus erythematosus	C3, IgG	EBMZ	Linear
Erythema multiforme	C3, IgM	EBMZ	Granular
Dermatitis herpetiformis	IgA	EBMZ	Granular

Abbreviation: EBMZ, epidermal basement membrane zone.

Table 3: Immunofluorescence pattern in different glomerulonephritis

Kidney disease	*Light microscopy*	*Electron microscopy*	*Immunofluorescence microscopy*
Minimal change GN	Normal, lipid in tubules	Loss of foot proceses, no deposit	Negative
Membranous GN	Diffuse capillary wall thickening	Subepithelial deposit	Granular IgG and C3, diffuse involvement
Focal segmental GN	Focal and segmental sclerosis and hyalinosis	Loss of foot processes epithelial denudation	IgM and C3, Focal
Membranoproliferative GN, Type I	Glomeruli are large and hypercellular	Subendothelial deposits	IgG, C3, C1q, C4
Membranoproliferative GN, Type II	Same	Dense deposits	C3 ± IgG, no C1q or C4
Good-Pasture syndrome	Extracapillary proliferations with crescent formation, necrois	No deposits GBM disruption	Linear IgG and C3, fibrin in crescents
IgA nephropathy	Mesangial widening and proliferation	Mesangial dense deposits	IgA ± IgG, IgM, C3 in mesangiurn
Post-streptococcal GN	Diffuse endocapillary proliferation, neutrophil infiltration	Subepithelial hump	Granular IgG and C3 in mesangium and GBM
Chronic GN	Hyalinized glomeruli	-	Negative or granular

Abbreviations: GN, glomerulonephritis; GBM, glomerular basement membrane.

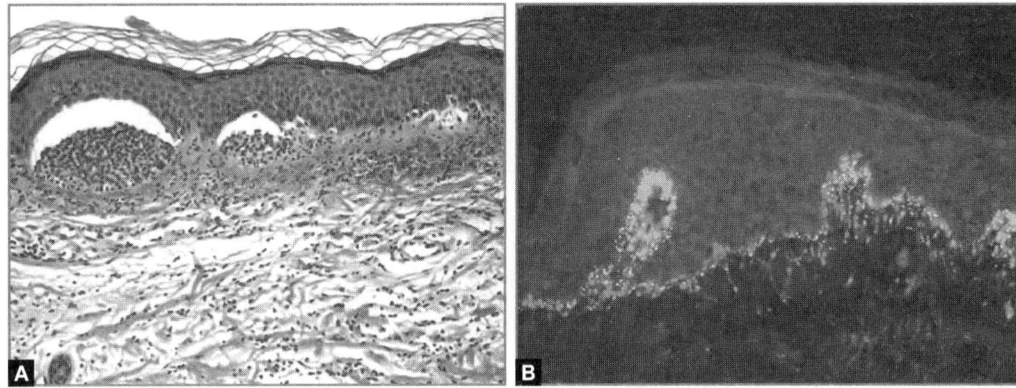

Figs 2A and B: Dermatitis herpetiformis. (A) Microphotograph showing microabscesses at the tips of dermal papilla which one forming a multilocular subepidermal bulla. Eosinophils are also present (H & E × 100). (B) Microphotograph showing immunofluorescence of granular and thready deposits of IgA at the epidermal basement membrane zone (EBMZ) *(For color version, see Plate 10)*

IF has made an important contribution to diagnosis of two medical areas, i.e. renal glomerular diseases and few immunological skin diseases. Renal biopsy samples are stained for IgG, IgM, IgA, k, λ, C1q, C3 and amyloid P. Renal transplant biopsies are examined for lymphocytic infiltration using CD3, CD4, CD8, CD19 and CD20. The skin biopsy samples are stained for IgG, IgM, IgA, kappa (k), lambda (λ), C3 and C1q (Figs 2A and B).

Different antibodies which may be present in the serum are antinuclear antibody (ANA), smooth muscle antibody (SMA), mitochondrial antibody, liver kidney microsomal (LKM) antibody, etc.

CHAPTER 20 Museum Technique

INTRODUCTION

The preservation of pathological specimens is important and a well-organized pathology museum fulfils many objectives:

- A permanent source for teaching and research
- A permanent exhibition for common pathologic disease for self-education of undergraduate, postgraduate and research scholars
- To display some rare pathologic conditions which may be of historical interest
- A permanent source for photography of gross findings which are needed for publications, presentations, etc.

The basic museum technique can be divided into following steps:

- Reception of the specimen
- Preparation of the specimen
- Fixation in fixatives
- Restoration of color.
- Preservation of the specimen in mounting fluid
- Presentation of the specimen.

RECEPTION OF THE SPECIMEN

The specimen may be from operation theaters of hospitals, research laboratories and from postmortem room. All specimen should be recorded in a reception book with all the relevant information. These will include the diagnosis or disease, name of the patient and operating surgeons, source (hospital, PM, research labs), biopsy/necropsy slide number. Each case should be given an accession number (case no, month and year). Remember liver and gallbladder specimens should be stored separately as the bile of these specimens will discolor other specimens.

PREPARATION OF THE SPECIMEN

The biopsy or necropsy specimens may be fresh or already in a fixative. The fresh unfixed specimen is obviously better for museum technique. Any gross trimming or dissection should be carried out immediately after arrival of specimens.

The fresh unfixed specimen should not be allowed to dry as it causes irreversibly discoloration. Again it should not be washed in water or tap water because the resultant hemolysis greatly reduces the specimen quality and causes discoloration. The specimen should be washed only with saline. But specimen should not be kept in saline for more than two hours, otherwise autolysis will start.

In case of necropsies, it should be performed as soon as possible after death. In some cases of necropsies, like stomach, intestinal tract or brain, 4% formal saline should be injected into the stomach, peritoneal cavity or carotid arteries respectively as soon as possible after death. For vascular system also this injection is necessary.

The cut surface of the specimen must be flat. In many cases, this is carried out by passing a glass rod into a structure such as large bronchus and cutting along the rod with a knife. For microscopical section, material should be selected at the time of mounting the specimen. One should also remember that, it is desirable to open hollow viscera or to dissect specimen until fixation is complete.

Gough and Wentworth in 1949, demonstrated a technique for lungs in cases of pneumoconiosis. The lungs are inflated and immersed in fixative, then thin slides of specimen are cut with a knife by hand. These thin slices are impregnated with increasing strengths of gelatin. After final embedding in formol gelatine, sections are cut at 600 μm thickness by a microtome. Then these sections are laid on sheets of "Perspex". Sheets of Whatman's No. 1 filter papers are queezed over the surface and allowed to dry. The sections adhere to the paper and now the paper can be peeled off. Finally the specimens are displayed.

The specimen should be photographed when it comes unfixed fresh because it retains its natural color. But if it is already fixed, then photography should be done only after restoration of color (which will be discussed in the later part of this section).

FIXATION IN FIXATIVE

Most specimens (surgical or necropsy) usually sent to laboratory by placing them in 10% formalin or formal-saline solution. This is ideal fixative for museum technique though color restoration is still possible with the use of this initial fixative.

There are several fixatives used for museum techniques but formalin based formula is still very popular. The most common fixative used for this purpose is one which was advocated by Kaiserling in 1897. Actually Kaiserling formulated three solutions. Kaiserling I for fixation, Kaiserling II for restoration of color, and Kaiserling III for preservation in mounting fluid. The original formula of Kaiserling I is as follows:

Kaiserling I Solution

- Formalin: 400 mL
- Potassium acetate: 60 g
- Potassium nitrate: 30 g
- Tap water: 2000 mL.

The pH of this solution is approximately 7. The specimen should be placed in a large container having fixative (Kaiserling I) which should be 3–4 times volume of the specimen. Specimens should be fixed for 3–14 days depending on their size. Small specimen will require 3 days while large specimen like liver, whole limb or lung will, require 14 days.

Certain **important general principles of fixation** should be kept in mind.

- Specimen undergoing fixation must not touch the other specimens or sides of the container.
- The specimen should lie washed fluffless lint or be suspended by linen thread. If the specimen has an undulating surface, then it should be supported with fixative-soaked cotton wool.
- Cystic cavities if opened, then it is packed with cotton wool soaked in fixative so as to maintain their natural shape. If cystic spaces are unopened, they are inflated with fixative.
- The specimen together with other attached structures must be fixed to display the original position of the specimen in relation to other structure. Skin, membrane, intestine and other structures may be pinned to cork board and then it is floated on the fixing fluid (specimen downwards).
- The hollow viscera (e.g. intestine, stomach, etc.) should be filled with cotton wool soaked in fixative, both ends tied off and immerse in the jar containing fixatives.
- Certains solid organs (e.g. brain, liver, spleen) should be fixed by vascular injection—for example, brain through basilar or cerebral artery. The lungs and limbs are also suitable for vascular injection. The spleen should be cut only after vascular injection and fixation. But unfortunately even after this treatment, there may be patchy fixation and cut specimen has to be fixed as in usual way.
- The specimen containing much blood should not be washed by water as it causes hemolysis. If excess blood or mucus is to be removed, it should be washed by saline or formal-saline.
- Bile-containing specimen or bile stained specimen must be fixed and stored separately, otherwise they will stain other specimens.
- The slice of solid organs is placed cut surface downwards on to the lint covered base of the container.
- The heart specimen is usually sent cut-open. For such specimen, in order to maintain the normal natural shape, the major vessels and cavities are filled with cotton-wool soaked with fixative. If the heart specimen is uncut, then it is placed in a large container of fixative. Through coronary ostia, additional fixative may be injected by a syringe.

RESTORATION OF COLOR

After fixation of the specimen, the color should be restored as close to its natural color in the next step. For this, Kaiserling II solution is used. But before placing the specimen into this solution, remove the specimen from fixative and wash in running tap water, then place them in Kaiserling II solution.

Kaiserling II Solution

Ethyl alcohol: 80%.

Some prefer using 95% ethyl alcohol, but Kaiserling himself used 80% ethyl alcohol. The specimen is kept in this solution for 1/2–12 hours, depending on the size of specimen. The specimen is watched carefully during this period as the color develops throughout the specimen. Once the optimum/near natural color develops, specimen should be taken out from this fluid as this alcohol has a permanent bleaching effect and the color so lost cannot be recoverd in the next step.

After color restoration in Kaiserling II solution (80% ethyl alcohol), the specimen is removed from the alcohol and it is bottled dry.

PRESERVATION IN MOUNTING FLUID

This is the last solution in which the specimen will be mounted for display. In the original Kaiserling III solution, 25% glycerine was used. But in later modification, it was raised to 30% and 0.5% formalin was added instead of arsenic and thymol.

Pulvertaft-Kaiserling III Solution

- Glycerine: 300 mL
- Sodium acetate: 100 g
- Formalin: 5 mL
- Tap water to 1,000 mL.

To this solution, 0.4% sodium hydrosulfite is added immediately before sealing the jar.

Preparation of the solution: First dissolve the sodium acetate in warm water, add the glycerine and formalin to it. Add cold tap water to make up the volume (1000 mL). The pH should be alkaline, i.e. pH 8. If it is not so or acidic (pH <7), then a few drops of 1N sodium hydroxide (NaOH) should be added.

If the solution is cloudy or not crystal clear, then the solution should be filtered by a paper (Whatman). Usually presence of impurities in sodium acetate make the solution cloudy. If even after paper filtration, the solution is cloudy, then 50 mL of saturated solution of camphor in alcohol should be added to 1,000 mL of the solution. Refilter as before. Addition of camphor will make the solution crystal clear. But the odd smell is a disadvantage. For rapid restoration of color 0.6% sodium hydrosulfite may be used (causes white precipitate and should be avoided).

Carbon monoxide has also been employed as a color retaining agent. Schultz (1931) introduced this method which gives brilliant color contrast but has the risk of poisoning and explosion.

Schultz's carbon monoxide technique:

- Bubble carbon monoxide (CO) through Kaiserling fluid I containing fixed specimen. This step should be carried out in a fume cupboard with a good draught.
- When the specimen regains its color, then it is placed in mounting fluid, i.e. Pulvertaft-Kaiserling III fluid (do not add sodium hydrosulfite) which has been saturated with carbon monoxide (CO).

Both the carbon monoxide method and hydrosulfite method produce brilliant color contrast but colors are not natural in any of these methods.

Aegerter (1941) prepared modified solution for color fixation and mounting which has some advantages.

Color Fixation Fluid (Aegerter)

- Sodium chloride: 14 g
- Sodium bicarbonate: 8 g
- Chloral hydrate: 62.5 g
- Formalin: 51 mL
- Distilled water: 2,000 mL

After immersion in this fluid for up to 20 hours specimen are placed in original Kaiserling I solution for 1–5 days without washing. Then again without washing placed in modified Kaiserling III solution for mounting.

- Potassium acetate: 200 g
- Glycerine: 400 mL
- Thymol: 0.5 g
- Distilled water: 2,000 mL.

Points to Remember

- Jars or containers must be sealed after mounting and the lids of the jars must not be perforated.
- Unsatisfactory results are due to inadequate fixation in fixative/Kaiserling I solution, washing with water before fixation, excess hydrosulfite, acid pH of mounting fluid (pH should be 8), delayed sealing of the jars, or due to use of impure formalin which contains paraformaldehyde as a white precipitate.
- Fragile specimen like embryos will shrink when kept in mounting fluid (Kaiserling III) due to osmosis effect of glycerine. This may be prevented by lowering the content in the mounting fluid and injecting gelatine into the cranial cavity.
- Wentworth (1942) omitted use of glycerine in the mounting fluid. This formulation makes the fluid cheaper but reduces the refractive index of the medium and hence causes a loss of brilliancy.

Some authors (Bancroft) advocated the use of Romhanyi's solution with regard to color preservation.

Romhanyi's Solution

- Formalin: 120 mL
- Pyridine: 10 mL
- Nicotine, crudum, 5% in water: 10 mL

- Crudum dithionite: 20 g
- Tap water: Up to 1,000 mL

This solution has few disadvantages:

- Nicotine is poisonous
- There is no use of glycerine in this solution. But 40% glycerine has far better in retaining the optical effect as nowadays the specimens are mounted in perspex.
- Pyridine has very bad pungent smell.

So, use of this fluid is limited. But partial replacement of Kaiserling III fluid with this Romhanyi's solution gives improved color, The method of choice is the original Kaiserling technique for fixing the specimen in Kaiserling I, restoring the color in Kaiserling II and mounting the specimen in Kaiserling III. By replacing some of the Kaiserling III with Romhanyi's solution to approximately 25% by volume gives better color restoration.

Romhanyi's solution may cause black deposits on some specimen like on bones. This can be removed by washing with 10% hydrochloric acid. This solution is avoided for specimens which have been previously preserved with alcohol, liquid paraffin or perfused with phenol-based solutions.

PRESENTATION OF THE SPECIMEN

In the past, specimens were mounted in glass jars. Nowadays perspex boxes or jars are used almost universally. These perspex plastic jars have many advantages:

- These jars can be completely filled with mounting solution.
- They are light but strong
- The specimen can be attached to rigid supporting plates within the jar.
- These museum jars can be constructed to any specifications or required measurements easily.

But if the specimens are preserved in alcohol or methyl salicylate, then perspex jars can not be used as these solution dissolve it. Glass jars are to be used in these cases.

The whole procedure of presentation of the specimen can be divided into following steps:

- Preparation of the museum jars or boxes (Perspex).
- Mounting in perspex jars or routine mounting.
- Mounting in glass jars
- Gelatin embedding for delicate or intricate structures.

PREPARATION OF MUSEUM JARS OR BOXES (PERSPEX)

Perspex plastic jars can be made simply by cutting four sides, a top and a bottom from a perspex sheets and cementing them together with perspex cement. Firstly, the height, width and depth (thickness) of the specimen is measured. For making perspex jar, an extra 3.75 cm for height, an extra 2.5 cm for width and depth are allowed to accommodate the specimen into the jar. These dimensions are based on inner dimensions of the jar and not outside dimensions. These are referred as: height × width × depth.

An alternative and better method was suggested by professor Dugwid. He made perspex jars by bending a strip of perspex to form the top and sides of jars. Then the sides and bottom was made. He used heat for bending perspex sheets. Perspex pieces can be joined by any of these things:

- By using commercial filling cement, e.g. Tensol cement Numbers 3 or 7.
- By using a solvent of perspex like chloroform or ethylene dichloride.
- By using home-made cement prepared like this:
  - Glacial acetic acid: 200 mL
  - 1:2 dichloroethane: 200 mL
  - Perspex clippings: 10 g.

These solvents dissolve perspex and the affected areas or sides are joined together. These areas or joint/affected areas become hard when the solvent evaporates.

Apart from the advantages mentioned above, the Perspex jars have other advantages:

- The inner and outer surfaces are parallel and free from ridges.
- They have no distortion
- Refractive index of perspex is 1.49 and light transmission is 92%.
- These plastic jars can be dropped 6 feet without breaking while the glass jars break easily.
- These jars do not break with change of temperature when sealed, but glass jars when sealed break with extreme temperature variation.

MOUNTING IN PERSPEX JARS OR ROUTINE MOUNTING

The specimen is placed on the plate which forms the top of the jar. This is called central plate. The polished edge of the central plate is at the top of the specimen (inner side). The specimen is supported within the jar by attaching it to specimen plate/central plate. This is done by tying it to the plate.

The plate is either drilled or pierced with a hot needle and holes are made 0.2 cm in diameter. The specimen is stitched by nylon thread or Japanese thread. Nylon thread has the advantage of being almost unbreakable and is hard for specimens. So, it can cut through soft specimens. For this reason, linen threads are used for all specimen except bone.

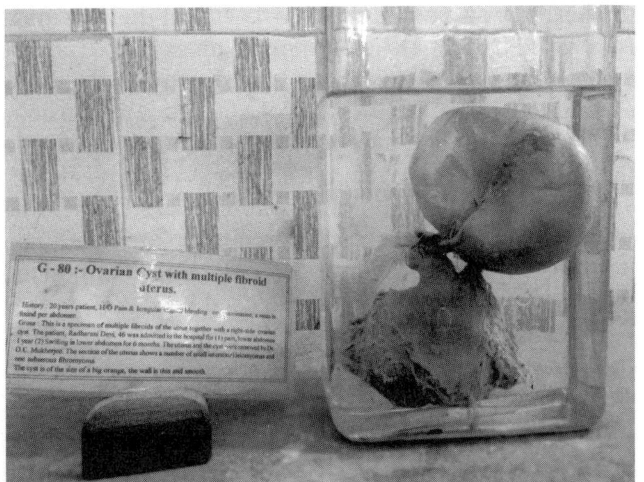

Fig. 1: Mounted specimen in a sealed glass jar in a pathology museum for display. It shows a specimen of uterus cervix and an ovarian cyst

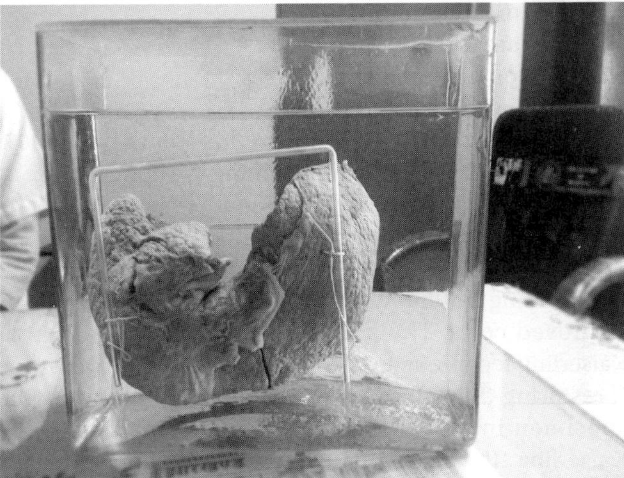

Fig. 2: Mounted specimen showing cirrhosis of liver

The number of stitches will vary depending on weight, size, consistency of specimen. As for example, half of a kidney is adequately supported with a stitch at each pole. Cystic or hollow organs or organs with attached other structures may require many stitches to hold the specimen in correct anatomical position and to provide enough support to the specimen. As for example, stomach, intestine or esophagus may require 10–12 stitches. Attached structure may be stitched to the main organ or to each other to keep them in anatomical position. Remember, the stitches should not pass through pathologic lesions or any other interesting points.

The central plate with attached specimen is placed into the perspex jar. When the specimen is in position, museum fluid to which 0.4% sodium hydrogen sulfite has been added is run into the jar. If there is entrapped air bubble in between specimen and central plate, these should be released with a broad-bladed spatula. A hole (diameter of 1/8th inch) is made in one corner of the lid and remaining mounting fluid is introduced through it.

After placing the specimen in proper position and filling the jar with mounting fluid, the jar is sealed. The top of the box is wiped dry and Perspex cement is applied by a Pasteur pipette. Alternatively ethylene dichloride can be used for sealing. The holes are sealed by using perspex plug and cement. Now the specimen is ready for cataloguing and placing in collection (Figs 1 and 2).

MOUNTING IN GLASS JARS

The specimens may be mounted in glass jars also. The sides and bottom are made of glasses. The top of the central plate may be made of perspex or made of glasses if the mounting medium dissolves perspex like alcohol, methyl salicylate or other fluid. The specimen are mounted as described above except that the holes are made by a metal rod with diamond-shaped end (hand drill) and camphor dissolved in turpentine as a lubricant. Glass jars are sealed with asphaltum-rubber compound (Picein) and is strictly applied on dry surfaces.

GELATIN EMBEDDING

Intricate or delicate structures like circle of Willis may be mounted by this technique as these structures are difficult to stitch. The specimen may be embedded in a thin layer of arsenious acid-gelatin on a central plate and then mounted in gelatin. For this a trough is made by applying sellotape around the edge of the central plate to a depth of 1/4–3/8 inch and the jar filled with gelatin through this trough. After the gelatin has set inside the jar, the sellotape is removed. Gelatin embedding was popular using glass jars. But the procedure has the disadvantages that gelatin becomes yellow with age and undergoes liquefaction with time with formation of air bubble. Use of perspex jars instead of glass jars solves this problem.

CHAPTER 21

Light Microscopy

INTRODUCTION

Visible light is the portion of electromagnetic spectrum that can be detected by human eyes. The range of wavelengths of light which can be detected is 400 nm (deep violet) to 800 nm (far red). But practically most of us cannot see light having wavelengths >700 nm (deep red) (Fig. 1).

- **Amplitude**: It refers to the strength or brightness of light.
- **Wavelength**: It is the distance between the apex of one wave and the apex of next wave. It determines the color of light measured in nm.
- **Frequency**: It refers to number of waves per second a light produces. Measured by Hertz (Hz).
- **Coherent rays**: It means individual rays of identical frequency from the same source.
- **Noncoherent rays**: These are the rays from different sources with different frequencies.
- **White light**: It is the mixture of light which contains some percentage of wavelengths from all of the visible portions of the electromagnetic spectrum.
- **Principal focus or focal point**: When parallel rays pass through a simple lens, they meet together at a single point due to refraction of light by the lens. An image will be formed of an object at this point. This point of convergence is called focal point or principal focus. The distance between the optical center of the lens and the principal focus is called the focal length.
- **Conjugate Foci**: Apart from the focal point, there are two points of lens which are located at opposite side of the lens. If one object is placed at one of these points, it will form a clear image of the object on the other point (opposite side of the lens). These points are called the conjugate foci.

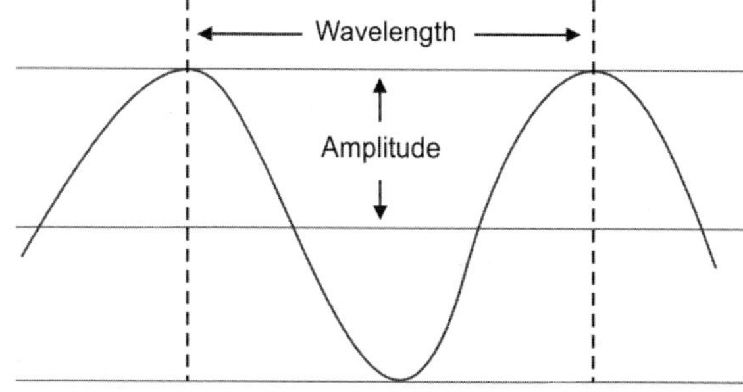

Fig. 1: A ray of light showing amplitude and wavelength

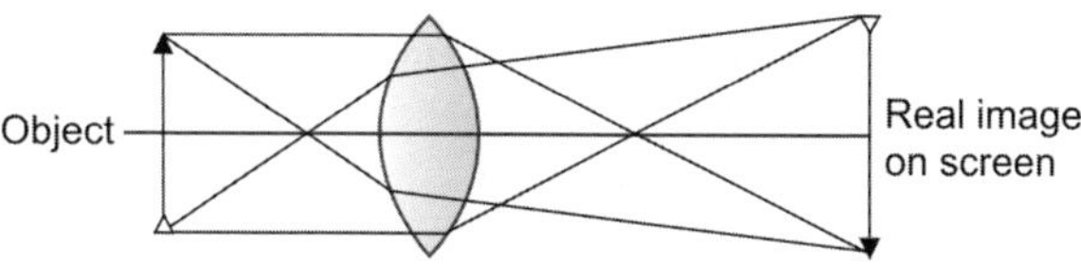

Fig. 2: Formation of real image

- **Real image**: The conjugate foci are not fixed unlike focal point and they vary in position. When an object is moved closer to a lens, the image will be formed further away on other conjugate point. This image has greater magnification and is inverted. This inverted image is called the "real image" and is formed by the objective lens of the microscope (Fig. 2).
- **Virtual image**: If the image is placed further close to the lens within focal point, then the image is formed within the same side. This image is enlarged and right way up (not inverted) and cannot be projected on the screen. This image is called the "virtual image" and is formed by the eye piece of a microscope (Fig. 3).

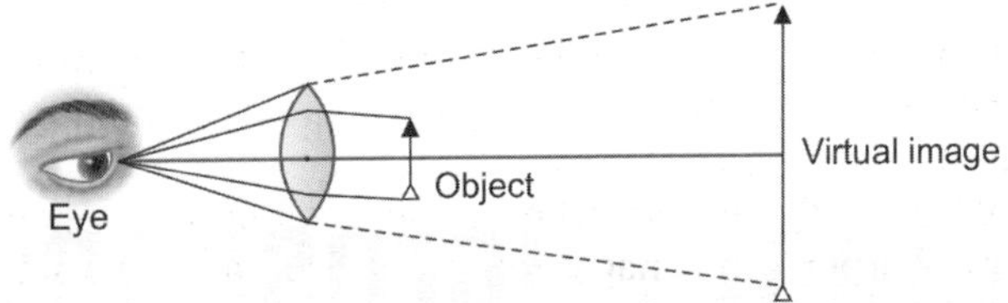

Fig. 3: Formation of virtual image

THE MICROSCOPE

Micro means "small" and scope means "to view".

A microscope magnifies the image of the object. Most of the laboratories use light microscopes (compound microscope) nowadays. The light microscope uses white light, source of which may be external sunlight or internal tungsten filament lamp.

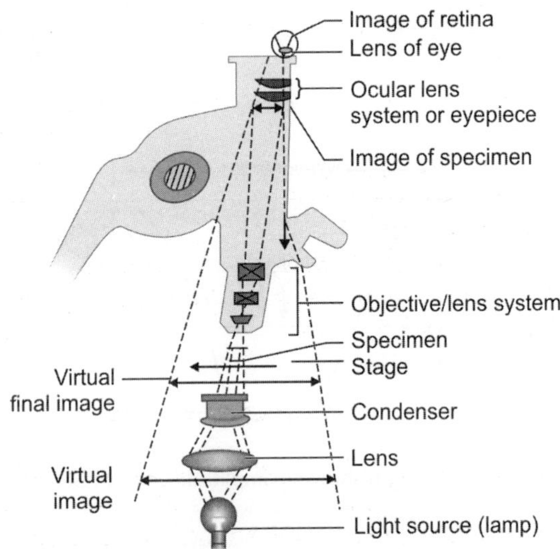

Fig. 4: Principle of light microscope

In case of a dark field microscope a special field condenser is used which lights up the object, like stars against a dark sky. The fluorescent microscope uses a special ultraviolet lamp as a source of illumination. When a fluorescent dye is attached to the object through laboratory procedures and exposed to ultraviolet radiation then it glows (Fig. 4).

COMPONENT OF A LIGHT MICROSCOPE

The light microscope has following major systems (Figs 5A and B):

1. **Support system:** Foot rest, tube, stage, arm, body, substage.
2. **Illumination system:** Mirror, filter, iris diaphragm, condenser.
3. **Magnification system:** Objective, eye piece.
4. **Others:** Coarse adjustment, fine adjustment.

Support System

- **The tube:** Supports eye piece and objective.
- **The body:** It gives support to the tube.
- **The arms:** It gives correct angulation and height to the body and tube.
- **The stage:** It has a pair of spring clips and it holds the object or slide this mechanical stage. It has an aperture of 1-1.5 inches in diameter.
- **The substage:** It holds the condenser lens with its iris diaphragm and a holder for light filter and stops.
- **The foot:** Other parts rest on it and it touches the surface on which the light microscope has been placed. The foot may be horseshoe shaped or tripod.

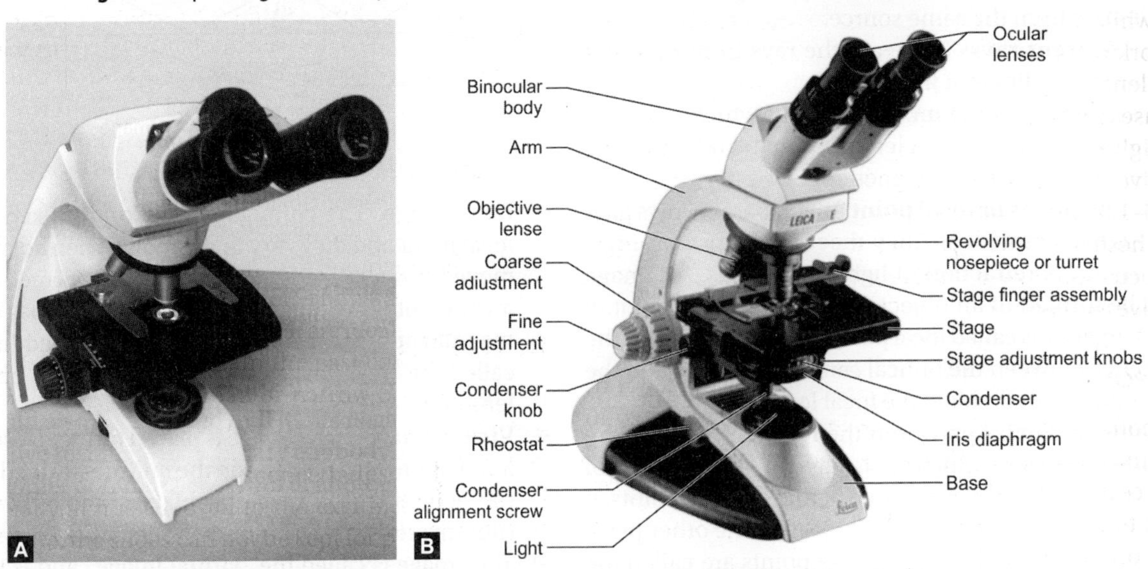

Figs 5A and B: (A) Photograph of a binocular light microscope; (B) Parts of binocular microscope

Illumination System

- **Mirror:** It is located under the condenser and it has two surfaces—plane and concave. The plane surface is required for the microscope with condenser and it concentrates the light which can pass through the narrow hole on the stage in order to illuminate the object placed over the opening. The concave side is used when the condenser is not provided. Most microscopes have a condenser, so use plane side of mirror. It is usually fitted about four inches below the stage.
- **Filter:** If the external light source is an electric lamp the filter takes away the yellow color of the incandescent lamp and creates a sky blue background.
- **Iris diaphragm:** It is located in between the mirror and condenser (nearest to the stage on the under surface). It regulates the amount of light that will illuminate the object. The diaphragm is closed for less light and is open for more light.
- **Condenser:** It concentrates light which is coming as parallel rays in such a way that it passes through the opening of the stage. Condenser is located immediately below the stage and can be raised for increased illumination. For maximum illumination, the condenser is raised (top position) and is regulated by iris diaphragm.

Magnification System

Objective

It is located at the bottom of the tube and is close to the object (just above the object). Four objectives are in use—scanner view (5×), low power (10×), high power (40×), and oil immersion (100×).

These objectives are attached to the revolving nose piece which helps in the selection of the objective for view. The working distance is the distance between the objective (front lens) and the object or slide. The working distance decreases as the magnification increases (higher objective). It is highest for scanner view objective. For low power objective (10×), it is 5–6 mm, for high power objective (40×) it is 0.5–1.5 mm and for oil immersion (100×), it is 0.15–0.20 mm. These objectives are **parfocal** (when an object/slide is in focus with one objective it will be focussed by other objective as well).

Eyepiece

It is another system of lenses which is attached to the top of the microscope tube and is located close to the eye. The eyepiece magnifies the real image (formed by the objective lens) into a virtual image which can be seen by eyes (cannot be put on a screen).

The most commonly used eye piece is known as Huyghen that has two lenses mounted at a correct distance apart with a circular diaphragm in between which gives a sharp edge to the image. The eyepieces are available in different magnifications. Lesser the magnification brighter and sharper is the image. For routine laboratory work 10X Huyghen eyepiece is good enough. Wide field and 15X eyepieces are also available.

Total magnification = magnification in the objective × magnification in the eyepiece

So scanner power gives 5 × 10 = 50X total magnification
Low power gives 10 × 10 = 100X total magnification
High power gives 40 × 10 = 400X total magnification
Oil immersion gives 100 × 10 = 1000X total magnification.

Others

- **Coarse adjustment:** It is controlled by a pair of large circular knobs, one on each side of the body. When the knobs are rotated the tube with lenses moves. Some microscope attaches this knob to the stage instead of tube. Coarse adjustment focuses objects for scanner view and low power lenses.
- **Fine adjustment:** It is controlled by two smaller circular knobs on each side of the body. Fine adjustment is necessary to focus the object for high power and oil immersion lenses.

LIGHT SOURCE

- **Daylight or sunlight**: If daylight is the only source of illumination, the microscope must be placed near the window. The microscope should be illuminated by subdued light and should not be placed under direct sunlight. Because use of direct sunlight is bad for eyes and microscope. But remember daylight/sunlight is not available in the night and it is not sufficient for use of oil immersion lenses.
- **Electric light**: Most modern microscopes have in built sources of illumination by providing electric bulbs in them. Alternatively a 60 Watt frosted electric lamp placed 20 cm away from the microscope is sufficient for illumination.

ROUTINE CARE AND MAINTENANCE

It should be remembered that the microscope is an exceedingly complicated and delicate piece of apparatus and a great deal of experience is required to maintain it. Dust and fungus are its worst enemies. Fungus growing on lenses and scratches caused by dust particles on the lens surface can destroy a microscope.

Routine Care of Microscope

- Always carry the microscope by holding its arm with one hand and the other hand will be under the foot rest. Do not swing the microscope while carrying it.
- Do not allow direct sunlight to fall on microscope. Put a plastic cover on the microscope. Before covering, remove the dust particles from microscope. Then keep it in warm dry place. Never store it in its wooden box.
- Never pull out the object-slide from the stage when oil-immersion lens is being used. The slide may cause scratches on oil-immersion lens. Also do not try to move the oil-immersion lens, when there is a slide on the stage. The slide may be taken out by using coarse adjustment knob or pulling down the stage, thus making wide gap in between oil immersion lens and slide.

Cleaning of Lenses

After day's work is over, the lenses should be cleaned daily.

- The lenses of the objectives should be cleaned with lens paper or tissue paper or well-washed silk. During cleaning, first blow off the dust particles from objectives with the help of a rubber bulb or a paint brush. While cleaning, a lens breathing on it by mouth is advisable.
- The oil immersion objective needs special attention and if requires frequent cleaning. After use, there should not be any oil left over the lens. Use clean tissue paper to remove oil by repeated gentle rubbing on the oil immersion lens surface. Move the cloth across and not circularly. Never use an organic solvent (e.g. ethanol, xylene, ether or toluene) to remove the oil from lens. This organic solvent may seep inside the socket and dissolve the cement holding the lens. If needed, tissue paper soaked with isopropyl alcohol lightly may be used and rub the paper gently and lightly on the oil immersion lens. Tissue paper soaked with xylene though not advisable, but may be used rarely (for emergency work).
- The top lens of eyepiece should be cleaned by tissue paper to remove dust or finger marks. Rotation of eyepiece will show if any dust is still present. If dust is present, dismantle the eyepiece and clean both lenses as well.
- The mirror and substage condenser may be cleaned in a similar way with a tissue paper.

CHAPTER 22

Molecular Diagnostic Techniques and its Applications

INTRODUCTION

The advent of molecular diagnostic techniques has a major impact on the practice of surgical pathology. These techniques were exclusive realm of research laboratories once upon a time. The entry of these techniques from research laboratories to diagnostic pathology, has resulted in the availability of indispensable tools for a multitude of uses in diagnostic laboratory.

Gene is the segment of DNA containing the codes for the amino acid sequence of a polypeptide and the regulatory sequences that control its expression. The exons (coding DNA sequences) of a gene are often interrupted by introns (noncoding DNA sequences). When mRNA (messenger RNA) is formed after translation, the noncoding nucleotides are removed during RNA splicing. The expression of genes is regulated by many factors, e.g. transcription factors, gene promoter and DNA methylation. Also, micro-RNA (a small RNA of 21–26 nucleotides long) can inactivate specific messenger RNAs in a sequence-specific manner.

SPECIMEN REQUIREMENTS

Specimen requirements are governed by the type of disease, including the type of tissue, amount of tissue and sample type (fresh or frozen tissue, FFPE or formalin-fixed paraffin-embedded tissue, cytology specimen). But irrespective of specimen type, two things in a tissue sample influence molecular assays.

- Firstly, there should have been sufficient quantity of the specific target cell containing target DNA or RNA in the tissue sample.
- Secondly, the nucleic acid degradation (heat, enzymatic, pH or mechanical forces) can reduce the sensitivity of test. So, size or integrity of the nucleic acids after isolation is important.

Tissue type: Fresh peripheral blood, bone marrow aspirates/biopsies, enriched cell populations (for example, from flow cytometry), surgical specimens or solid tissue biopsies, and FFPE are all sources of nucleic acid (DNA or RNA) for molecular diagnostic techniques. Any type of specimen should be collected and transported to the molecular diagnostic laboratory using aseptic techniques. If possible, transport on ice should be done which reduces cell lysis, minimizes nuclease activity and cause less nucleic acid degradation.

Tissue quality: Solid tissue should be preserved immediately by freezing or fixation as it minimizes nucleic acid degradation. Peripheral blood, bone marrow or hemorrhagic fluid should be collected either in EDTA (ethylene diamine tetra acetic acid) or ACD (acid-citrate dextrose). Heparin is unsuitable as an anticoagulant in this regard because heparin carryover after nucleic acid isolation may inhibit subsequent molecular diagnostic step. Freezing of hematologic specimens is not recommended.

Formalin-fixed paraffin-embedded (FFPE) tissue has few advantages. Fixation in formalin suspends the degradation of nucleic acids and fixed specimens can easily be transported and stored. But fixed tissues have disadvantages as well as advantages. Quality of extracted nucleic acid is highly variable because all fixatives, including formalin, chemically degrade nucleic acid to some extent.

Tissue quantity: minimum sample requirement may vary as per the molecular diagnostic technique. As for example, in conventional genomic Southern hybridization, approximately 10 μg of DNA (approximately 10^6 cells) is required per enzymatic digestion to detect a single copy of genomic DNA targets. But PCR (polymerase chain reaction) based assays require only 20–200 ng of DNA (10^3–10^4 cells), though multiplex-PCR requires a bit more DNA.

DNA ANALYSIS

Southern Blot (Filter Hybridization)

After DNA digestion and separation of the fragments by size, the DNA sample is bound to the membrane. Then identification of specially sized DNA fragments is carried out. The name comes from its inventor EM Southern.

In addition to denaturation (usually done by alkali or NaOH treatment of the gel), it is often necessary to partially hydrolyze the DNA to facilitate the transfer of the larger DNA fragments. This step is called **depurination** and is achieved by incubation of the gel in a mild acid solution (like HCl). The depurinated and denatured DNA fragments are carried by capillary action from the gel to the membrane. After this, the DNA is fixed onto the membrane by baking (nitrocellulose) or with ultraviolet light. Now, probes can be applied to the membrane (Figs 1 and 2).

Slot and Dot-blots (Filter Hybridization)

For slot-blot and dot-blot hybridization, there is no prior DNA digestion and electrophoresis. The DNA sample is directly bound to the membrane. But denaturation of DNA is necessary, so that hybridization with probe can occur.

Both the Southern blot and dot-blot hybridization techniques together is called filter hybridization. The filter hybridization technique is ideally suitable for:

- Gene rearrangements

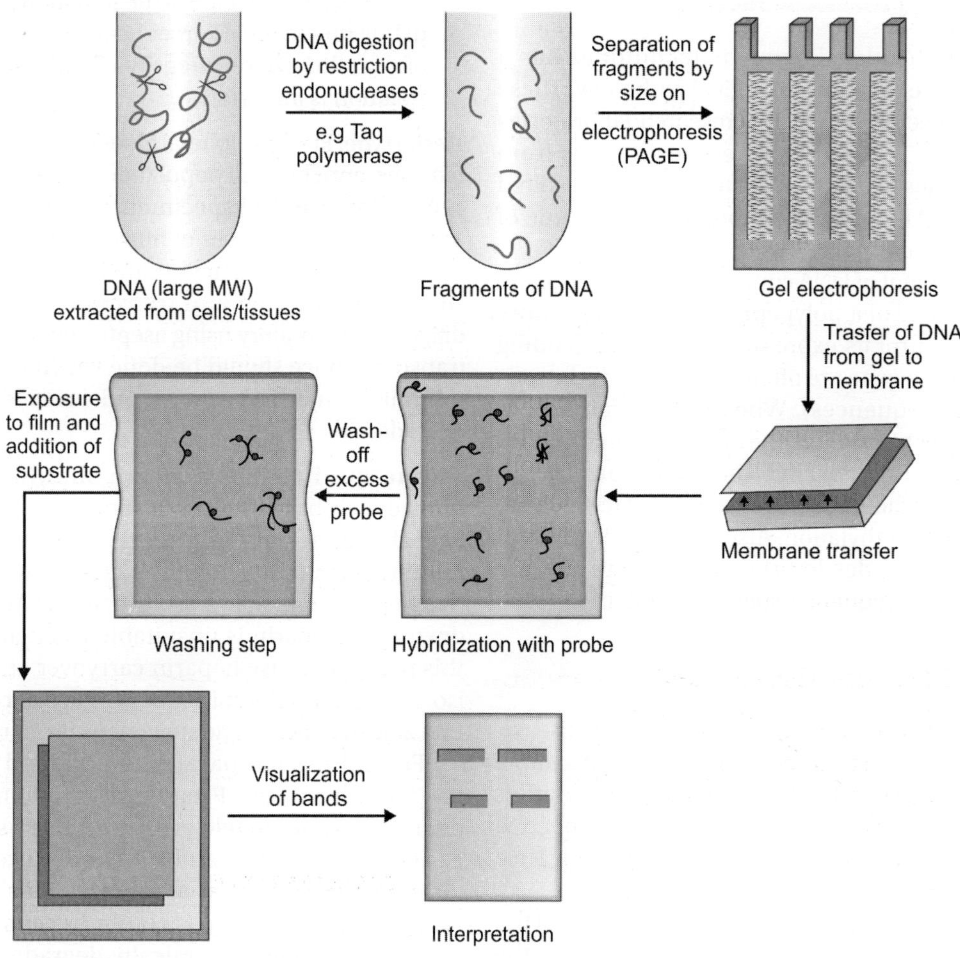

Fig. 1: Different steps of Southern blot technique

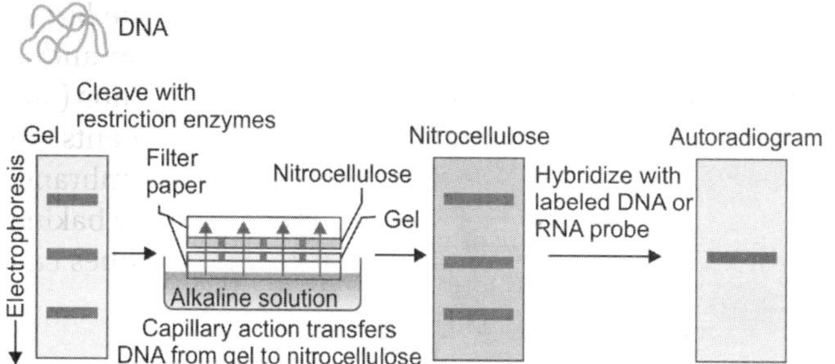

Fig. 2: Schematic diagram of Southern blot
(For color version, see Plate 11)

- Point mutations
- Gene deletions
- Gene amplifications.

Though, it is powerful molecular diagnostic tool, but it has some disadvantages. It needs prolonged time, it is susceptible to various artifacts and it needs radioactive substances. So, it is being replaced by other method like PCR.

Linkage Analysis

An **allele** is defined as being linked to the disease-causing gene and it is found at a greater frequency than that is expected by chance alone in affected persons. The use of linked probes is known as linkage analysis. Linkage analysis is useful to study inherited diseases. But one has to remember that the marker allele itself is not the cause of that inherited disease, rather it acts indirectly to track the disease causing gene or allele. But it has certain limitations:

- There must be a family with several affected individuals and all of them should be available for study.
- Linkage analysis can be performed only when polymorphism exist at a particular locus.
- All affected families will not be informative for a particular linked-polymorphic marker.

Restriction Fragment Length Polymorphisms (RFLP)

It can detect polymorphism at DNA level. RFLP may be due to single base mutations or to **variable number of tandem repeats (VNTRs).** An RFLP points to a particular fragment of DNA, created by enzymatic digestion (restriction endonuclease) of genomic DNA and it differs from one individual to another or at the two alleles of the gene in the same individual.

Genomic DNA or DNA produced from a PCR reaction undergoes enzymatic digestion and the fragments are analyzed by Southern blot with a site-specific probe. Changes in the sequence of the DNA may result in alteration of the recognition sequence of restriction endonuclease enzyme. This alteration in DNA may introduce additional cut sites, remove cut sites, or delete or insert sequences between cut sites. These changes in DNA will be reflected in a change in the band size hybridizing to the site-specific probe. But all changes will not be reflected in an altered recognition sequence, so unchanged band size should be interpreted in the context of marker and known frequency of polymorphism in the region (Fig. 3).

Polymorphisms in DNA closely linked to a disease gene may be used to predict inheritance of the altered allele. Many markers are locus specific and chromosomal maps of these markers are also available. Those regions with the most variations, having the most polymorphisms, are easiest to use to established allelic markers. The VNTRs can result in a complex banding pattern or genetic fingerprint. RFLP is useful in:

- Establishing association of region of genome to disease.
- Family studies of inherited diseases (classical genetics).
- Identifying regions of the genome altered in neoplasia (somatic mutation).

RNA ANALYSIS

Northern blotting is done for RNA analysis whereas Southern blotting is done for DNA analysis. But there are some fundamental differences between the two procedures. As for example, no restriction enzyme (endonuclease) is used for digestion in northern blotting. As RNA is single stranded unlike DNA, one may think that denaturation would not be required. But practically denaturation is required for RNA analysis also, because of the complex secondary structure of RNA molecules. But unlike heat or alkaline solution (NaOH) in DNA analysis, formaldehyde or formamide is used for RNA analysis. Formaldehyde is usually included in the gel during electrophoresis whereas formamide is added to the RNA sample before loading for electrophoresis.

In case of electrophoresis of DNA sample, known size markers must be used to determine the size of the band, produced after use of probes. But during RNA electrophoresis, the RNA sample has its own internal size-marker control, especially if it is rich in ribosomal RNA or rRNA. There is also another difference between northern and Southern blotting. In case of a diploid cell, the amount of DNA is constant, but the amount of RNA is highly variable. The northern blot analysis is used to assess the RNA in whole tissue.

PROTEIN ANALYSIS

Protein analysis is a broad area which encompasses fields including monoclonal antibody-determined expression of proteins and different electrophoretic analyses. Proteins are

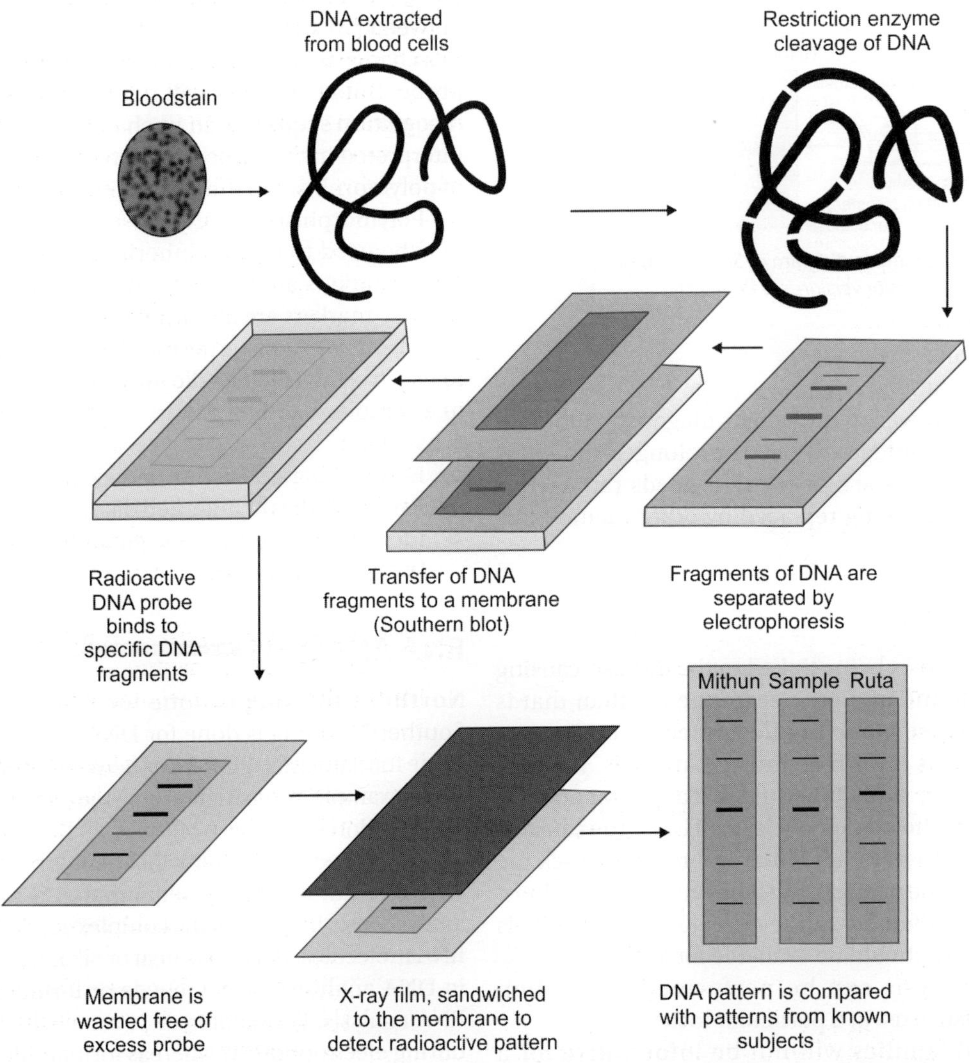

Fig. 3: Schematic diagram of RFLP procedure: Step 1: DNA extracted from sample (like blood cells). Step 2: Restriction enzyme cleavage of DNA. Step 3: Fragments of DNA are separated by electrophoresis. Step 4: Transfer of DNA fragments to a membrane. Step 4: Radioactive DNA probe binds to specific DNA fragment. Step 5: Membrane is made free of excess probe. Step 6: X-ray film sandwiched to membrane to detect radioactive pattern. Step 7: DNA patterns to compare with patterns with known subjects

usually extracted from tissues by mechanical methods or by using detergents or lysozyme. The extracted proteins are then analyzed in polyacrylamide gels. The dissociation of proteins is achieved with the use of a strong anionic detergent (SDS) along with heat and a reducing agent. Conventional polyacrylamide gel electrophoresis (PAGE) separates different peptides of proteins based on their size whereas two dimensional gel electrophoresis analyses many more peptides.

Like northern and Southern blotting, the protein extracts are transferred onto a solid support (western blotting) for analysis. In case of western blotting (protein analysis), antibodies are used like probes but in case of northern and Southern blotting, nucleic acid probes are used. These antibodies attach with specific antigenic epitopes within the target protein. This bound antibody is then detected by another reagent (anti-immunoglobulin or protein A, coupled with an enzyme like horseradish peroxidase or alkaline phosphatase) (Figs 4 and 5).

The advantage of western blotting or protein electrophoresis is that, it is highly sensitive and can detect as little as 1 nanogram of protein.

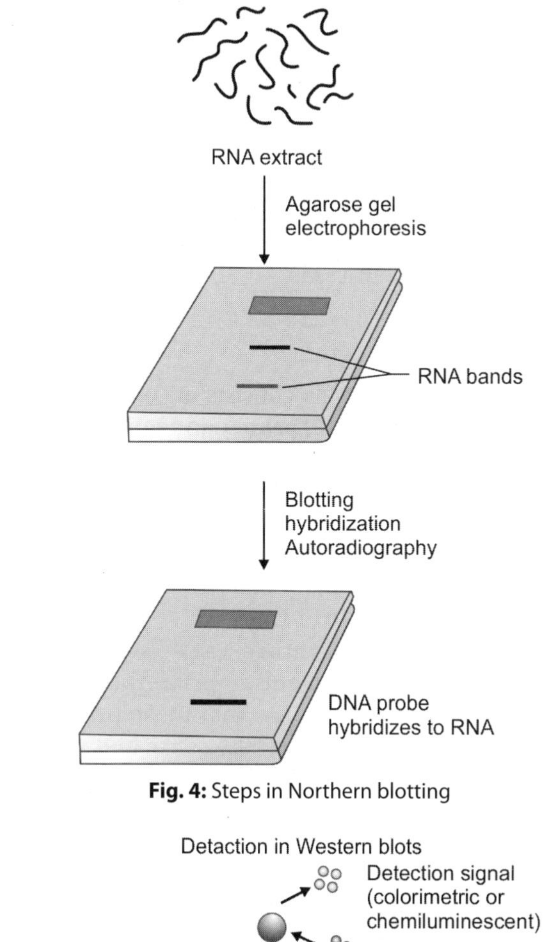

Fig. 4: Steps in Northern blotting

Fig. 5: Steps in Western blots for protein analysis

INTERPHASE CYTOGENETICS

It is the analysis of chromosomes in nondividing cells of **interphase (G_0 phase).** But in conventional chromosomal analysis, it is done in **metaphase (M phase).** But conventional chromosomal analysis has some limitations though it is very successful in right circumstances. The specimen should be fresh, in vitro culture is needed, dividing cells may not be representative of the original sample and chromosomes in metaphase spread may be of inferior quality.

Interphase cytogenetics has the advantage that it is free from these limitations. Also, it is very sensitive test and many chromosome-specific DNA probes are available for this. FISH (fluorescent in situ hybridization) has gained wide acceptability because of its great sensitivity and rapidity. But FISH need fluorescence microscopy set-up and unsuitable for light microscopy. On the other hand, **silver ISH (SISH)** and **chromogenic ISH (CISH)** are alternative methods which can be visualized under light microscopy. So, these methods correlate well with morphology when compared with positive signals (Fig. 6).

Interphase cytogenetics is ideal for cytologic preparations. Paraffin sections can also be studied, but the procedure is very cumbersome and morphologic assessment cannot be done. Two types of DNA probes are used: (1) **Centromeric probes** (used for enumeration of chromosomes, i.e. decrease or increase in number of chromosomes); (2) **Locus-specific probes** (used to hybridize specific genes of interest like HER2 genes, EWS gene). When two or more probes are used simultaneously, the probes should be labeled with different fluorochromes.

Interphase cytogenetics has many diagnostic applications:

- For the diagnosis of congenital anomalies (including sex chromosome abnormalities).
- For the detection of recipient's cells in the allograft of donor.
- For the detection of different hematologic malignancies and solid tumors (neoplastic diseases). Examples are:
  - Demonstration of gene fusion/chromosomal translocation in different hematolymphoid malignancies, soft tissue sarcomas and other tumors.
  - Detection of gene amplification like HER2 in breast and gastric cancer.
  - Detection of MDM2 amplification to diagnose dedifferentiated liposarcoma and atypical lipomatous tumor.
  - Detection of loss or gain in whole chromosome, as seen in renal cell carcinoma.
  - Detection of loss of specific locus or gene or chromosomal region (e.g. loss of 19q and 1p in oligodendroglioma).

MICRODISSECTION

In ancient time, microdissection was carried out with a pair of needles. Now, microdissection can be performed with the help of a scalpel or needle (for target region on the tissue sections). Very recently, sophisticated instruments employing laser technology has been used for this purpose. It dissects a pure cell population or single cells or even chromosomes. After microdissection, the material is captured and can be studied with different molecular techniques (Figs 7 to 9).

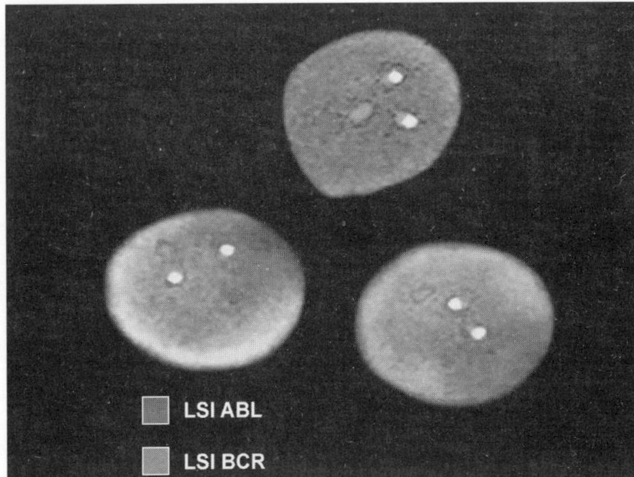

Fig. 6: Interphase cytogenetics, ABL-BCR transfusion in Philadelphia chromosome in chronic myeloid leukemia (CML). Normally, ABL gives red signal and BCR gives green signal. But when they are translocated and transfused to make a chimeric protein (in Philadelphia chromosome) they impart yellow signal *(For color version, see Plate 11)*

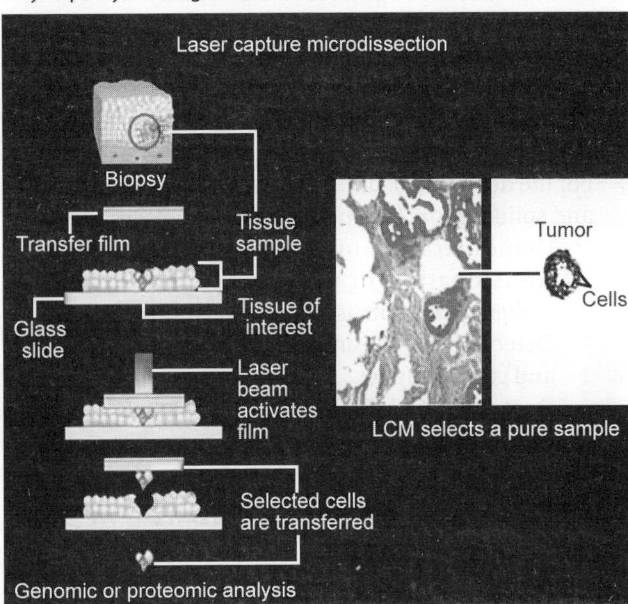

Fig. 7: Schematic diagram of laser capture microdissection technique *(For color version, see Plate 11)*

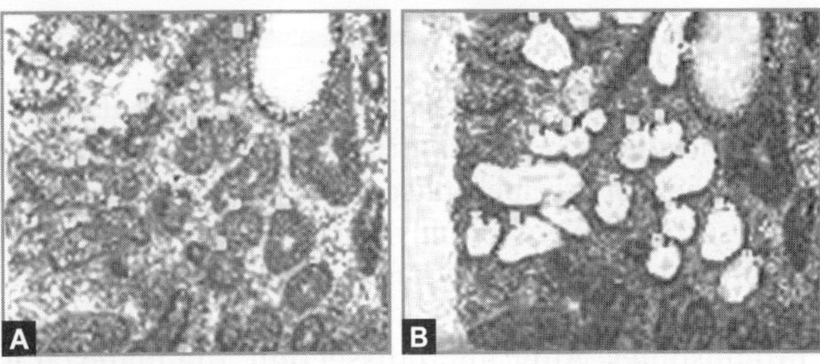

Figs 8A and B: (A) Before microdissection and (B) after microdissection. Note, areas marked in the left photographed have been taken out (microdissection) in the right photograph *(For color version, see Plate 11)*

POLYMERASE CHAIN REACTION (PCR)

Polymerase chain reaction (PCR) which was first introduced in 1985, revolutionized molecular diagnosis. PCR can amplify enormously target DNA or RNA (in the form of cDNA) sequences, enhancing diagnostic sensitivity or specificity. PCR was developed in the 1980s by Kary Mullis, who won Nobel Prize in 1994.

Procedure

A typical PCR reaction cycle consists of (i) **denaturation** for 30-90 seconds at 94°C, (ii) **primer annealing** for 30-120 seconds at 55°C, and (iii) **extension** for 60-180 seconds at 72°C. PCR relies on the ability of DNA polymerases like Taq polymerase with the help of a mixture of deoxynucleotide triphosphates (dATP, dCTP, dGTP, dTTP), to copy a DNA strand using a short complimentary DNA fragment as an initiating template (Figs 10 to 12).

The time and temperature vary as per specific application. The oligonucleotide primers are needed to flank a specific sequence, so that these primers will hybridize to the 3' ends of both the sense and antisense strands of the two denatured DNA strands.

After this annealing, extension of primers is done by adding free nucleotides (dNTPs) by the action of DNA polymerase. It generates a second target molecule which now acts as a template for second/next cycle. Thermostable DNA polymerases are required, otherwise they will be destroyed by the high denaturing temperature. These **DNA polymerase** are derived from microorganisms like hot springs or from bacteria like **Thermus aquaticus (Taq), Thermotoga maritima (Tma)** and **Thermus thermophilus (Tth).**

Repeated PCR reaction cycles result in enormous number of target sequence (target sequence 2^n, where n is the number of cycles). So, a reaction that runs for 20 cycles will produce 2^{20} copies and reaction which runs for 30 cycles will produce 2^{30} copies or one billion copies. Though theoretically, PCR reaction can be run for many cycles,

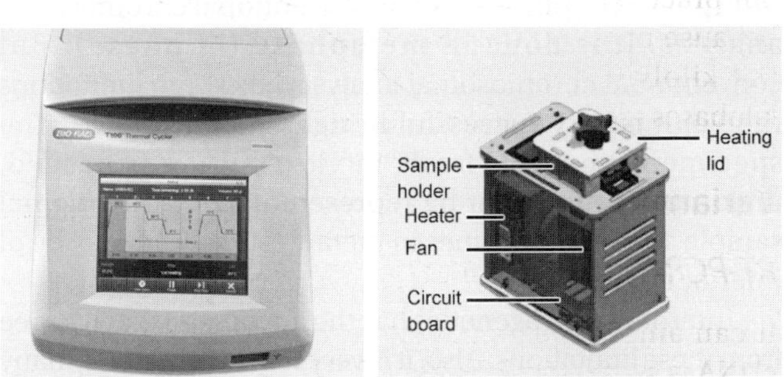

Fig. 9: PCR machine and its parts *(For color version, see Plate 11)*

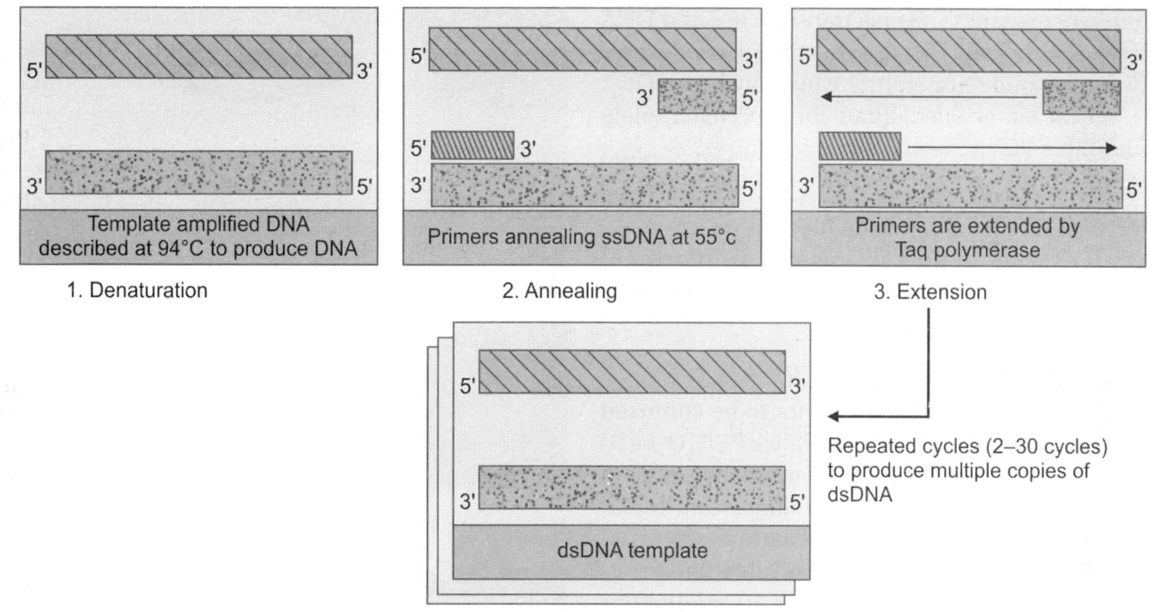

Fig. 10: Different steps in PCR

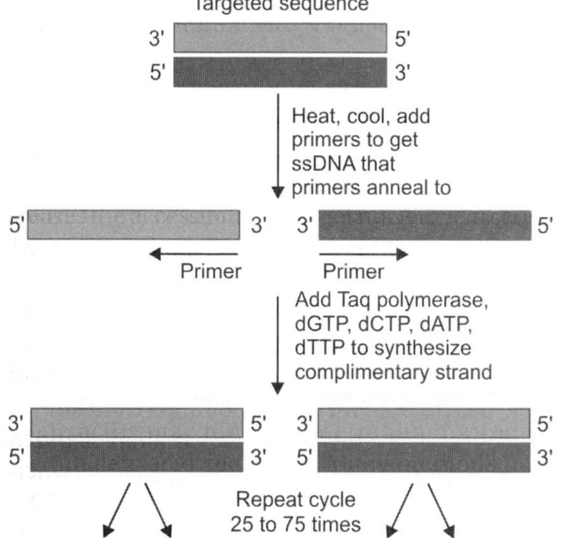

Fig. 11: Denaturation, annealing and extension; three important steps in PCR *(For color version, see Plate 12)*

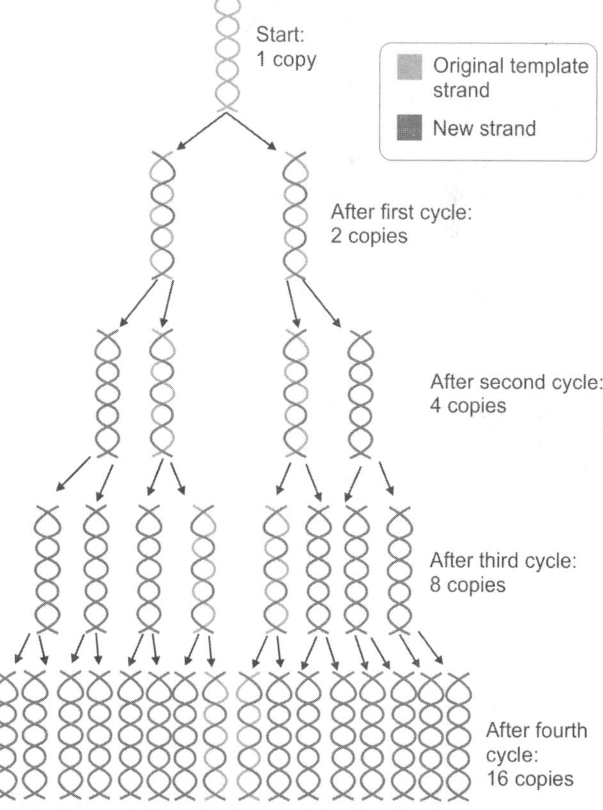

Fig. 12: Schematic diagram of different steps in a PCR *(For color version, see Plate 12)*

but practically, most PCR assay plateaus after 30 cycles, because of substrate excess. Smaller fragments of DNA (≤4 kilobases) are optimal and DNA fragments > 10 kilobases are unsuitable for PCR.

Variants of PCR

RT-PCR (Reverse Transcriptase PCR)

It can amplify RNA extracted from a tissue sample. A cDNA is synthesized from the RNA template with the help of enzyme reverse transcriptase. After the production of cDNA, it is then amplified by conventional PCR. The Tth DNA polymerase is ideal for RT-PCR because it has reverse transcription (RT) activity in the presence of manganese (rather than magnesium) and it overcomes the requirement for two different enzymes (reverse transcriptase and DNA polymerase). Another advantage is that the Tth can reverse transcribe at elevated temperature which improves DNA synthesis, as heat acts as a denaturant for the RNA template (Fig. 13 and Table 1).

Use:

- RT-PCR well suited for detection of RNA viruses.
- Molecular cytogenetic analysis of chromosomal translocation where there is formation of chimeric/fusion mRNAs.

Quantitative PCR (or Real-time PCR)

Some people also call it RT-PCR and not to be confused with reverse-transcriptase PCR. Quantitative PCR (Q-PCR) or real time PCR uses real time measurements of DNA accumulation, usually with the help of fluorescent-based markers. Many different chemical reactions are used for Q-PCR. Among them are **TaqMan** (also known as 5-exonuclease or hydrolysis real time PCR), **molecular beacon** (differentiates targets with only one single nucleotide difference), **scorpion** (also known as self-probing amplicons), hybridization probe and intercalating dye method. Whatever the chemistry in the reaction, change in fluorescence occurs due to amplification of targets. This change in color/fluorescence occurs due to amplification of targets. This change in color/fluorescence is measured by a detector during each cycle of reaction and is calculated by a computer. Then an amplification plot of fluorescence versus the cycle number is prepared and quantification of input target DNA sequence is done. The fluorescent composites used are TaqMan and SYBR green (Tables 2 and 3 and Figs 14 to 16).

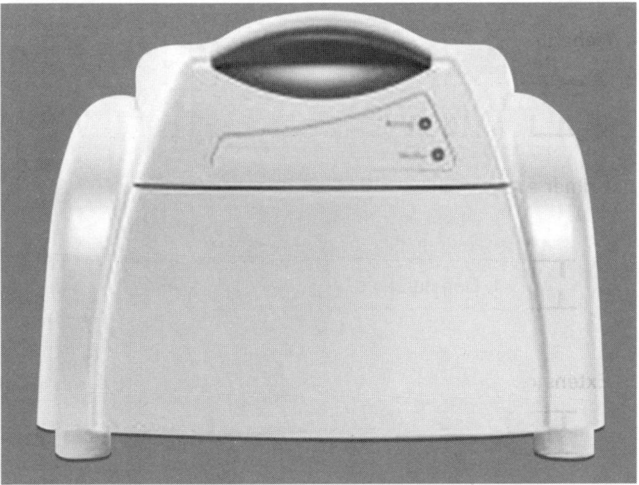

Fig. 13: RT-PCR machine

Table 1: Advantages and disadvantages of RT-PCR

Advantages of RT-PCR	*Disadvantages of RT-PCR*
1. Direct amplification of multiexon sequences by removing intervening introns 2. Simplifies mutation scanning methods 3. Demonstrate chromosomal translocations which create fusion genes easily 4. Detect change in mRNA structure which results from alternative splicing 5. Detect aberrant splicing due to mutation 6. Can evaluate the level of gene expression through quantitative PCR or Q-PCR	1. RNA is less stable than DNA, so PCR based on RNA is technically more demanding 2. As mRNA degrades quickly, tissue samples must be processed quickly 3. If target RNA is low in quantity, RT-PCR cannot be performed. A nested PCR is better 4. There is a chance of contamination and amplification of undesirable sequences, resulting in failure

Table 2: Advantages and disadvantages of Q-PCR

Advantages of Q-PCR	*Disadvantages of Q-PCR*
1. It can be applied to both fresh tissue and formalin fixed paraffin embedded tissue (FFPE)	1. Result may be erroneous due to amplification bias
2. It can be combined with reverse-transcriptase—PCR (Q-RT-PCR) which is a robust analytic approach	2. In case of Q-RT-PCR, due to lack of completion of the reverse transcription reaction, additional variables may be introduced into the analysis
3. Phenotype-genotype correlation can be done by analyzing-specific cell population (collected via microdissection or laser capture microdissection)	

Table 3: Differences between real-time PCR and conventional PCR

Real-time PCR	*Traditional/conventional PCR*
1. Detection time—shorter	1. Relatively longer
2. Quantification of bacterial or viral load—possible	2. Not possible
3. Contamination—no	3. May occur
4. Processing steps—easy	4. Laborious and time consuming
5. Positive result—detect as little as two-fold change	5. Requires at least 10-fold change
6. Accuracy of result—precise	6. Not very precise
7. New applications: a. Monitoring drug therapy b. Genotyping for drug resistance c. Identification of species/sub-species of different organisms	7. Not possible

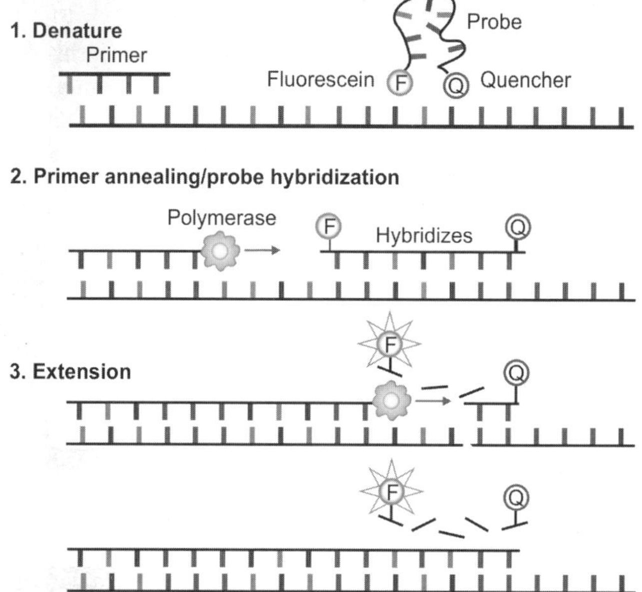

Fig. 14: Schematic diagram (TaqMan® probe method) of real-time PCR (RT-PCR) or quantitative PCR (Q-PCR) *(For color version, see Plate 12)*

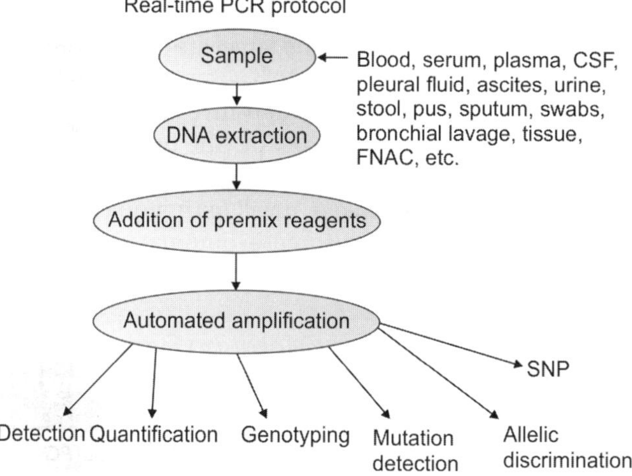

Fig. 15: Schematic diagram of real-time PCR protocol

Multiplex PCR

Multiplex PCR is the simultaneous amplification of multiple target sequences in a single reaction which is accomplished by simultaneous use of multiple pairs of probes. It can be applied to nested PCR and Q-PCR . It is ideal for conserving templates which are in short supply. Multiplex PCR saves lots of time as well money.

Nested PCR

In this method, two consecutive PCRs are performed on the same DNA template and second PCR is done on the

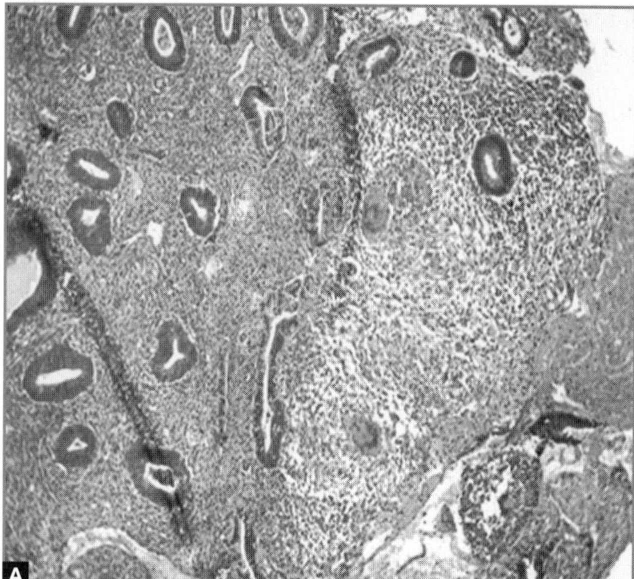

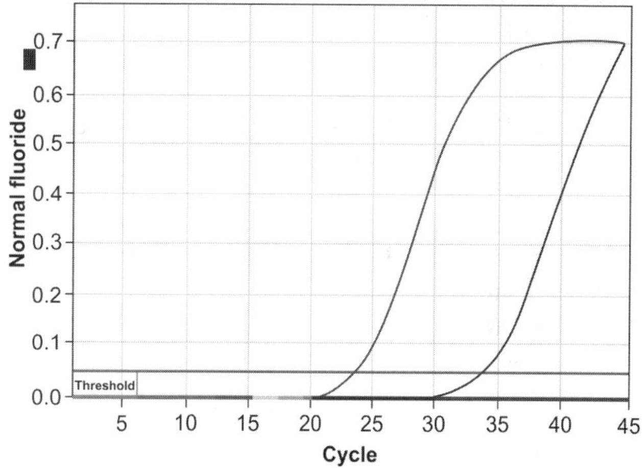

No.	Co-lor	Name	Type	Ct	Given Conc (copies)	Calc Conc (copies)	% Variation
1		C2	NTC				
2		C1	Standard	23.67	250,000	250,000	
3		Manibha Kumar	Unknown	33.89		Detected	

Legend: 1. C2 (NTC) – Negative control
2. C1 (Standard) – Positive control
3. Unkown – Patient sample

B

Figs 16A and B: (A) Photomicrograph showing few epithelioid granulomas of tuberculosis in the endometrium. The endometrium is in proliferative stage (H&E, × 100); (B) Real-time or RT-PCR detecting the *Mycobacterium tuberculosis* and its quantity/concentration *(For color version, see Plate 13)*

Table 4: Advantages and disadvantages of PCR techniques

Advantages	*Disadvantage*
1. PCR has high sensitivity and specificity. It can detect a single abnormal cell admixed with 10^5 normal cells	1. Amplification bias can be present. PCR bias refers to the fact that few DNA templates are preferentially amplified while other templates are not. It may be due to variation in template length, variation in template number and random differences in PCR efficiency with each cycle
2. PCR technique is simple, quick and inexpensive. A single PCR cycle consists of melting (denaturation), annealing and extension. It is completed within 3 minutes and required number of multiple cycles (25–35, average 28–30) can be done in few hours	2. PCR gives information about the target region in a gene only. Apart from target gene, information about other genes is not obtained
3. It can detect many genetic abnormalities resulting from structural abnormality, translocation, deletion or single base pair changes	3. It can amplify the target gene only when it is intact. If there is damage in the target region due to mutation (like deletion, insertion or point mutation), then primer cannot bind to the region of interest or primer binding site. So, it will give erroneous result
4. Phenotype -genotype correlations can be made. For this, microdissection from FFPE (formalin fixed paraffin embedded) tissue block, laser capture microdissection, flow cytometry and immunogenetic methods are used	4. Fresh tissue is better than fixed tissue in many cases. Degradation of DNA and mRNA (messenger RNA) may occur prior to and during fixation. Degradation of nucleic acids (DNA and mRNA) causes lowering of the sensitivity and specificity especially when it is necessary to use nested PCR or to amplify shorter target sequence
5. PCR products can be easily conjugated (labeled) and detection becomes easy. Conjugates or labels are usually attached to the 5' end of either or both oligonucleotide primers	5. There may be cross-contamination and presence of inhibitors which lowers the sensitivity and specificity

shorter sequence of the same DNA template. The primers used for the second PCR may be internal to those used for the first PCR reaction **(fully nested)**. If one primer is internal and the other primer is orginal primer, then it is called **seminested** PCR.

Nested PCR can be applied when the copy of target sequence is present in very low number or when nucleic acids (DNA or RNA) have been degraded due to tissue fixation or reverse transcriptase PCR (RT-PCR) when target mRNA is expressed at a very low level (Table 4).

Telomerase Repeat Amplification Protocol (TRAP)

For maintenance of chromosomal stability and integrity, the hexanucleotide TTAGGG repeat sequence of telomeres is essential. So, if there is any change in the telomere length, it will lead to development abnormalities and malignancies. The PCR-based TRAP assay is a simple, sensitive and reproducible method which measures telomerase activity. The protein extract used for testing can only be derived from fresh tissue or cells. Both false positive and false negative result may occur. If there is heterogeneity in a tumor, then test result may vary.

Ligase Chain Reaction (LCR)

In this method, a pair of adjacent oligonucleotide primers are used along with an additional enzyme called DNA ligase. This DNA ligase catalyzes the joining or ligation of adjacent DNA strands, in contrast to complimentary DNA strands. One of the two primers acts as the **"capture" probe** while the other primer acts as the **" reporter " probe**. The first or capture probe is allele specific. This technique (LCR) distinguishes normal alleles from the mutated alleles (single mutation), as ligation (joining) occurs only when exact matches between the primer and target are present. Usually, short sequence of DNA (with <50 base pairs) is analyzed in this method. The product gives positive result only when the sequence of interest is present. The two primers can be attached with different conjugates and when ligated, they will be covalently linked. It will permit quantification of LCR product, when measured in automated laboratory analyzers.

Amplification Refractory Mutation System (ARMS)

This technique also detects mutations using PCR. This technique is based on the fact that the most critical region for amplification to occur in the primer is its 3-end. So, if there is a mismatch in this 3-end, amplification will not occur. In this method, two primers which are identical in sequence, except at their 3-nucleotides are used. One primer has 3-nucleotide that is complimentary to the wild type gene (normal gene), while the 3-nucleotide of other primer is complimentary to the mutant gene. Amplification will occur when there is a perfect match between the primer and gene (3 nucleotide end) and it will produce positive signal. Hence, wild type or normal gene can be distinguished from the mutant or abnormal gene.

APPLICATIONS OF PCR

Medical Applications

- The first application of PCR was **genetic testing**, where a DNA sample is analyzed to detect genetic disease mutations. The parents can be tested for being genetic carriers while their children might be tested for actually affected by a disease process (like thalassemia).
- DNA samples for **prenatal diagnosis** can be obtained by amniocentesis, chorionic villus biopsy or even by analyzing the rare fetal cells circulating in the mother's blood stream.
- PCR analysis can also be done for **preimplantation genetic diagnosis**, where individual cells of a developing embryo are tested for mutations.
- PCR can also be used for **tissue typing, before organ transplantation**.
- Neoplasia or many forms of cancer alter the oncogenes. By using PCR-based test to study these **mutations in different cancers**, specific therapy regimen can be started.

Infectious Disease Applications

- **Detection of bacteria:**
  - ***Helicobacter pylori*:** Detection of *H. pylori* by PCR can be done from either fresh or FFP tissue (including the coccoid form which is nonculturable). The most common target regions are 16 S rRNA gene, Urease gene or arbitrarily choose genetic segment of the bacterial genome.
  - **Mycobacteria:** PCR-based analysis has allowed detection of small numbers of disease organisms (both live or dead). The targets are highly conserve gene that encodes the 65 kd heat shock protein (hsp). Other targets are repetitive insertion element IS6110 and genes encoding 16S ribosomal RNA (rRNA).
  - **Other bacteria** like bacillus anthracis can be detected by PCR.
- **Detection of viruses:**
  - **Human immunodeficiency viruses:** It is a difficult virus to find and eradicate. PCR test can detect as little as one viral genome of HIV among the DNA over 50,000 host cells.
  - **Human papilloma virus:** Most PCR protocols target the viral L1 gene and use consensus primers. After amplification of target region using consensus primer, the particular type of HPV (low-risk type 1, 2, 4, 7, or high-risk type 16, 18, 31, etc.) can be determined by either DNA sequence analysis or membrane hybridization with type specific probes.
  - **Respiratory viruses:** A multiplex RT PCR assay can detect 7 common respiratory viruses. These are adenovirus, respiratory syncytial virus, parainfluenza virus type 1, 2, 3 and influenza virus type A and B. corona virus (severe acute respiratory syndrome or SARS) can be detected by nested RT PCR.
  - **Epstein-Barr virus:** Five highly conserved segments of this virus or targets can be amplified and measured by Q-PCR. The test result gives highest sensitivity when all those five marker loci are analyzed. it can be done on FFP tissue also.
  - **Hepatitis C virus:** RT PCR can detect this virus in liver biopsies and focus on the 5-noncoding region which is highly conserved between the six genotypes and more than 90 subtypes of this virus. Highest sensitivity is achieved when RT-PCR is done via a nested RT PCR protocol or PCR products are analyzed by Southern blot hybridization.
- **Detection of protozoans:**
  - **Leishmaniasis:** Target regions for PCR analysis are genes encoding r-RNA, repetitive nuclear DNA sequences and kinetoplast DNA. PCR which amplify a 120-bp fragment of kinetoplast DNA has the highest sensitivity.
  - **Toxoplasmosis:** Many different PCR- based assays can detect the organisms, *Toxoplasma gondii* either from fresh or FFPE tissue. During active infection, immunoglobulin M level always does not correlate with recent infection and serologic diagnosis is unreliable. Also, reactivation of the disease is not always accompanied by change in antibody level. PCR does not have this drawback and PCR detection has clinical utility
  - **Intestinal parasite:** PCR which targets genes encoding 18 s rRNA or oocyst wall protein can detect Cryptosporidium. A nested PCR can detect microsporidia and targets the genes encoding the small subunit rRNA gene.
- **Detection of fungi:** Fungi can be detected by PCR in two ways. PCR can be performed using universal primers which bind to highly conserved sequences in the region, followed by direct or indirect DNA sequence analysis of PCR product to detect the specific fungal pathogen. In the second method, sequence differences in 18 s rRNA gene can be used to make primers which are specific for particular fungus. Most PCR protocols target sequence within the fungal rRNA genes. *Pneumocystis jiroveci*

(previously called *Pneumocystis carinii*) and *Aspergillus* species are detected by PCR.

Forensic Applications

- **Genetic fingerprinting** can uniquely identify any person from entire population of the world. Minute amount of DNA sample (like blood, saliva, semen, hair, etc.) can be isolated from a crime scene and is compared with the sample of suspects. It can also be done from a DNA database of convicts or earlier evidence.
- DNA finger printing can also be used for DNA **paternity testing**, in which an indivual is matched with their close relatives. DNA from unidentified person can be tested and compared with possible parents, siblings or children. The real biological father of a newborn can be confirmed (or ruled out). Also, similar tests can be adopted to confirm the biological parents of an adopted or kidnapped child.

Research Applications

- PCR augments many other molecular techniques such as generating **hybridization probes** for Southern or Northern blot hybridization. PCR supplies large amount of pure DNA, sometimes as single strand to these methods, enabling analysis even from very small amounts of starting material.
- **DNA sequencing** can also be assisted by PCR.
- PCR can be utilized for **DNA cloning**. It can extract DNA segments for insertion into a vector from a large genome. By using a single set of 'vecror primers', PCR can analyze or extract fragments which have been inserted into vectors.
- Another common application of PCR is the study of **gene expression**. Tissues (or even indivual cells) can be analyzed at different stages to assess which genes have become active or which have been inactive. Q-PCR can assess the actual level of expression.
- PCR is useful for **genetic mapping** by studying chromosomal crossovers after meiosis. PCR's ability to simultaneously amplify several loci from individual sperm has revolutionized genetic mapping and can detect rare crossovers, unusual deletions, translocations, inversion, etc.
- One interesting applications of PCR is the **phylogenic analysis of DNA** from ancient sources like frozen tissues of mammoth or recovered bones of dinosaurs or other ancient animals.

DNA MICROARRAYS

DNA microarray ('chip') is a technique of scientific revolution and it can analyze thousands of gene in a single step but require very small amount of nucleic acids. One should not confuse DNA microarray with tissue microarray, in which many cores of tissues from different cases are placed in the same paraffin block. Tissue microarray allows immunohistochemistry (IHC) or fluorescent in situ hybridization (FISH) to diagnose different cases from single block, and thus saves a lot of money and time. DNA microarray are applied in genotyping for point mutations, gene expression profile (GEP), single nucleotide polymorphism (SNP) and array-based comparative genomic hybridization (CGH) (Fig. 17).

Gene Expression Profile

It is based on hybridization of nucleic acid between free targets derived from biologic sample and an array of DNA fragments (probes) that have anchored to a solid surface. The targets are generated by reverse transcription and at the same time labeling of RNA molecules is done which are part of a complex mixtures of a distinct cDNA fragments that hybridize with the corresponding probe. A reference control is also used. The signal generated for each probe reflex the mRNA expression level of the corresponding gene in comparison to reference control. After detection of the signals, quantification

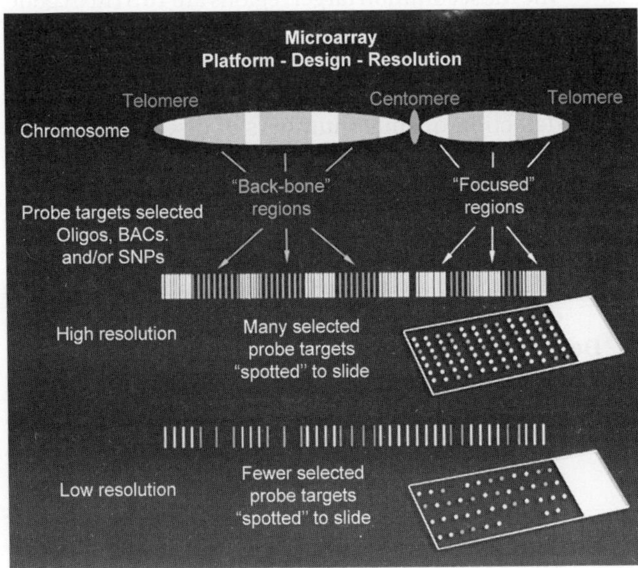

Fig. 17: Schematic diagram of DNA microarray
(For color version, see Plate 14)

and integration are done using specialized software. Thus our gene expression profile is made.

Application of GEP

- Tumor classification (Breast cancer, subtypes of large B cell or diffuse lymphomas).
- Validation and definition of tumor entities (translocation of t8:14 in Burkitt lymphoma).
- Determination of the site of origin of a tumor due to existence of organ-related gene expression.
- Identification of signaling pathways which is important in tumorigenesis.
- Prognostication or prediction of response of tumor to a particular therapy.

Single Nucleotide Polymorphism (SNP)

This is a DNA sequence variation which may be seen when a single nucleotide in the genome differs between the paired chromosomes in an individual or between members of a species. SNP may be seen in coding sequences of genes, noncoding regions of genes or in the intergenic regions. In entire human genome about 1.8 million SNPs are present.

The study of variation in DNA or polymorphism explains how humans develop disease (e.g. mental illness, diabetes, vascular disease) and respond to pathogens, drugs or chemicals. As for example, two SNPs are present in apolipoprotein (Apo E) resulting in three alleles, E2, E3 and E4. Each of these alleles differs by one DNA base and the protein product of each gene differs by single amino acids. The E2 allele appears to be protective for Alzheimer's disease while E4 allele increases the risk of developing the disease.

Array-based Comparative Genomic Hybridization (CGH)

In this technique, arrayed DNA probes (made from bacterial artificial chromosomes, cDNA or oligonucleotides) are used on a slide instead of metaphase spread of normal cells in conventional CGH. These arrayed DNA probes, cover-selected regions along all the different chromosomes. There is a competitive binding of tumor DNA and reference DNA for the indivual probes. This will indicate gain or loss of a particular chromosome segment. The resolution of the array or ability of the method precisely define the gain or loss of region, increases as the number of probes increases in the array CGH.

CHAPTER 23

In Situ Hybridization and Fluorescent In Situ Hybridization

IN SITU HYBRIDIZATION

INTRODUCTION

In the field of molecular diagnostics, most techniques are hybridization-based assays directed at the detection of specific DNA or RNA sequences, which have been extracted from a cellular sample. **Hybridization** refers to the binding or annealing of complementary DNA or RNA sequences. The **in situ hybridization (ISH)** technique permits the detection of nucleic acid targets within a micro anatomy context. So, ISH can detect specific nucleic acid sequences in morphologically preserved chromosomes, cells or tissue sections.

All nuclei acid hybridization tests are based on the fact that two antiparallel single-stranded nucleic acid molecules will recognize one another and Hybridize (bind to each other). This binding or hybridization is due to hydrogen bonding and hydrophobic base-stacking interactions of complementary base pairs. Adenine (A) binds to thymine (T) or uracil (U) if it is RNA. Likewise, guanine (G) binds to cytosine (C). Thus DNA:DNA, RNA:RNA and DNA:RNA duplexes may be formed.

ISH techniques were described by Gallan an Purdue, who used labeled 18s and 28s rRNA (ribosomal RNA) probes to detect genes of *Xenopus laevis* (an African frog). Previously, radioisotopes were used as labels for nucleic acids and detection of hybridization sequences was done by autoradiography. As technology of ISH advances, enzymatic and fluorescent methods become available, which are quick and safe for analysis. Haptenated probes (labeled with digoxigenin, biotin, dinitrophenol) may be detected with one of the three sets of distinguishable fluorophores, viz. green emitting light (fluorescein), red emitting light (rhodamine or Texas red) and blue (7-amino-4-methyl coumarin-3-acetic acid or AMCA, or Cascade blue).

Simultaneous hybridization with two or more of this different haptens and flurophores allows for simultaneous detection of two or more sequences of gene (or whole chromosome) of interest. Combinational use or labeling of multiple probes with two or more different reporters (such as fluorescein with rhodamine) further increases the number of distinguishable target. Furthermore, there is marked increase in the sensitivity and it permits the detection of small unique or low copy-number gene sequences (as small as 500 base pairs).

A major limitation of ISH compared to PCR and filter hybridization is its relatively low sensitivity (Table 1).

METHODS OF IN SITU HYBRIDIZATION

Laboratory

For RNA studies, a clean, dust-free work space or laboratory is essential and it must be ribonuclease (RNAse) free. The

Table 1: Different molecular techniques and their sensitivity

Tests/assay	*Sensitivity (detection threshold)*	*Specimen type*
1. Polymerase chain reaction (PCR)	10 copies/tissue	Fresh or fixed
2. In situ hybridization (ISH)	10 copies/cell	Fresh or fixed
3. PCR in situ hybridization	1 copy/cell	Fixed
4. Filter hybridization (Southern blot or slot blot)	1 copy/ 100 cells	Fresh

glasswares should be washed and treated with 0.1% diethyl pyrocarbonate (DEPC), autoclaved and then wrapped in aluminum foil. Then baked in an microwave oven at 180°C for 4 hours to overnight to eliminate residual RNAase. All solution must be treated with 0.1% DEPC before autoclaving is done. Plastwares must be RNAse free and should be sterile and disposable. In case of formalin fixed tissue, it is less problematic as formalin cross-linking protects RNA from degradation.

Glass Slides

Coating glass slides with an organosilane solution improves tissue adherance from about 10%–99%. Nowadays, silane-coated slides are available in the market. Other adhesives which may be used are gelatin, poly-L-lysine glue or Denhardt's solution. But silane coated slides are better.

Tissue Fixation

ISH may be performed on cell smears, or frozen sections or on fixed tissue. Buffered formalin (pH 7.0) is an excellent fixative for ISH. Unbuffered formalin, fixatives containing heavy metals (mercury in Zenker's solution) or picric acid (Bouin's solution) reduce the intensity of hybridization signal.

Frozen sections are not ideal for ISH because of its core morphology compared to fixed paraffin embedded tissue. Pretreatment with a protease (usually proteinase K) increases the accessibility of target nucleic acid sequence in gene and signal quality. But in frozen sections, proteinase K pretreatment degrades morphology.

Protease Digestion

Fixatives like formalin, which cross-links proteins and nucleic acids may hinder penetration of probes to the target nucleic acid sequence. Many methods have been adopted which facilitate probe entry, like treatment with HCl, Sodium sulfite and photo fluor. But pre-treatment with protease is superior. Different types of protaeses (Pepsin, proeteinase K, trypsin, Pronase) are available. Too much pre treatment with protease will destroy tissue morphology.

Generally, pepsin pre-treatment (2 mL/ml) for 12–25 minutes is good for tissues fixed for 8–24 hours in 10% buffered formalin. Proteinase K may be used at concentration 0.25–1.0 mg/mL depending on the type of tissue. In fact, the optimal concentration of protease and incubation time of particular tissue should be determined by titration using a positive control probe for hybridization.

Probe Labels

Probes may be labeled with a radioisotope (^{35}S, ^{32}P,^{3}H, ^{125}I) and detected by autoradiography. ^{35}S is the best radioisotope because it yields the best compromise between speed, resolution, background labeling and sensitivity.

Nonradioisotope labeling (Biotin or Digoxigenin) is safer, easier to use and gives faster signal detection. Biotin labeled probes may be detected by use of a streptavidin-alkaline phosphatase conjugate method. Digoxigenin labeled probes are detected with alkaline phosphatase conjugated antidigoxigenin antibody.

Probes

There are two types of probes used in ISH: **genomic probes** and **oligonucleotide probes (oligoprobes).** Genomic probes are derived from DNA segments (>1000 base pairs in length). Eventually genomic probes with 50–250 base pairs have been developed. The length of genomic probe is determined by the amount of DNase in the reaction for probes or by concentration by primer. Genomic probe synthesis and its labeling is usually done by PCR, nick translation or random priming (Table 2).

Oligoprobes are shorter in length (20-40 bp). They may be produced commercially or synthetically without the need of cloning technique (PCR, etc). Oligoprobes are less sensitive compared to genomc probes. It can be labeled for better specificity with terminal deoxy nucleotidyl transferase (TdT) at 3' end tailing.

Addition of formamide and low concentration of salt facilitate denaturing of the probe and target DNA. For genomic probes higher concentration (40–50%) of formamide is used compared to oligoprobes (10%). Dextran sulfate is commonly used to increase the effective concentration of the probe as well as the rate of hybridization.

Post-hybridization Wash

Post-hybridization wash is very important especially for radioactive probes. These probes have a tendency to nonspecifically bind to the membranes and nontarget nucleic acids producing too much background color. For nonradioisotope labeling, this is less problematic. This wash removes the probes which are bound to nontarget molecules and membranes.

For genomic or oligoprobes, different salt concentrations and temperature are used during post hybridization wash.

Table 2: Requirement of genomic and oligo probe

Requirement for genomic probe	*Requirement for oligo probe*
1. Salt concentration: 15 mM NaCl	1. 150 mM NaCl
2. Albumin: 0.1% bovine serum albumin	2. 0.1% bovine serum albumin
3. Temperature and time: 55–65°C for 10 minutes	3. 45–55°C for 10 minutes

Detection System

After post-hybridization, a probe-target complex is produced. A wide range of chromogens are used to localize and visualize the alkaline-phosphatase target-probe complex. The chromogens may be blue, red, yellow or other color. Fluorescent chromogens are also available. Many prefer to use the chromogen 5-bromo-4-chloro-3-indolylphosphate in the presence of nitroblue tetrazolium (NBT-BCIP). When NBT-BCIP is used as chromogen, the counterstain nuclear fast red gives good nuclear identification (pale pink).

Troubleshooting

- **Background staining**: This is the most commonly encountered problem and is due to nonspecific binding. If the probe to undesirable targets. By two ways, the problem can be sorted out: decreasing the concentration of salt during post-hybridization wash and increasing the wash time by 10 minutes intervals or decrease the concentration of probe. One may also do both if required.
- **Poor tissue morphology:** This is due to over treatment with protease. Decreasing the protease concentration (5–10 times) or by decreasing the time of protease digestion (2–3 minute interval) will solve this problem.
- **Silane-coating/adhesive:** Tissue must stick to the silane/adhesive. A loss of more than 5% means incorrect silanization and will produce poor/absence of hybridization signal.

IN SITU HYBRIDIZATION (ISH) PROTOCOL

- Tissue preparation.
  - Place the paraffin-embedded sections (4–5 μm) on glass slides.
  - Wash these slides with xylene for 5–10 minutes, then 100% ethanol for 5 minutes and then air dried.
- Probe cocktail: Genomic or oligoprobes as per requirements.
- Denaturation of probe and target DNA
  - Add 10 μL of the probe on to tissue section.
  - Cover it with a coverslip (little larger than the tissue section).
  - Now, place the glass slide on hot plate at 95–100°C for 5 minutes.
  - If there is any bubble, remove it with a toothpick.
- Hybridization and washing
  - Keep the slides in humidity chamber at 37°C for 2 hours.
  - Remove the coverslips and place the slides in wash solution (refer to post-hybridization wash).
  - Remove/wipe off excess wash solution.
  - Place the slides in a humidity chamber so that slides do not dry out.
- Detection
  - Add digoxigenin-alkaline phosphate conjugate (1:200 dilution) to the tissue sections, which are in humidity chamber.
  - Incubate for 30–40 mins at 37°C.
  - Wash the slides for 3–5 minutes at room temperature [by a solution of 0.1M Tris HCl (pH 9–9.5) and 0.1M NaCl].
  - Place the slides in detection reagent solution with added chromogen (NBT-BCIP)
  - Incubate the slides for 1/2–2 hours and check under microscope for optimal result.
- Counterstain and coverslip
  - Wash the slides in distilled water for 1–2 minutes.
  - Counterstain with nuclear fast red solution for 5–7 minutes.
  - Again wash the slides in distilled water for 2 times.
  - Place the slides in 95% ethanol first, then in 100% ethanol (each 1 minute duration).
  - Keep them in xylene for 1–2 minutes.
  - Cover the slides using permount and coverslip.
  - View under microscope.

RESULT

- Blue Signal: Positive
- Red: Negative (nuclear fast red as counterstain).

APPLICATIONS OF ISH

- Detection of Viral infections: Human papilloma virus, JC virus (which causes progressive multifocal leukoencephalopathy or PML), Cytomegalovirus, Epstein- Barr virus, Human Immunodeficiency Virus or HIV-1, adenovirus, herpes simplex virus and measles virus.
- Identification of chromosomal disorder.
- Analysis of certain human tumors and sensitive assay for the study of oncogenes.

FLUORESCENT IN SITU HYBRIDIZATION (FISH)

INTRODUCTION

Fluoroscent in situ hybridization (FISH) uses tagged probes which bind to chromosome-specific DNA

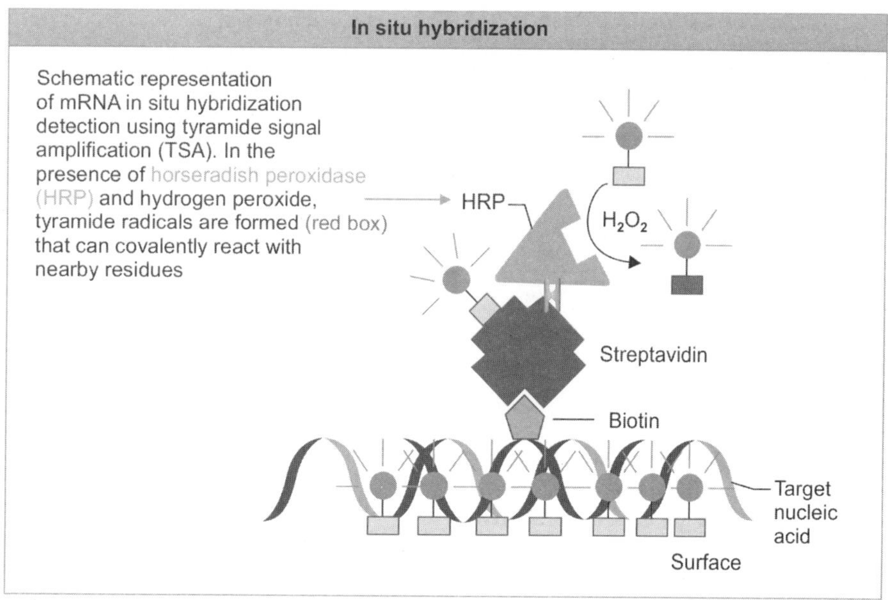

Fig. 1: Schematic diagram of mRNA in situ hybridization (ISH) *(For color version, see Plate 14)*

sequences of interest and detect structural as well as numerical aberrations in different tumors/malignancies. FISH can be performed **on dividing cells (metaphase)** as well as in **nondividing cells (interphase).** Also it can be performed on formalin fixed paraffin-embedded tissue (FFPE) or air-dried smears. In surgical pathology, FISH is used primarily to detect somatic cancer-associated alterations with known diagnostic, therapeutic and prognostic implications. It can detect four common chromosomal abnormalities, e.g., gene deletion, aneusomy (gain or loss of a chromosome), translocation and gene amplification (Fig. 1).

BASIC STEPS OF FISH

It includes fixation of the DNA (in metaphase or interphase nuclei) on slides and denaturation of DNA in situ to make DNA single stranded. Then target DNA sequence is hybridized to specific DNA probe sequences that are conjugated or labeled with fluorochrome for their easy detection. Excess of probe is added. So that binding of probe to target DNA happens. For visualization, fluorescent microscope is used. Analysis of probe signals includes gain of signals, loss of signals, fusion of signals and positioning of signals.

PROBES

Usually they are of three types:

1. Unique sequences probes (size less than 1kb to greater than 1 Mb of DNA).
2. Repetitive sequences probes (e.g, centromeres and alpha-satellite regions of chromosome).
3. Whole chromosome sequences probes (that includes short arm, long arm and the centromere).

LABELING IN FISH

Probes can be labeled directly or indirectly. Directly labeled probes are available commercially and fluorochrome is directly bound to proble nucleotides. The probes can also be indirectly labeled with addition of a hapten (biotin or digoxigenin) into DNA via nick translation for example. Then the probes are detected with the help of fluorescent labeled antibody (streptavidin and antidigoxigenin).

Probes may be labeled in green (e.g. spectrum Green or fluorescein), in red (spectrum Orange or Texas Red), in blue (Sperteim Aqua) or in gold (Specteim Gold). **Fusion** of green and red signals in FISH is visualized as **yellow signal** under fluorescent microscope (Table 3).

TISSUE TYPES

- **Dividing cells (in metaphase)**: Cultured cells like amniocytes, chorionic villi, lymphocytes, bone marrow aspirates or from solid tumors. Metaphase spreads are routinely used in cytogenetics also.
- **Nondividing cells (in interphase)**:Peripheral blood smears, uncultured amniocytes (used for rapid prenatal diagnosis) or bone marrow aspirate smears.
- **Fixed tissues**: FISH can also be performed from paraffin block sections, touch/imprint preparations from solid

Table 3: Symbols and abbreviations used in interphase FISH

Symbol or abbreviation	Description
Plus sign (+)	Present on a specific chromosome
Minus sign (-)	Absent on a specific chromosome
WCP	Whole chromosome paint
SCP	Separated signals (usually close in normal cells).
PCP	Partial chromosome paint
NUC ISH	Nuclear or interphase in situ hybridization
ISH	In situ hybridization
CON	Connected or adjacent signals
PERIOD (.)	Separate cytogenetic results from ISH results

tumors or lymph nodes, disaggregated cells from paraffin blocks.

FISH PROCEDURES (GENERAL/COMMON THINGS)

- Fixed metaphase or interphase chromosome on a glass slide are required. To obtain good signals slides should be aged because it hardens the DNA, removes the water and increases signal intensity.
- If slides are prepared and FISH analysis to be performed on the same day then artificial aging should be done by keeping slides in a oven at 37°C for at least 2–3 hours.
- Other method of artificial aging (for slides kept at room temperature for <3 weeks) is to place them in 2 X SSC (sodium chloride-sodium citrate solution) at 73°C for 2–3 minutes. It can also be done by placing the slides in 37°C for 1 hour followed by dehydration in ethanol.
- For metaphase FISH, (using metaphase probes) at least 15 metaphases/22–22 mm area should be present (Fig. 2).

REAGENTS

Preparation of SSC Solution

20 X SSC buffer

- Sodium chloride: 87.66 g
- Sodium citrate: 44.10 g
- Distilled water: 400 mL

Make the pH of the solution 7.0 with 1M HCl. Make the volume to 500 mL with addition of distilled water. Filter it (0.4 μm filtration unit) and store at room temperature. Discard after 6 months.

2 × SSC buffer

- 20 × SSC: 25 mL
- Distilled water: 225 mL

Store at room temperature. Discard after 6 months.

Graded Alcohol

70%, 80%, 95%, and 100% ethanol.

Denaturing Solution (70% Formamide/2x SSC)

- Formamide: 17.5 mL
- 20 × SSC: 2.5 mL
- Distilled water: 5.0 mL

With 1M HCl, make the pH to 7.0. Store at 4°C. Discard after 7 days.

Post-wash Solution I

- 20 × SSC: 50 mL
- Distilled water: 449.5 mL
- NP-40–0.5 mL [Nonidet P-40]

Make the pH to 7.0 ± 0.2 with the help of 1M NaOH. Mix well. Can be stored for 6 month at room temperature.

Post-wash Solution II

- 20 × SSC: 10 mL
- Distilled water: 488.5 mL
- NP-40 –1.5 mL [Nonidet P-40]

Make the pH to 7.5 ± 0.2 with the help of 1M NaOH. Mix well. Can be stored for 6 month at room temperature.

DNA Counterstain

DAPI (4', 6-diamildino-2-phenyl-indole) and propidium iodide fluoresencent dyes are used to counterstain DNA. There are two type of DAPI (DAPI I and DAPI II). DAPI I is used when a more intense counterstain is desired while DAPI II is used for weaker counterstain.

Next the FISH procedure can be performed **in two days** (though same day procedure is also available).

Day-1

- Denature the slide in denaturing solution in water bath at 37°C.
- Examine for optimal target area on a glass slide prepared for FISH.
- Dehydrate in cold graded ethanol/alcohol (70%, 85%, and 100%) each 2 minutes duration.
- Dry the slides.
- Store the dried slides for aging (>3 week at room temperature) to obtain good signals.
- Probes should be pre-warmed to room temperature for 5 minutes. If probes need denaturation, then aliquot 7 μL hybridization butter, 2 μL distilled water and 1 μL probe into a centrifuge tube. If probes do not require denaturation, then aliquot 10 μL of probes for 22 × 22 mm target area [Keep the probes in dark area and return to refrigeration as soon as possible].

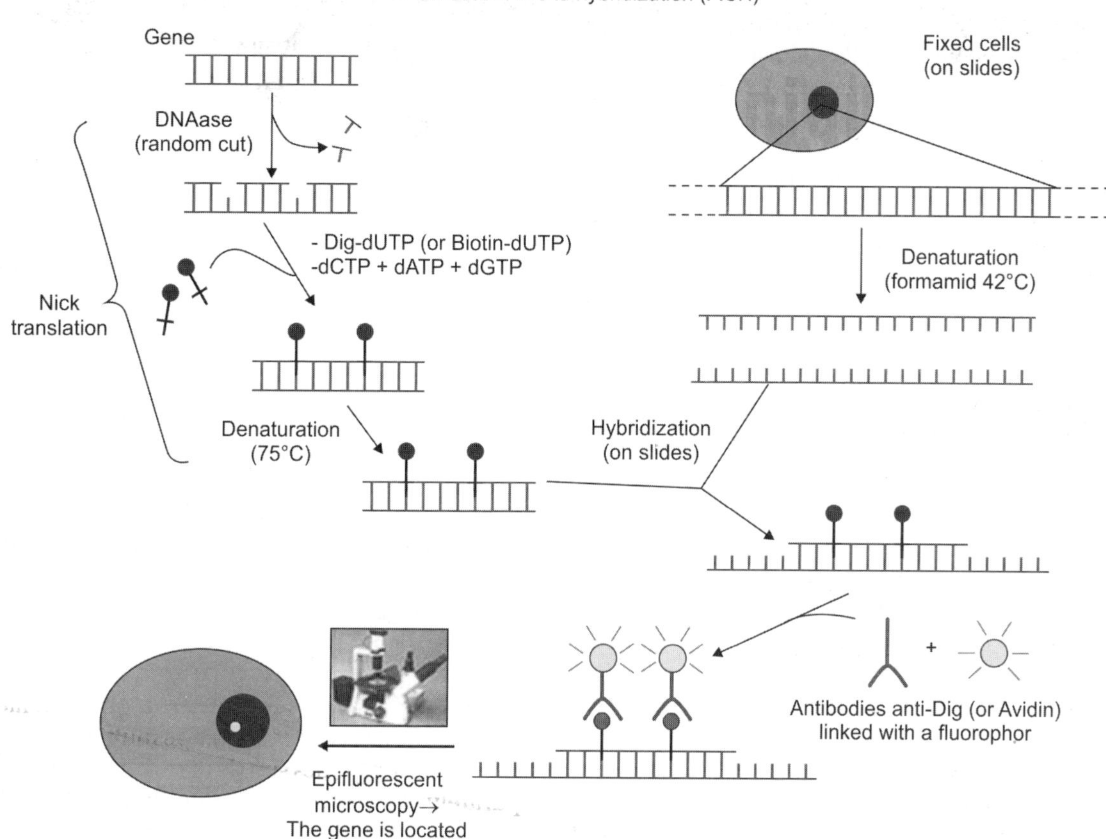

Fig. 2: Scheme of the principle of the FISH (fluorescent in situ hybridization). Experiment to localize a gene in the nucleus
(For color version, see Plate 15)

- Vortex the probe for brief period.
- Centrifuge for 2–3 seconds.
- Denature the slides in the pre-warmed denaturant at 73°C for exactly 2 minutes [A maximum of 3 slides should be denatured at one time to maintain correct denaturation temperature].
- After denaturation keep the denatured probes and slides in an humidified chamber for overnight at 37°C [Use moist paper towels or sponge in an airtight, opaque container].

Points to remember

- If denaturation of probes and slides are not performed separately, they can be co-denatured (denaturation of both probes and slides simultaneously). As for example; Hybridization system from Abbott molecule Inc. and Thermobrite™ Denaturation at 73°C for 2 minutes.
- Following denaturation of probes and slides (either form mentioned above), they should be placed in a humidified chamber, so that slides are not dried out.
- Slides may be left in the Thermobrite™ instrument for hybridization of probes with targets at 37°C for 4–12 hours.

Day-2

- Warm glass Coplin containing **post-wash solution II** to 73±1°C. To maintain correct temperature, do not wash more than 3 slides at a time.
- Remove the coverslips or rubber cement from the hybridized slides. The slides (hybridized) were kept in dark and covered as much as possible.
- Wash the slides in **post-wash solution II** at room temperature for 2 minutes. Agitate slides for 1-3 seconds.
- Wash the slides in **post-wash solution I** at room temperature for 1 minute. -Agitate slides for 1-3 seconds.
- Let the slides be dried and protect it from light.
- Incubate with 2 µl of DAPI I or DAPI II to slides and cover the slides with glass coverslip (approximately sized).

Interphase Scoring Criteria

- A minimum of 200 individual interphase cells should be analyzed.
- Only monolayered cells with distinct borders are considered for analysis. Overlapping cells are unsuitable.

- Signals are considered fusion signals if two signals are on top of each other (e.g. fusion of orange and green signals when fused impart yellow signals).
- An orange signal and a green signal with discrete border are regarded separate signals and not a fusion (yellow) signal.
- Signals should be discrete and not diffuse; signals are counted as two signals if they are more than one-signal-width apart. If the signals are closer than one signal-width apart, it should be counted as one signal (Tables 4 and 5).

Table 4: Different chromosomal abnormalities in tumors/cancers by FISH and their significance

Chromosomal abnormality	*Tumor/cancer type*	*Chromosomal alteration/ probes*	*Significance*
Translocation	• CML	• BCR-ABL	• Diagnostic, MRD
	• AML	• AML1-ETO,CBFB-BA,PML-RARA,BCL-ABL	• Diagnostic, predictive, prognostic
	• ALL	• TEL-AML1,BCR-ABL,MLL-BA	• Diagnostic, predictive, prognostic
	• Multiple myeloma	• IGH-CCND1, IGH-BA	• Prognostic
	• Burkitt lymphoma	• MYC-IGH, MYC-BA	• Diagnostic
	• Synovial sarcoma	• SYT-SSX, SYT-BA	• Diagnostic
	• EWS/PNET	• EWS-FLI1,EWS-BA	• Diagnostic
	• Follicular lymphoma	• IGH-BCL2	• Diagnostic
Amplification	• Medulloblastoma	• MYCN, c-myc	• Diagnostic, prognostic
	• Breast carcinoma	• HER-2/neu	• prognostic, predictive
	• Neuroblastoma	• N-myc	• Diagnostic, prognostic
Aneusomies/ Deletions	• CLL	• 13q-, 11q-, 17q-	• Diagnostic, prognostic
	• Prostatic carcinoma	• 8p-, 8q+	• Prognostic
	• Oligodendrio-glioma	• 1p- with 19q-	• Diagnostic, predictive
	• Lung carcinoma	• 8q,5p, +7p	• Diagnostic
	• Urothelial carcinoma	• +3,7 or 17;9p-	• Diagnostic
	• Multiple myeloma	• RB1 (13q-), TP53 (17p-)	• Prognostic
	• Leukemia/MDS	• +8,+12,-5,-7	• Diagnostic, prognostic

Abbreviations: CML, chronic myeloid leukemia; AML, acute myelogenous leukemia; ALL, acute lymphoblastic leukemia; EWS/PNET, Ewing's sarcoma/primitive neuroectodermal tumor; MDS, myelodysplatic syndrome.

METAPHASE SCORING CRITERIA

- A minimum of 10 metaphase cells should be analyzed. Only complete metaphases (with all 46 chromosomes in metaphase) should be scored.
- If the analysis is normal, only one image capture is required. But if the analysis is abnormal, then at least two images should be captured.

Reasons for False-negative (Wrong) Results

- Incomplete staining of tissue
- Wrong tissue sent
- Slide mountant not solid before taking to pathologist.
- Coverslip moves after being marked.
- Tissue sections fall off during pretreatment during FISH.
- Different orientation of tissue on side to H&E which affects transfer of target area.
- Marked area on H&E does not match that on FISH slide.

Though FISH has wide clinical applications, one disadvantage is signal fading as the slides become old. Capturing digital images for permanent record is done. Otherwise, chromogenic in situ hybridization (CISH) may be done to bypass this problem of signal fading. But multicolor CISH is not as simple as multicolor FISH. Some commercial companies supply the test and reference probes separately, so that instead of on dual-color FISH assay, two single-color CISH assays are performed (Flowchart 1) (Figs 3 to 5).

SINGLE DAY FISH PROTOCOL (SIGMA–ALDRICH)

Reagant and Equipment Required

- 20x saline-sodium citrate buffer (SSC:3 M NaCl, 0·3 M sodium citrate, pH 7 or product No. S6639).

Table 5: Fish and diagnostic tests

1. Prenatal testing for chromosomal disorders a. Trisomy 13, 18 and 21. b. XY aneusomies.
2. Microdeletion syndrome a. Cri-du-chat (5p-) b. Prader-Willi/Angelman (15q-) c. Di George syndrome (22q-)
3. Oncology (diagnostic predictive and prognostic markers) a. Translocation in different tumors/cancers b. Chromosomal aneusomies c. Gene amplifications d. Gene/locus deletions
4. Transplant pathology a. Disease relapse using known genetic alterations in primary tumor b. XY FISH on sex-mismatched organ transport

Flowchart 1: FISH and CISH

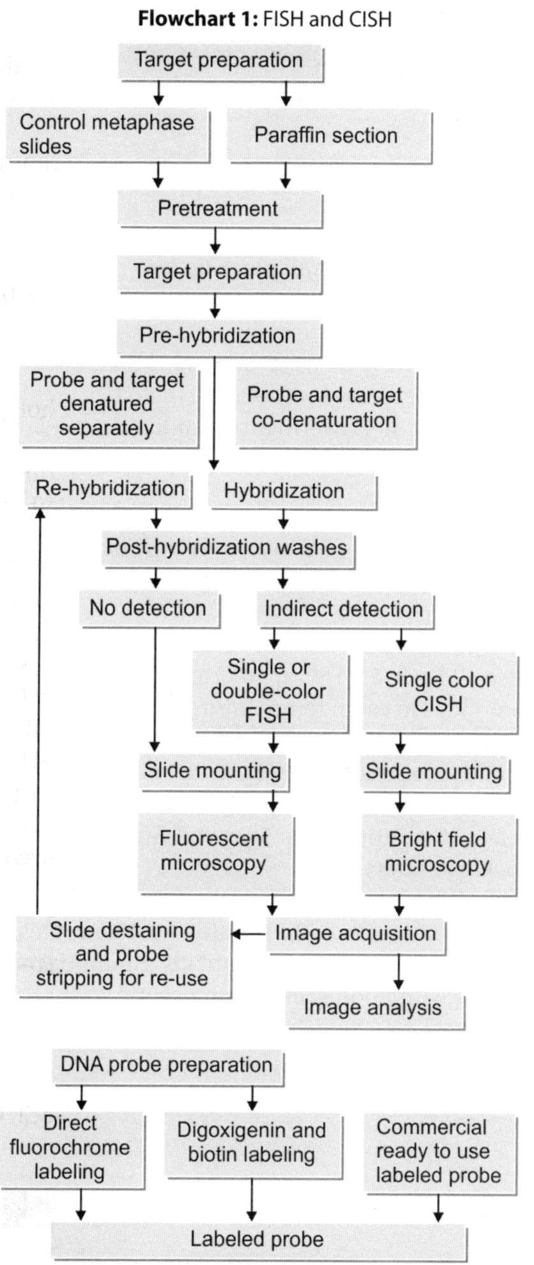

Abbreviations: FISH, fluorescent in situ hybridization; CISH, chromogenic in situ hybridization

- RNase (product No. R4642) 100 µg/mL in 2xSSC.
- Pepsin (product No. P6887) 40 units/mL in 10 mM HCl.
- Paraformaldehyde, EM grade (product No. P6148), freshly depolymerized, 4% w/v in water.
- Ethanol.
- Labeled probe. Plasmid DNA is labeled with biotin-II-dUTP using nick translation random priming or the PCR (e.g. ADVENCE™ Nick Translation Kit).
- Hybridization mix solution: 50% formamide (product No. F7508), 10% dextran sulfate (product No. D8906),

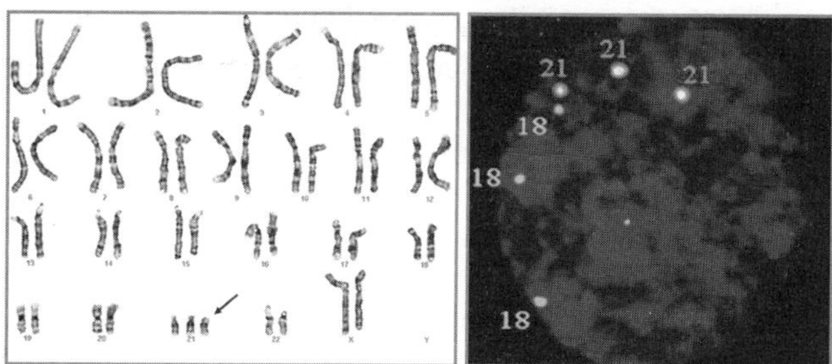

Fig. 3: Conventional cytogenetic G-banded karyotype demonstrating trisomy 21. The arrow indicates the third copy of chromosome 21. Trisomy 21 detected by FISH. An extra chromosome of 21, which gives red signal. Do not be confused about the chromosome 18 in the lower left corner which is part of a pairs of other chromosome 18 and is not part of chromosome 18 pair above it *(For color version, see Plate 15)*

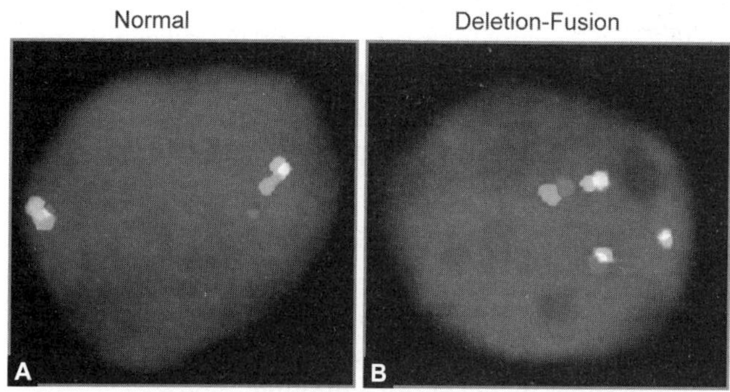

Figs 4A and B: Four-color FISH assay after probe hybridization in a normal (A) and prostate tumor cell (B). In the normal cell, all four of the probes (red, yellow, green, and blue) exist within close proximity to one another (in two four-colored foci corresponding to a diploid nucleus) since the probes recognize a distinct chromosomal locus containing two adjacent genes, TRMPRSS2 and ERG. The tumor cell on the right has had two deletion-fusion events at the TRMPRSS2 and ERG loci, as evidenced by two blue/red dimeric probe signals and the loss of the other two-colored signals (lower right side of nucleus) *(For color version, see Plate 16)*

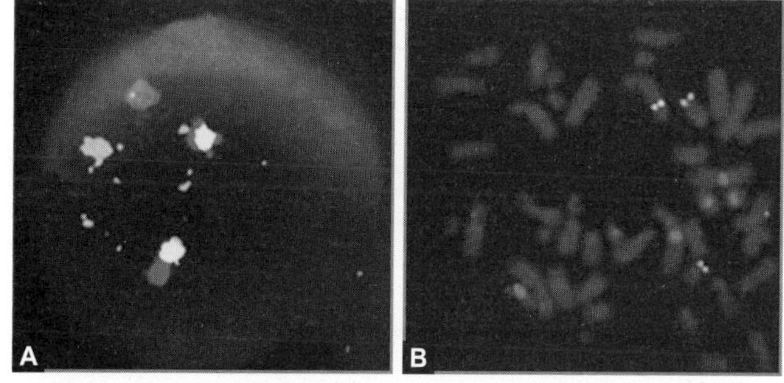

Figs 5A and B: Fluorescence in situ hybridization (FISH) analysis on interphase (A) and metaphase nuclei (B), using the ***LSI IGH/CCND1*** XT dual-color probes. Dual-fusion translocation DNA probe identifying the presence of the t (11;14) (q13;q32) chromosomal translocation. One orange (CCND1 on chromosome 11q13), one green (IGH on chromosome 14q32), and two fusion signal patterns [der (11) and (der14)], indicating the chromosomal rearrangements produced by the translocation can be observed *(For color version, see Plate 16)*

0.1% SDS (product No. L4390), 0.5-1.5 ng/μL labeled probe and 300 ng/mL Salmon sperm DNA (product No. D7656) in 2×SSC.

- Wash buffer: 20% formamide (product No. F7508) in 0.1×SSC
- Detection buffer: 0.2% Tween 20 (product No. P1379) in 4×SSC
- Block buffer: 5% bovine albumin (product No. A3803) in detection buffer
- Antibody or detection compound (e.g. streptavidin-Cy 3, product No. S6402) in blocking buffer.
- DAPI (product No. D9542) 2 μg/mL in antifade mounting medium.
- Fluoresence microscope, filters and optional triple band pass filter (x58, Omega optics).
- Glass slides (product No. S8400).
- Plastic coverslips for incubation and hybridization steps (cut from autoclave waste bags, e.g. product No. B4408).
- Heat block/modified thermocycler.
- Coplin jars for washing steps (product No. S6016, S5641 or S5891).

Procedure

- Start with chromosome preparation from any cell type.
- Incubate with 200 μL RNase for 1 hour at 37°C.
- Wash slides in 2× SSC for 5 minutes, repeat.
- Rinse slides in 10 nM HCl.
- Incubate with 200 μL pepsin for 10 minutes at 37°C.
- Rinse slides in deionized H_2O.
- Wash slides in 2 × SSC for 5 minutes, repeat.
- Stabilize slides in paraformaldehyde for 10 minutes.
- Wash slides in 2 × SSC for 5 minutes, repeat.
- Dehydrate slides in an ethanol series: 70%, 80%, 95%; 2 minutes each.
- Air dry.

Hybridization

- Prepare 30 μL hybridization solution per slide. Heat to 70°C for 10 minutes and place on ice.
- Place 30 μL of hybridization solution on each slide and cover with a plastic coverslip.
- Denature slide at 65–70°C for 5 minutes on heat block.
- Gradually decrease temperature to 37°C.
- Hybridize at 37°C overnight humidity chamber.

Detection

- Wash slides in 2 × SSC to remove coverslip.
- Wash slide in wash buffer at 40°C for 5 minutes, repeat.
- Wash slides in 0.1 × SSC at 40°C for 5-15 minutes.
- Wash slides in 2 × SSC at 40°C for 5-15 minutes.
- Cool slides to room temperature.
- Equilibrate slides in detection buffer for 5 minutes.
- Block in blocking buffer for 20–30 minutes.
- Incubate with 50 μl antibody or detection compound for 30–60 minutes (e.g. 5 μg/mL Streptavidin-Cy3 in blocking buffer).
- Wash slides in 2 × SSC for 5–15 minutes, repeat twice.
- Counterstain with DAPI solution for 10 minutes.
- Rinse briefly and mount in antifade mounting medium.
- Analyze with fluorescence microscope.

Appendix

LENGTH

The basic unit is meter (m).

Unit Meter	Abbreviation m	Size
Centimeter	cm	10^{-2} m
Milimeter	mm	10^{-3} m
Micrometer	µm	10^{-6} m
Nanometer	nm	10^{-9} m
Picometer	pm	10^{-12} m

MASS

The basic unit is kilogram (kg) and working unit is gram (g).

Unit	Abbreviation	Size
Kilogram	Kg	1,000 g or 10^{3} g
Miligram	mg	10^{-3} g
Microgram	µg	10^{-6} g
Nanogram	ng	10^{-9} g
Picogram	pg	10^{-12} g

PREPARATION OF SOLUTION

The most common fixative used in histology is 10% formalin or 10% neutral buffered formalin. To make 10% formalin add one part of formalin (concentrated formaldehyde, which contains 40% w/v formaldehyde) to 9 parts of water. This 10% formalin contain 4% solution of formaldehyde. If a solution of solid solute is to be prepared, then add solute in the solvent water by weight. If 10% solution of NaCl (sodium chloride) is to be prepared then, add 10 g of NaCl in 100 mL of water (aqueous solution). If solvent other than water is used, then it is non-aqueous solution (Tables 1 and 2).

MOLAR SOLUTION (M)

A 1 molar solution or 1M solution is the molecular weight (MW) in grams of the solute dissolved in 1 liter (1000 mL) of solvent or water. Molecular weight of sodium chloride

Table 1: Volume to volume preparation for making 100 mL solution

% Aqueous solution	mL of solute	mL of water
0.1%	0.1 mL	99.9 mL
1%	1 mL	99 mL
10%	10 mL	90 mL
50%	50 mL	50 mL
90%	90 mL	10 mL

Table 2: Weight to volume preparation for making 100 mL solution

%Weight	Solute	Solvent (water)
1%	1 g	100 mL
5%	5 g	100 mL
10%	10 g	100 mL
50%	50 g	100 mL
0.1%	10 mL of 1%	90 mL
0.01%	1 mL of 1%	99 mL

(NaCl) is 23 + 35.5 = 58.5. So to make 1M solution of NaCl, 58.5 of sodium chloride is to be dissolved in 1000 mL of water.

Solution	Weight of solute	Volume of solvent
1 molar or 1M	Molecular weight (MW) in grams 1,000 mL	
0.1 molar or 0.1M	0.1×MW in grams	1,000 mL
0.01 molar or 0.01m	0.01×MW in grams	1,000 mL
	Or	
	10 mL of 0.1 molar (0.1 M)	90 mL of solvent

Normal Solution (N)

This depends on molecular weight (MW) and number of positive charges present in the solute. For example, in case of NaCl, there is only one positive charge. So to make a normal solution (1N), 58.5 g of NaCl is to be dissolved, which is the same amount to prepare 1M solution of NaCl.

But in case of $CaCl_2$, the calcium ion has two positive charges (valency 2). So, molecular weight is to be divided by 2 and this amount of $CaCl_2$ is to be dissolved in 1,000 mL. This weight is called equivalent weight. If the valency or number of positive ions is 3, then MW is to be divided by 3. Suppose positive molecules is X and negative molecule is Y then:

Normality	*Species*	*Equivalent weight*
1N	$X^{+1}Y^{-1}$	Molecular weight (MW)
2N	$X^{+1}Y^{-1}$	2XMW
1N	$X^{+2}Y^{-2}$	½ X MW
1N	$X^{+3}Y^{-3}$	1/3 X MW
0.1N	Any solution	1 part 1N + 9 parts water

PREPARATION OF SOME USEFUL SOLUTIONS

- *Scott's tap water*
  - Magnesium sulfate: 20 g
  - Potassium bicarbonate: 2 g
  - Distilled water: 100 mL
- *Lugol's iodine*
  - Iodine: 1 g
  - Potassium iodide: 2 g
  - Distilled water: 100 mL
- *Gram's iodine*
  - Iodine: 1 g
  - Potassium iodide: 2 g
  - Distilled water: 300 mL
- *Alcian blue (with different pH)*
  - pH 0.2—1 g dissolved in 100 mL 10% sulfuric acid
  - pH 0.5—1 g dissolved in 100 mL 0.2 M hydrochloric acid
  - pH 1.0—1 g dissolved in 100 mL 0.1 M hydrochloric acid
  - pH 2.5—1 g dissolved in 100 mL 3% acetic acid
  - pH 3.2—1 g dissolved in 100 mL of 0.5% acetic acid
- *Acid alcohol*
  - 70% alcohol: 99 mL
  - Concentrated hydrochloric acid: 1 mL
- *Saturated picric acid solution*
  - Dry picric acid is hazardous. So it is commercially available as hydrated picric acid containing 30–35% water.
  - Hydrated picric acid: 1.6 g
  - Distilled water: 100 mL

This solution of picric acid should be kept in air tight container, so that it does not evaporate and picric acid becomes dry. Dry picric acid may cause explosion.

PREPARATION OF SOME USEFUL BUFFER SOLUTIONS

Buffers

They are chemical solutions, which prevent changes in hydrogen ion concentration or pH. So addition of small amount of acid or bases will cause no or little change in the pH. Buffers are composed of inorganic acid and organic acids or base plus salts. These absorb free hydrogen or H+ (coming from acid) and free hydoxyl or OH- (coming from base or alkali) to prevent change in pH.

pH—It is defined as the logarithm to base 10 of 1 divided by the concentration of the free hydrogen ion in the solution.

So, $pH = \log_{10} 1/[H^+] = -\log_{10} [H^+]$.

Neutral $pH = -\log_{10} [10^{-7}] = 7$

Phosphate Buffer

Preparation of stock solution:

- **Stock solution A: 0.2 M sodium dihydrogen orthophosphate (MW 156):** 3.12 g of sodium dihydrogen orthophosphtate in 100 mL of distilled water.
- **Stock solution B: 0.2 M disodium hydrogen orthophosphate (MW 142):** 2.83 g of disodium hydrogen orthophosphate in 100 mL of distilled water.

To make 100 mL of solution of desired pH; mix X mL of A with Y mL of B stock solution and make up to 100 mL with ditilled water.

pH of phosphate buffer	*X mL of A*	*Y mL of B*	*Distilled water*
5.8	46.0	4.0	50 mL
6.0	43.8	6.2	50 mL
6.2	40.7	9.3	50 mL
6.4	36.7	13.3	50 mL
6.6	31.2	18.8	50 mL
6.8	25.5	24.5	50 mL
7	19.5	30.5	50 mL
7.2	14.0	36	50 mL
7.4	9.5	40.5	50 mL
7.6	6.5	43.5	50 mL
7.8	4.2	45.8	50 mL
8.0	2.6	47.4	50 mL

Citrate Buffer (Sorenson's I)

Preparation of stock solutions:

- **Stock solution of A:** 0.1 M disodium citrate (MW 210.0)-2.1 g citric acid dissolved in 20 mL of normal (1N) sodium hydroxide and made up to 100 mL with distilled water.

- **Stock solution of B:** 0.1 M hydrochloric acid (MW 36.46)–0.85 mL hydrochloric acid in 100 mL of distilled water.

To make 100 mL of citrate buffer of desired pH; mix x mL of A+ (100-×) mL of B.

pH of citrate buffer	*X mL of A solution*	*(100-x) mL of B solution*
2.2	33.3	67.0
2.4	34.6	65.4
2.6	36.4	63.6
2.8	38.4	61.6
3	40.5	59.5
3.2	42.8	57.2
3.4	46	54
3.6	48.5	51.5
3.8	52	48
4	55.8	44.2
4.2	61.2	38.8
4.4	67.8	32.2
4.6	76.6	23.4
4.8	88.2	11.8

Tris-HCL Buffer

- **Stock solution A:** 0.2 M Tris (MW 121.0) 2.42 g of Tris (hydroxymethyl) aminomethane in 100 mL of distilled water.
- **Stock solution B:** 0.2 M HCl (MW 36.46) 1.7 mL of hydrochloric acid in 100 mL of distilled water.

To make 100 mL of buffer, mix 25 mL of A with Y mL of B and make up to 100 mL with distilled water.

pH of Tris-HCl buffer	*Y mL of solution B (stock)*
7.2	22.1
7.4	20.7
7.6	19.2
7.8	16.3
8	13.4
8.2	11.0
8.6	6.1
9.0	2.5

Phosphate Citrate Buffer

Preparation of stock solutions:

- **Stock solution A:** 0.2 M disodium hydrogen orthophosphate (MW 142.0) 2.83 g of disodium hydrogen orthophosphate in 100 mL of distilled water.
- **Stock solution B:** 0.1 M citric acid (MW 210.0) 2.1 g of citric acid in 100 mL of distilled water.

To make 100 mL of buffer solution, mix X mL of A with (100-×) mL of B.

pH of citrate phosphate buffer	*X mL of A*	*mL of B*
3.6	32.2	67.8
3.8	35.5	64.5
4.0	38.5	61.5
4.2	41.4	58.6
4.4	44.1	55.9
4.6	46.7	53.3
4.8	49.3	50.7
5.0	51.5	48.5
5.2	53.6	46.4
5.4	55.7	44.3
5.6	58.0	42.0
5.8	60.4	39.6
6.0	63.1	36.9
6.2	66.1	33.9
6.4	69.2	30.8
6.6	72.7	27.3
6.8	77.2	22.8
7.0	82.3	17.7
7.2	86.9	13.1
7.4	90.8	9.2
7.6	93.6	6.4
7.8	95.7	4.3

Glossary

Absorption	The penetration and coloring of a tissue element without chemical charges or reactions.
Acetone	An inorganic metabolite coming from incomplete degradation of fat. It is one of the components of ketone bodies.
Acid	A sour substance like lemon juice (contains citric acid). Acid neutralizes alkali (bases). It turns litmus paper red and carries hydrogen ion (H^+). It makes the Ph below 7. Common acids are nitric acid (HNO_3), sulphuric acid (H_2SO_4) and hydrochloric acid (HCl).
Acidic dye	A negatively charged dye that easily stains acidophilic or eosinophilic elements like cytoplasm, muscle and collagen.
Acid fast	Not decolorized easily by acids (H_2SO_4) after staining. Acid fast bacteria like Mycobacteria and Nocardia retain the red dye after acid-alcohol treatment. Other bacteria lose the red color after acid treatment and takes the counter stain (methyl blue) to be become blue colored.
Acidophilic	A substance or tissue element, usually basic in nature, which is usually stained with acid dyes, e.g. methylene blue.
Aldehyde	A reactive organic compound containing carbon, hydrogen and oxygen.
Analytical reagents	Pure chemicals of known composition.
Anhydride	A form of a substance where the water molecule is chemically removed.
Anhydrous	The chemical form of a salt without water molecule.
Anion	Negatively charged ion attracted to the anode (positively changed) during electrolysis.
Argentaffin	A reaction in which silver impregnation and subsequent reduction result in visualization of tissue elements.
Argyrophilic	The ability to bind or be impregnated with silver ions.
Artefact	An element that is not normally present but that is produced by an external action.
Autolysis	Spontaneous disintegration of cells or tissues by autologous enzymes, as occurs after death and in some pathologic conditions.
Background	All nonspecific staining, which result to from procedural artefacts.
Basic dye	A positively charge dye, which easily stains basophilic elements.
Basophilic	A substance or tissue element, usually acidic in nature, that is easily stained with basic dyes.
Birefringence	The splitting of light wave into two waves that are refracted in different directions.
Biopsy	A diagnostic procedure which comprises of microscopic examination of tissue removed from the living body.
Carbohydrates	Compounds, including sugar, starches and cellulose which contain carbon, hydrogen and oxygen only.
Calorie	Amount of heat required to raise the temperature of water to 1°C.
Catalyst	A substance which alters the rate of chemical reaction without apparently participating in it. It is required in small quantity.
Cation	Positively charged ion, which is attracted to the cathode (negatively in electrolysis).
Cholesterol	A monohydric solid alcohol, a widely distributed sterol in animal tissues. It serves as a precursor of various steroid hormones, e.g. sex hormones and adrenal corticoids.
Chromophilic	Capable of being stained readily with dyes.
Chromophore	The specific chemical grouping that bestows the property of a color on a background.
Clearing	The process of replacing alcohol with a reagent that can be mixed with paraffin.
Counterstain	A secondary stain that is applied to provide a visual contrast to the primary stain. For example, safranin in Gram stain or methylene blue in acid-fast stain.

Decolorization	The removal of color from tissue.
Dehydration	The removal of water from tissue.
Deparaffinization	The removal of paraffin from a tissue section.
Differentiation	The removal of excess stain from a tissue section so that only the desired element remains stained.
Enzyme	A special protein produced by living cells, which acts as a catalyst and accelerates biochemical reactions, e.g. amylase enzyme converts starch into glucose.
Eosinophilic	A substance or tissue element, usually basic in nature that is easily stained with dyes.
Epitopes	In the antibody sites of antigens, there are highly specific regions which are antigenic determinal groups, called epitopes.
Ester	A compound formed from an alcohol and an acid by removal of water. Fat is an ester of glycerol (alcohol) and fatty acids.
Fixation	The stabilization of protein.
Fluorescence	A property of few substances to emit light when exposed to certain types of light radiation, usually ultraviolet. It is caused by the absorption of high energy shorter wavelengths of light (<400 nm) and emits longer wavelengths of light simultaneously (yellowish-green).
Hematin	The oxidation product of hematoxylin; the active ingredient in hematoxylin solutions.
Histology	The study of the structure of the tissues or tissue elements.
Impregnation	The deposition of metals on or around a tissue element of interest.
Incubation	To maintain tissue sections at optimal environments or temperature for a desired chemical reactions occur.
Isotonic	Having the same salt concentration as the cell cytoplasm.
Isotonic solution	A solution of sodium chloride in distilled water, that has the same osmotic pressure as red blood cells. This is 0.85% solution which is also called physiological saline.
Lake (in staining)	The combination of a mordant with a dye.
Lipid	A fat-like substance easily stored in body as a reserve fuel. Fat is also a lipid.
Lipoprotein	A complex lipid in conjugation with protein, the form in which lipids are transported in blood.
Mordant	A reagent used to link stain to the tissue.
Monosaccharide	A simple sugar, like glucose, which cannot be further broken down into other sugars.
Mucoprotein	A protein combines with carbohydrate. A substance present in all connective and supportive tissues.
Neutral buffered formalin (10%)	4% formaldehyde in phosphate buffered saline.
Oxidation	A chemical reaction involving the removal of electrons from a molecule.
Osmosis	A process whereby liquids of different concentrations, separated by a semi-permeable membrane percolate and mix until their concentrations are equal.
Osmolality	Solute concentration of a fluid measured in terms of osmotic pressure, which increases with increased solute concentration.
Parafocal	Objectives (Scanner view, low power or high power) are said to be parafocal, when an object or slide is focussed by an objective, it will be focussed by other objectives also.
Pepsin	A gastric proteolytic enzyme which converts proteins into peptone in acid medium.
pH	It depends on free hydrogen ion concentration in the solution. pH 7 is neutral, pH <7 is acidic and pH >7 is alkaline.
Polychromasia	Multi-coloration in the same cell (usually in RBC)
Progressive staining	Staining to the desired intensity and stopping the stain. No differentiation is required.
Proteins	Characteristic constituent of animal and plant tissues formed by the linkage of amino acids.
Regressive staining	Over staining followed by decolorizing or differentiation.
Reduction	A chemical reaction involving the addition of electrons to a molecule.
Ripening	Oxidation of chemical to make good stains.

Index

Page numbers followed by *t* indicate tables and *f* indicate figures

A

B

H

I

J

K

L

P

Q

R

S

T

U

V